The Office Management of Digestive Diseases

The Office Management of Digestive Diseases

Edited by

JOSEPH T. DANZI, MD

Vice President for Professional Affairs
United Health Services Hospitals
Johnson City, New York

Associate Dean for Undergraduate and Graduate Affairs
Clinical Campus
Health Science Center
Syracuse, New York

JOSEPH A. SCOPELLITI, MD

Associate, Section of Gastroenterology
Guthrie Clinic
Sayre, Pennsylvania

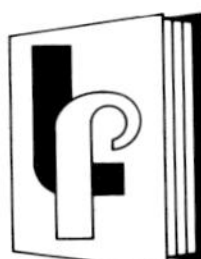

Lea & Febiger • Philadelphia • London • 1992

Lea & Febiger
200 Chester Field Parkway
Box 3024
Malvern, Pennsylvania 19355-9725
U.S.A.
(215) 251-2230

Executive Editor—Carroll C. Cann
Project Editor—Lisa Stead
Production Manager—Michael DeNardo

Library of Congress Cataloging-in-Publication Data

The Office management of digestive diseases / edited by Joseph T.
Danzi, Joseph A. Scopelliti.
c. pm.
Includes index.
ISBN 0-8121-1436-1
1. Gastrointestinal system—Diseases. 2. Ambulatory medical care.
I. Danzi, J. Thomas. II. Scopelliti, Joseph A.
[DNLM: 1. Ambulatory Care. 2. Digestive System Diseases—therapy.
WI 100 032]
RC801.033 1992
616.3—dc20
DNLM/DLC
for Library of Congress 92-6916
CIP

Reprints of chapters may be purchased from Lea & Febiger in quantities of 100 or more. Contact Sally Grande in the Sales Department.

PRINTED IN THE UNITED STATES OF AMERICA

Print number: 5 4 3 2 1

preface

The concept for this textbook arose from the authors' participation in annual seminars for primary care physicians dealing with the office management of common medical conditions. The preparation for our lectures helped us realize that the majority of texts written about digestive diseases are directed at inpatient, rather than outpatient, management. The impetus of recent medical practice has resulted in an increase in the delivery of health care in the ambulatory setting. The intent of this textbook is to be a source of information for primary care physicians and gastroenterologists on the office management of common gastrointestinal diseases.

The authors wish to acknowledge the well written chapters of the contributing authors. Their participation gives the text both national and international approaches to therapy. Finally, the authors wish to thank Mr. Carroll Cann, the executive editor, for his support and advice.

contributors

Romulo M. Bunao, MD
Associate, Section of Gastroenterology
Guthrie Clinic
Sayre, Pennsylvania

Faculty in Medicine
Hahnemann University Hospital
Philadelphia, Pennsylvania

Kevin V. Carey, MD
Chief, Section of Gastroenterology
Guthrie Clinic
Sayre, Pennsylvania

Eugene F. Cassone, MD
Champlain Valley Physicians Hospital
Plattsburgh, New York

Joseph T. Danzi, MD
Vice President for Professional Affairs
United Health Services Hospitals
Johnson City, New York

Associate Dean for Undergraduate and Graduate Affairs
Clinical Campus
Health Science Center
Syracuse, New York

Richard G. Farmer, MD
Chairman, Division of Medicine, Department of Gastroenterology
Cleveland Clinic Foundation
Cleveland, Ohio

Richard J. Fastiggi, MD
Associate, Section of Gastroenterology
Guthrie Clinic
Corning, New York

James Ferenzi, MD
Department of Surgery
Guthrie Clinic
Sayre, Pennsylvania

Mark Christian Flemmer, MD
Associate, Department of Medicine
Guthrie Clinic
Sayre, Pennsylvania

Philip G. Holtzapple, MD
Associate Dean of Curriculum
Health Science Center
SUNY-Syracuse College of Medicine
Syracuse, New York

Talley I. Parker, MD
Assistant Professor of Clinical Medicine
Center for Liver Diseases
University of Miami School of Medicine
Miami, Florida

Eugene R. Schiff, MD, FACP
Professor of Medicine
Chief, Division of Hepatology
Center for Liver Diseases
University of Miami School of Medicine

Chief, Hepatology Section
Veterans Administration Medical Center
Miami, Florida

Melanie L. Swartz, RN
MSN/MBA Candidate
State University of New York at Binghamton
Binghamton, New York

Head Nurse, Gastrointestinal Endoscopy Suite
Robert Packer Hospital
Sayre, Pennsylvania

Joseph A. Scopelliti, MD
Associate, Section of Gastroenterology
Guthrie Clinic
Sayre, Pennsylvania

Dame Sheila Sherlock
Professor of Medicine
Royal Free Hospital School of Medicine
University of London
London, England

Steven Y. Villanueva, MD
Fellow, Section of Gastroenterology
Guthrie Clinic
Sayre, Pennsylvania

contents

chapter

1

THE DIAGNOSIS AND TREATMENT OF REFLUX ESOPHAGITIS

Eugene Cassone
Joseph A. Scopelliti

Gastroesophageal reflux was first described as a pathologic entity by Winklestein in 1935.[1] It encompasses various symptoms, is frequent, and may be the most common intestinal complaint seen in the outpatient setting. It occurs as a recurrent and common problem in up to 10% of the population, and may occur in as much as 60% of the adult population at one time.[2]

CLINICAL MANIFESTATIONS

The common clinical symptom of gastroesophageal reflux disease (GERD) is "heartburn." This is generally described as a retrosternal burning sensation that radiates from the epigastrium to the throat. It is generally considered worse after meals and during recumbency. In patients with severe gastroesophageal reflux, nocturnal symptoms awakening them at night are present. It can be associated with severe chest pain which mimics that of angina, but this does not have the characteristic burning sensation and is often difficult to differentiate from cardiac chest pain. Previous relief of the above symptoms obtained with antacids taken on a prn basis is helpful in identifying GERD.

Occasionally, patients present with spontaneous reflux of a bitter-tasting liquid. This regurgitation of gastric contents usually occurs with straining or bending over, but may also occur when the patient is recumbent. It is clearly worse after a large meal. An associated symptom is that of "water brash," which is a mucoid saliva associated with reflux esophagitis. This hypersalivation appears to be stimulated by the reflux of acid into the esophagus. The patient also notes that this fluid is extremely bitter tasting.

Rarely, in patients with severe esophageal ulceration, the symptom of odynophagia may be present. The possibility of an infectious esophagitis must be considered with this finding, but it also occurs with GERD.

Dysphagia is a symptom that can be present with reflux esophagitis, both as a primary symptom and as a complication of the disorder. Often, patients with symptomatic reflux esophagitis describe intermittent solid food dysphagia in which no mechanical, fixed obstruction is found. This may represent a concomitant motor disorder or may simply be a stiff-walled esophagus, the result of inflammation. It is generally not progressive in nature and its severity usually parallels that of other reflux symptoms. More importantly, it resolves with typical medical therapy, and does not require esophageal dilation.

Finally, a more difficult situation revolves around the pulmonary symptoms associated with reflux esophagitis. As many as 10% of patients with GERD may have pulmonary symptoms.[3] These may present as recurrent pneumonia or just a paroxysmal cough, particularly at night. In children with recurrent asthma or nocturnal coughing, reflux esophagitis appears to be common. Pulmonary symptoms in adults are less clearly understood, but adult recurrent asthma may be a result of "silent gastroesophageal reflux." The pulmonary complications of GERD can nonetheless be severe, and can result in bronchiectasis as an end-stage event. An atypical presentation of asthma in the adult or child should raise the consideration of reflux-related problems.

PATHOPHYSIOLOGY

Although GERD is usually considered a peptic disorder, it is more properly regarded as a motility defect. Certainly, it appears that it is the result of the reflux of acid, as well as of pepsin, bile and alkaline intestinal secretions, which result in mucosal injury. Some degree of gastroesophageal reflux occurs in normal individuals, particularly after meals. These episodes have been termed "physiologic reflux" and are of short duration, occur rarely at night, and are generally asymptomatic. In contrast, reflux with pathologic consequences seems to involve several other factors. A defective lower esophageal sphincter is thought to play an important role in the pathogenesis. The lower esophageal sphincter is the barrier against reflux between the higher pressure of the abdominal cavity and the negative pressure of the thoracic cavity. Most patients with gastroesophageal reflux disease have idiopathic sphincter incompetence, with or without the presence of a hiatal hernia. Some authors believe that a decrease in basal competence of the lower esophageal sphincter leads to reflux, whereas others believe that the basal pressure is normal but inappropriate relaxation occurs, leading to reflux episodes.[4–6]

Several other factors may also be operative, including poor esophageal clearance of acid material and delayed gastric emptying.[7] The former serves as a protective mechanism, particularly at night. As noted, physiologic reflux does occur, and this secondary peristalsis is meant to prevent physiologic reflux from causing mucosal injury to the esophagus. In patients with GERD, esophageal clearance appears to be diminished.[8] In addition, primary peristalsis (swallowing) is a normal method for clearing refluxed material. Deep sleep significantly diminishes the frequency of swallowing, and secondary peristalsis thus becomes important. Patients with GERD have less frequent and ineffective secondary peristalsis.

Delayed gastric emptying has been proposed by several authors as the potential initiating factor in some patients with GERD.[9] Certainly, this has been shown to play a major contributing role in some subsets of patients. The complete definition of this factor appears to be heterogeneous, and the usual causes of gastroparesis must be considered. Negative changes in gastric emptying would result in higher intragastric pressures. Larger volumes of gastric content would predispose the patient to reflux of larger quantities during the so-called "physiologic" episodes of reflux, as well as initiate pathologic episodes.

MEDICAL TREATMENT

In most patients, a careful history correctly makes the diagnosis of gastroesophageal reflux disease. Generally, in uncomplicated cases (i.e., no dysphagia, odynophagia, or respiratory symptoms), no further testing is needed. Therapy may be initiated without confirmatory testing, and used as a therapeutic trial. Depending on the severity of complaints, response to previous medication, and the resistance to therapy, further diagnostic or therapeutic measures would be considered.

The treatment of gastroesophageal disease is often broken down into different phases. Phase I involves lifestyle modifications (Table 1–1). These

TABLE 1–1. PHASE I THERAPY FOR GASTROESOPHAGEAL REFLUX DISEASE
Lifestyle Modifications
Elevate head of bed 4 to 8 inches.
Use a wedge if you cannot elevate the bed.
Avoid eating at bedtime or taking the supine position after meals; allow at least 3 hours between eating and assuming the recumbent position.
Lose weight if overweight.
Stop smoking.
Avoid fatty, spicy or irritating foods, including chocolate.
Do not drink coffee or alcohol.
Medical Therapy
Antacids, 10 to 20 ml, 1 hour after meals and at bedtime.
Consider decreasing or stopping other ulcerogenic medications (e.g., nonsteroidal anti-inflammatory drugs, Theophylline, anticholinergics.)

include simple measures that all GERD patients should follow. Often, they alone are adequate for patients with mild, uncomplicated symptoms, but should also be followed by patients under intensive medical therapy. They have been proven effective in many studies.[10,11]

After a period of 2 to 4 weeks, the patient should be re-evaluated. If patients are refractory to phase I modification, the next phase of therapy should be initiated. Phase II therapy involves different medical options that have been shown to be effective. First-line therapy includes histamine-2 (H_2) antagonists, which reduce the secretion of acid by the stomach. Cimetidine (Tagamet), the first H_2 antagonist released, has consistently been shown to improve symptoms, although endoscopic and histologic outcomes have varied.[12–14] In these studies, however, less than optimum doses were sometimes used, and phase I measures were not uniformly instituted. Another consideration in the use of cimetidine is its potential for altering the hepatic metabolism of such drugs as warfarin, phenytoin, and theophylline. These effects may not be a problem with newer H_2 antagonists.

Studies published to date have revealed significant symptomatic improvement with ranitidine.[9,11,15,16] Four of these six studies also indicated histologic improvement.[15]

Data on famotidine, a newer and more potent H_2 antagonist, are still limited, but two studies have shown it to be effective for the symptomatic relief of GERD.[16,17] Data on nizatidine, the latest H_2 antagonist to be released, are still forthcoming.

After an initial treatment period of 6 weeks, maintenance therapy is begun. A high relapse rate is noted for gastroesophageal reflux, as for peptic ulcer disease. The use of a low-dose therapeutic regimen can prevent symptomatic relapses from occurring.

For the patient who continues to have symptoms despite medical therapy, as described above, the next step involves the addition of prokinetic drugs. These constitute the second line of medical therapy and are used if the patient does not respond to the protocol outlined above. Bethanechol is a cholinergic agent that has been shown to increase lowered esophageal sphincter pressure, promote salivation, and therefore improve esophageal clearance. It also can help increase gastric contractions and thereby aid in gastric emptying.[18,19] It has been shown to be significantly better than placebo in improving symptoms, endoscopic findings, and decreasing antacid use in those with GERD.[20] The usual dosage is 25 mg qid, to be taken before each meal and at bedtime. A single bedtime dose has also been shown to be effective.[21] This latter effect is probably related to the amount of reflux damage occurring at night. Side effects of a cholinergic drug such as bethanechol include abdominal cramps, diarrhea, urinary frequency, and blurred vision. It is also relatively contraindicated in patients with asthma.

Metoclopramide, another prokinetic drug, is a peripheral and central dopamine antagonist that also functions as a cholinomimetic drug by augmenting acetylcholine released from postganglionic nerve terminals. Metoclopramide, however, has no effect on gastric acid secretion. Studies have shown that its major effect in GERD is a dose-dependent rise in lower esophageal sphincter (LES) pressure, although this effect is decreased in patients with LES incompetence. Also, it increases the rate of gastric emptying.[22]

Metoclopramide has been shown to be as effective as cimetidine in terms of symptom improvement, but side effects may limit its therapeutic usefulness.[22] The most common side effects are psychotropic, with fatigue, drowsiness, anxiety, nightmares, and extrapyramidal manifestations. Most of these effects are reversible with cessation of the drug, but tardive dyskinesias may persist. Most of the side effects are dose-dependent and, in most studies, 10 to 20 mg qid have been used. We generally recommend adding metoclopramide to an H_2 antagonist if the patient's symptoms persist after 6 weeks. A nightly dose of 10 to 20 mg is used. Only if the patient has severe, continuing symptoms is the dosage increased to 10 mg qid.

Two new prokinetic agents not yet released for general use are cisapride[23] and domperidone. Both may have significant beneficial affects, but definitive data are not yet available. Another agent is sucralfate (Carafate), in which a slurry is used. Its exact role in gastroesophageal reflux disease has not been determined, but preliminary studies have shown it be of benefit.[24–26]

A newly released agent, omeprazole, has been extremely successful in the treatment of GERD. It represents a new class of drug for the treatment of acid peptic disorders. It acts as a specific hydrogen-potassium ATPase inhibitor, which is the final pathway of hydrogen release by the parietal cell. It is a potent acid suppressor with a long half-life, about 2 to 3 days. In a double-blind, randomized trial, omeprazole was markedly superior to ranitidine, 150 mg bid, in the rapidity of symptom response and endoscopic healing.[27] The major drawback of omeprazole therapy is the seemingly increased frequency of carcinoid tumors in animal studies. This is thought to be caused by secondary hypergastrinemia and its tropic affect on gastric mucosa. A high relapse rate has been noted when omeprazole is discontinued, but maintenance dosing has been shown to be effective, with only mild elevations of serum gastrin levels.[28] Omeprazole's role at present is only for those patients with refractory symptoms. In the future, it may play a more general role in the treatment of GERD, but, for now, it remains to be used only in this subset of patients.

DIAGNOSTIC TESTING

The use of diagnostic testing in patients with GERD is generally reserved for those patients with the following: (1) a questionable diagnosis; (2) severe refractory symptoms, despite phases I and II therapy; (3) odynophagia, dysphagia, or other major complications. Various diagnostic tests are available.

Barium Esophagography. This was once the study of choice, but it is insensitive in diagnosing esophagitis. It identifies barium reflux, but the validity of this is questioned. It is primarily helpful in identifying strictures, motor function, and esophageal clearance.

Upper Gastrointestinal Endoscopy. This allows direct visualization of the esophagus and affords the opportunity for mucosal biopsy. It is the test of choice in patients with refractory or complicated symptoms. It is also helpful in evaluating atypical chest pain and in following the response to therapy.

Bernstein Test. This is useful only in assessing whether the patient's symptoms are identifiable as a result of acid reflux. It was formerly used frequently, but 24-hour ambulatory pH monitoring has replaced it.

Ambulatory pH Monitoring. This technique allows continuous, intraesophageal pH recording over a period ranging from 8 to 24 hours. It has been shown to be an accurate test for identifying acid reflux. Patients keep a diary and symptoms are correlated with a decrease in the esophageal pH, indicating a reflux episode. It is particularly useful in those patients with atypical chest pain syndromes. It can help determine whether reflux does occur, and whether acid reflux is the source of the patient's symptoms.

Esophageal Manometry. This has a limited role in the management of gastroesophageal reflux disease. Its aim is to measure lower esophageal sphincter pressure in a resting setting. As noted, lower esophageal sphincter might be abnormal in patients with GERD, so abnormalities identified on esophageal manometry might not be helpful. One specific indication for the use of esophageal manometry is the perioperative evaluation of patients who have had antireflux surgery. Certainly, these patients should undergo esophageal manometry preoperatively to ensure that motility in the esophageal body is normal.

COMPLICATIONS

Major complications of GERD include bleeding, ulceration, stricture, and Barrett's esophagus. Other, less common complications include recurrent aspiration pneumonia, asthma, and laryngeal irritation leading to hoarseness.

Significant hemorrhage from an esophageal source may represent 6 to 8% of all cases of significant upper gastrointestinal bleeding. Less than 50% of patients with hemorrhage from an esophageal source have a history compatible with that of GERD.[29] The bleeding may be hemodynamically unstable and require large numbers of transfusions, as well as endoscopic or surgical intervention. Bleeding in these patients is believed to originate from vessels situated in the dernal pegs of the mucosa, which become exposed in reflux disease. In the case of an esophageal ulcer, the underlying arterioles in the submucosa are responsible, and result in a pumping artery, or "visible vessel," which is observed at endoscopy. Hemorrhagic esophageal ulcers might be malignant, and proper follow-up with re-endoscopy and biopsy should be performed, as indicated. Nonsteroidal anti-inflammatory drugs also cause hemorrhage secondary to ulceration, especially when a pill is lodged at a stricture. Therapy for hemorrhage is stabilization, as for all gastrointestinal bleeding, and prompt endoscopy for a diagnosis. Nasogastric tube placement alone for diagnosis may be negative in up to one-third of patients.[29,30]

Approximately 10% of patients with severe reflux develop a stricture. The most common complaints of a stricture are solid food dysphagia. Occasionally, an individual presents for the first time with a food impaction. Patients usually give a long history of reflux symptoms, but up to 25% of patients give no prior history of heartburn.[31]

Most peptic strictures (non-Barrett's) usually occur within 2 cm of the gastroesophageal junction, and are easily recognized by barium swallow or endoscopy. We recommend that endoscopy be the first test performed in all patients with dysphagia; only if endoscopy is not readily available does fluoroscopic study suffice.

Treatment of peptic strictures is usually effective using esophageal dilators. For simple strictures, mercury-filled rubber dilators (Maloney type) are commonly used. In tortuous or tight strictures, fluoroscopically guided dilators or balloons may be used for added safety. Overall, the complication rate is generally less than 1 to 2%. Patients should be maintained on antireflux programs indefinitely, and this may minimize the need for repetitive dilations. Approximately two-thirds of all patients require additional dilation, despite medical therapy. A small percentage of strictures require surgical intervention.[32]

The incidence has been debated, but Barrett's esophagus may occur in up to 10% of patients with chronic GERD.[33] Symptoms are usually of heartburn and regurgitation, but dysphagia also occurs commonly. Half of all benign strictures occur in Barrett's esophagus, and the characteristic feature of these strictures is their midesophageal location. Barrett's mucosa is columnar and is believed to be a metaplastic change, the result of chronic reflux. Three types of columnar mucosa may be seen: cardiac (or junctional), fundic, and intestinal (specialized mucosa). It is the latter that is thought to be the most frequently associated with a premalignant state. Diagnosis of Barrett's esophagus is made endoscopically, with the squamocolumnar junction noted to be at least 3 cm proximal to the esophagogastric junction. The diagnosis should be confirmed with mucosal biopsies above and below the squamocolumnar junction.

The increased incidence of adenocarcinoma arising in Barrett's esophagus has long been recognized. Unfortunately, the prediction of an increased incidence has been flawed. Many studies have been retrospective and have used incomplete patient populations. A more recent study has placed the incidence at about one case in 56 patient-years of observation.[34] The question of surveillance for patients with Barrett's remains unanswered. Periodic endoscopy with biopsy costs about $20,000 for each cancer diagnosis. It still remains to be proven whether finding the cancer early changes the survival rate. Present recommendations for surveillance include upper gastrointestinal endoscopy, with multiple biopsies at 1-year intervals. If dysplasia is seen in a Barrett's mucosa, especially if it is high grade, repeat endoscopy should be performed to confirm this within 3 months. A decision must then be made regarding surgery. In the case of severe or high-grade dysplasia, even though frank adenocarcinoma is not visualized, an underlying adenocarcinoma may be present and require surgery.

Therapy for Barrett's esophagus in the absence of a malignancy requires standard reflux therapy. This includes both lifestyle modifications and medical therapy. Medical therapies, although they have been shown to improve symptoms, have never prevented the occurrence of Barrett's or caused a regression in a pre-existing Barrett's esophagus. Treatment of esophageal ulcers in Barrett's esophagus (which may occur in 20 to 40% of patients) includes standard medical therapy (see above). Strictures in Barrett's esophagus, as noted, are usually midesophageal in location, and generally respond well to esophageal dilation. In refractory cases surgery may be required to alleviate the stricture, and the Barrett's esophagus should be excised at this time.

SURGICAL THERAPY

A small percentage of patients with GERD, despite maximum medical therapy, require surgical intervention. General indications for surgery include the following: (1) failure of adequate medical therapy to alleviate symptoms; (2) refractory hemorrhagic esophagitis; (3) refractory strictures; and (4) recurrent pulmonary disease caused by GERD. Barrett's epithelium alone is not an indication for elective surgery.

Current surgical procedures used for GERD involve a gastric fundoplication to restore sphincter competence. The three most commonly used are the Belsey-Mark IV, Hill, and Nissen procedures. They all involve plication or wrapping of the distal esophagus with the gastric fundus. Satisfactory results have been noted with all these procedures, especially the Nissen fundoplication. Failure rates in this group have ranged from 10 to 20% in most studies.[35] Side effects, in addition to those related to surgery, include dysphagia and "gas bloat" syndrome, which is the inability of the patient to belch. They are usually indicative of a fundic wrap that is too tight, and this may actually require esophageal dilation.

Patients with reflux esophagitis are a common sight in a physician's office. Medical management of this problem is generally straightforward, but clear-cut steps can be taken in the management of those patients with refractory symptoms. This chapter has outlined some of these decision-making points and clarified the management of this problem.

REFERENCES

1. Nebel OT, Fomes MF, Castell PO: Symptomatic gastroesophageal reflux incidence and precipitating factors. Dig Dis Sci, 21:955, 1976.
2. Winklestein A: Peptic esophagitis: A new clinical entity. JAMA, 104:906, 1935.
3. Skinner DB, Roth JLA, Sullivan BH, et al: Reflux esophagitis. *In* Bockus Gastroenterology. 4th Ed, Vol 2. Edited by JE Berk, WS Haubrich, MH Kalser, et al. Philadelphia, WB Saunders, 1985, pp 717–768.
4. Dodds WJ, Dent J, Hogan WJ, et al: Mechanism of gastroesophageal reflux in patients with reflux esophagitis. N Engl J Med, 307:1547, 1982.

5. Dent J, Dodds WJ, Friedman RH, et al: Mechanism of GER in recumbent asymptomatic human subject. J Clin Invest, 65:256, 1980.
6. Dodds WJ, Hogan WJ, Helm JF, et al: Pathogenesis of reflux esophagitis. Gastroenterology, 81:376, 1981.
7. Stancio L, Bennett JR: Esophageal acid clearing: One factor in the prevention of reflux esophagitis. Gut, 15:852, 1974.
8. Booth DJ, Kemmer WT, Skinner DB: Acid clearing from the distal esophagus. Arch Surg, 96:731, 1968.
9. Sherbanuils R, Wensel R, Bailey R, et al: Ranitidine in the treatment of symptomatic GER disease. J Clin Gastroenterol, 6:9, 1984.
10. McCallum RW, Berkowitz DM, Cerner E: Gastric emptying in patients with GER. Gastroenterology, 80:285, 1981.
11. Robinson MG: Management of reflux esophageal disease. Am J Med, 77(Suppl 5B):106, 1984.
12. Wesdorp E, Bartelsman J, Pope K, et al: Oral cimetidine in reflux esophagitis: A double-blind controlled trial. Gastroenterology, 74:821, 1978.
13. Behar J, Brand DL, Brown FL, et al: Cimetidine in the treatment of symptomatic gastroesophageal reflux: A double-blind controlled trial. Gastroenterology, 74:441, 1978.
14. Fiasse R, Hanin C, Lepet A, et al: Controlled trial of cimetidine in reflux esophagitis. Dig Dis Sci, 25:750, 1980.
15. Hire KR, Holmes CK, Melikian V, et al: Ranitidine in reflux esophagitis. A double-blind placebo-controlled study. Digestion, 29:119, 1984.
16. Sekigochi T, Nishokia T, Kogura M, et al: Once-daily administration of famotidine for reflux esophagitis. Scand J Gastroenterol, 22(Suppl 134):51, 1981.
17. Orr WC, Robinson MG, Humphries TJ, et al: Dose response effects of famotidine on gastroesophageal reflux (GER). Gastroenterology, 92:1562(A), 1978.
18. Farrell RL, Rolins GT, Castell DO: Stimulation of the incomplete lower esophageal sphincter. Am J Dig Dis, 18:646, 1973.
19. Hollis JB, Castell DO: Effects of cholinergic stimulation on human esophageal peristalsis. J Appl Physiol, 40:40, 1976.
20. Thanik KD, Chey WY, Shah AN, Gutierrez JG: Reflux esophagitis: Effect of oral bethanechol on symptoms and endoscopic findings. Ann Intern Med, 93:805, 1980.
21. Thanik KD, Chey WY, Shah AN, et al: Comparative studies on effects of cimetidine and bethanechol in the treatment of reflux esophagitis. Gastroenterology, 78:1277, 1980.
22. Cohen S, Morris DW, Schoen HJ, et al: The effect of oral and intravenous metoclopramide on the human lower esophageal sphincter pressure. Gastroenterology, 70:484, 1976.
23. Janisch HD, CISRAN Study Group: A double-blind multicenter trial to compare the efficacy of cisapride in the treatment of Grade II and III esophagitis. Gastroenterology, 92:1501(A), 1987.
24. Williams RM, Orlando RL, Bozymski EM, et al: Multicenter trial of sucralfate suspension (SS) in the treatment of reflux esophagitis. Gastroenterology, 92:1696(A), 1987.
25. Laitinen S, Stahlberg M, Kairalooma M, et al: Sucralfate and alginate/antacid in reflux esophagitis. Scand J Gastroenterol, 20:229, 1985.
26. Haneeteman W, Boomgavel DM, Dekker W, et al: Sucralfate versus cimetidine in reflux esophagitis. A single-blind multicenter study. J Clin Gastroenterol, 9:390, 1987.
27. Klinkenberg-Knol EC, Jansen JM, Festen HP, et al: Double-blind multicenter comparison of omeprazole and ranitidine in the treatment of reflux esophagitis. Lancet, 1:349, 1980.
28. Dent J, Hetzel DJ, Reed WD, et al: Healing of peptic esophagitis with omeprazole. Gastroenterology, 90:1392(A), 1986.
29. Silverstein FE, Gilbert DA, Tedesco FJ, et al: The national ASGE survey on upper gastrointestinal bleeding. II. Clinical prognostic factors. Gastrointest Endosc 27:80, 1981.
30. Silverstein FE, Gilbert DA, Tedesco FJ, et al: The national ASGE survey on upper gastrointestinal bleeding. III. Endoscopy in upper gastrointestinal bleeding. Gastrointest Endosc, 27:94, 1981.

31. Palmer ED: The hiatus hernia—esophagitis-esophageal stricture complex: A twenty-year prospective study. Am J Med, 44:566, 1968.
32. Glick ME: Clinical course of esophageal stricture managed by bougienage. Dig Dis Sci, 27:884, 1982.
33. Spechler SJ, Goyal RF: Barrett's esophagus. N Engl J Med, 315:362, 1986.
34. Robertson CS, Mayberry JF, Nicholson DA, et al: Value of endoscopy in Barrett's esophagus. Br J Surg, 75:760, 1988.
35. Negre JB, Markkula HT, Keryrilainen O, et al: Nissen fundoplication results at 10-year follow-up. Am J Surg, 146:635, 1983.

chapter

2

THE APPROACH TO THE PATIENT WITH DYSPHAGIA

Joseph A. Scopelliti

Dysphagia, or difficulty in swallowing, is a manifestation of various medical problems. Its evaluation may require investigation of the oropharynx, upper esophageal sphincter, esophageal body, or gastric cardia, depending on the patient's presentation. This chapter focuses on the basic approach to this symptom.

OROPHARYNGEAL DYSPHAGIA

Symptoms associated with disorders of the oropharyngeal musculature and nervous system are known as transfer dysphagia. They are the result of the ineffective transfer of food from the mouth into the upper esophagus. This complex process requires coordination and strength of various neuromuscular structures, almost any of which can be the source of a problem.

HISTORY AND PHYSICAL EXAMINATION

History taking for this disorder should focus on a clear description by the patient of problems in swallowing. Usually, they can clearly ascribe the location of the dysphagia to the cervical region. Associated symptoms are important. The presence of aspiration or nasal regurgitation is a hallmark of this problem. More importantly, oropharyngeal dysphagia is significantly worse with liquids, rather than solid foods. The musculature of the oropharynx grasps solid foods and propels them into the esophagus more easily than liquids. A mixture of solid and liquid foods invariably creates the worst symptoms for the patient. An unexplained cough or disturbances of the voice should also be elicited.

The physical examination in this process focuses primarily on the cranial nerves. Close observation for any cranial nerve dysfunction is a necessity. Disorders that can result in oropharyngeal dysphagia include pseudobulbar palsy or bulbar palsy, polio, myasthenia gravis, myotonic dystrophies, and disorders of the skeletal musculature. All these produce neuromotor dysfunction of the oropharynx. In addition, mechanical processes can produce this symptom. Cricopharyngeal achalasia and Plummer-Vinson syndrome are two mechanical problems that should be considered. Zenker's diverticulum represents another problem. It must be remembered that, when a mechanical process is present, the patient has more problems with solid foods than with liquids, and that they note a cervical location for their dysphagia.

DIAGNOSTIC TESTING AND EVALUATION

The first step involves a simple observation of the patient drinking a glass of water. The patient with neuromuscular problems may try several times to initiate swallowing. An inexact swallow may occur, and the patient may even evidence a small degree of aspiration. The next step in the evaluation of oropharyngeal problems should be a detailed evaluation of cranial nerve function.

Radiologic Studies. Barium swallow is the most helpful study for the evaluation of neuromuscular function. Ideally, this should be performed and videotaped so that a detailed analysis of muscular coordination and strength can be made. Simple evaluation by fluoroscopy is helpful, but is best when it can be reviewed. This study can also be performed with barium tablets and barium liquid to assess variations in swallowing between these two. Finally, the addition of a barium-soaked marshmallow can be extremely helpful, because this is often a challenge for the patient to swallow when a neuromuscular process is involved.

Esophageal Manometry. Esophageal manometry is somewhat limited in evaluating the oropharynx and cervical esophagus. Motor abnormalities are often identified on radiologic studies and can be defined further with manometry. This requires a high-speed evaluation of the oropharynx with transducers located within the oropharynx, upper esophageal sphincter, and cervical esophagus. The examination must demonstrate normally propagated peristaltic waves through these areas, which is a more subjective assessment. Absolute normal values for the amplitude of peristaltic pressures in this area have great variability within the normal range. In addition, as these waves are propagated through the upper esophageal sphincter, asymmetry of the radial pressures is noted, further hindering the differentiation of normal from abnormal. Inadequate propagation of a peristaltic wave, however, can be identified. Sphincter relaxation should be complete and of adequate duration. It should also be timed appropriately with the peristaltic wave.[1]

DISORDERS OF THE ESOPHAGEAL BODY

Symptoms of problems originating in the esophageal body are those of mechanical dysphagia. They revolve around the inability to swallow solid foods. Liquids are rarely a problem in this area. The patient can often note a location for the source of dysphagia, but this could be referred distally. The source of the dysphagia is never above the area noted by the patient, although it can be more distal to this. This is often useful in making the initial steps in evaluation. Two symptoms that are helpful in assessing the mechanical nature of dysphagia are the presence of self-induced vomiting to clear the food bolus and of weight loss. Both of these indicate a mechanical narrowing of the esophageal lumen. There are basically three causes for this—neoplasms, peptic strictures, and rings (or webs).

Solid food dysphagia, which is intermittent in nature and present for many years, is typical of an esophageal web or ring. This is usually located at the esophagogastric junction. Progressive solid food dysphagia with associated chronic pyrosis is typical of a peptic stricture. Finally, progressive solid food dysphagia of fairly short duration (i.e., less than 6 months) in an older patient is indicative of a neoplasm. Typically, peptic strictures have symptoms for a longer period and have a slower progression than neoplasms, which progress from minimal difficulty in swallowing to a near-inability to eat at all, usually over a course of 6 months.

Motor disorders of the esophageal body also cause dysphagia. These can be generally separated into those that affect the body of the esophagus and those that affect the lower esophageal sphincter. Symptoms include difficulty in swallowing both solids and liquids. These may have a highly variable course, from occasional symptoms to significantly progressive difficulty in swallowing. Patients with motor disorders usually have associated chest pain when the problem is diffuse esophageal spasm, a disorder of the esophageal body. Conversely, those with diffuse neuromuscular diseases, such as achalasia and scleroderma, have no associated chest pain, (Table 2–1).

TABLE 2–1. DIFFERENTIAL DIAGNOSES FOR OROPHARYNGEAL DYSPHAGIA
Diseases of striated muscle (e.g., polymyositis, myasthenia gravis)
CNS disease, including diseases of the brain stem and of the nuclei of cranial nerves V, VII, IX, X, and XII
Mechanical processes (e.g., cervical webs, thyroiditis, thyroid masses, Zenker's diverticulum)
Peripheral neuropathies, including amyotrophic lateral sclerosis, multiple sclerosis, Parkinson's disease

DIAGNOSTIC TESTING AND EVALUATION

Testing should be carried out on the basis of the patient's history. Upper gastrointestinal endoscopy is routinely used for any patient with symptoms of mechanical dysphagia. This requires an inspection of the esophageal mucosa to rule out neoplasms and strictures. Regardless of the duration or progression of symptoms, this is the first step in the evaluation of symptoms of mechanical dysphagia.

Barium esophagrams can be helpful in evaluating disorders of the esophageal body. Both mechanical problems and motor disorders can be evaluated. Upper gastrointestinal endoscopy can miss causes of mechanical dysphagia and, in the work-up of such a process, barium studies are indicated if endoscopy is not diagnostic. Generally, however, specific causes can be identified more precisely with upper gastrointestinal endoscopy or esophageal manometry.

Esophageal manometry is the test of choice when a motor disorder of the esophagus is suspected. Pressure recordings of the lower esophageal sphincter can thereby be obtained. In addition, coordination and relaxation of the lower esophageal sphincter can be determined. Dysmotility of the esophageal body can also be identified in its various forms.

MECHANICAL DISORDERS

Esophageal Cancer

Carcinoma of the esophagus is a disorder of the elderly. It is rarely present in patients under the age of 50 years, and increases in frequency with each decade of life.[2] It is characterized by progressive solid food dysphagia over a period of months, which is often associated with the need for self-induced vomiting to clear a food impaction. Patients may have substernal, aching discomfort between meals. Occasionally, the symptom of odynophagia is present. Weight loss is a prominent feature of this disorder.

Pre-existing heartburn of a severe nature suggests the diagnosis of Barrett's esophagus, with subsequent adenocarcinoma. A long history of alcohol and tobacco use predisposes the patient to squamous carcinomas. In addition, lye ingestions in the past, achalasia, celiac sprue, and tylosis are conditions thought to predispose to esophageal cancers.[3]

Diagnostic testing is best carried out by upper gastrointestinal endoscopy, which allows delineation of the exact location of the neoplasm. In addition, biopsies can be obtained to confirm the diagnosis.

Peptic Esophageal Strictures

Peptic esophageal strictures are the result of chronic reflux esophagitis, and develop over the course of many years from acid reflux into the esophagus. Often, the patient with this type of stricture does not give a pre-existing history of heartburn. This unusual finding is often explained as some abnormal sensation. Its exact basis is unclear, but patients with heartburn experience it frequently before they progress to an esophageal stricture. These strictures can be irregular in nature and symptoms can mimic those of carcinoma on barium swallow. Patients usually note symptoms of slowly progressive solid food dysphagia over a period of months to years. Self-induced vomiting is occasionally present, but weight loss is rare.

Evaluation of this disorder requires upper gastrointestinal endoscopy. As noted, these strictures can be irregular and mimic carcinoma on barium esophagography.

Esophageal Webs

Esophageal webs come in various forms. They can be present within the upper esophagus and at the squamocolumnar junction. Those present within 2 to 4 cm of the pharynx are known as Plummer-Vinson syndrome.[4] Many patients with esophageal webs have an associated iron deficiency anemia. Dysphagia of a cervical origin for solid foods is the hallmark. This disorder is best identified by testing with barium swallow.

Esophageal webs at the lower esophageal sphincter are called Schatzki's rings,[5] and are the result of chronic acid reflux. Patients with this disorder note intermittent solid food dysphagia, which may have been present for many years. Typically, patients often go for months between episodes of dysphagia, and then note that food gets stuck for no apparent reason. These patients often do not have self-induced vomiting, as they usually can wash down the food impaction. Invariably, a history of heartburn is present. This abnormality is best identified on barium swallow, although upper gastrointestinal endoscopy can be a useful diagnostic test.

MOTOR DISORDERS

Achalasia

This disorder results in a hypertensive, lower esophageal sphincter, and generally occurs in 40- to 60-year-olds. Most patients complain of dysphagia, which in the early stages of disease occurs intermittently. Solid foods may seem to pass more readily than liquids. Occasionally, some variation in swallowing is noted between warm and cold foods. Over time, the patient progresses to worsened swallowing problems, which usually takes 1 to 3 years to evolve. Several symptoms are helpful in this diagnosis. The first is the sensation of a substernal fullness or pressure while eating. The esophagus gradually dilates in patients with achalasia and becomes a reservoir for food, which is sensed as a fullness while eating. The second symptom is regurgitation. Often, patients note an unusual type of regurgitation, in which they passively bring up food after a meal whenever they bend over or perform a Valsalva maneuver. Weight loss is variable in achalasia, but tends not to be a problem.

Endoscopy usually reveals the esophageal body to be dilated, and without evidence of peristalsis. Often, food or liquid is retained within the esophageal body. The endoscope passes through the lower esophageal sphincter region with gentle pressure. Radiographically, the esophageal body is dilated and atonic, with a "bird beak" appearance of the lower esophageal sphincter. Again, retention of food and liquid within the esophageal body is noted.

Esophageal manometry is the test of choice to confirm this diagnosis. Characteristics include a hypertensive, nonrelaxing lower esophageal sphincter. Aperistalsis or greatly diminished peristaltic pressures in the esophageal body are noted. A variation, vigorous achalasia, results in high-amplitude contractions within the esophageal body.

Diffuse Esophageal Spasm

This disorder is characterized by high-amplitude but uncoordinated contractions in the esophageal body. Patients present variably with complaints of chest pain and difficulty in swallowing. Their swallowing problems may involve difficulty with both solids and liquids, and some variation in swallowing hot and cold foods is noted. This is generally a disorder of those in younger age groups.

When findings of diffuse esophageal spasm are identified in the elderly, it is often called presbyesophagus. This is a commonly identified abnormality on routine upper gastrointestinal roentgenography in the elderly. It is characterized by tertiary contractions in the esophageal body. This disorder is rarely symptomatic, but can be a cause for dysphagia. Initially described in patients with neuropathic diseases, such as diabetes mellitus and tabes dorsalis, it can be found incidentally in the elderly population.[6] It increases in frequency with age, although it rarely requires therapy.[7] If dysphagia is present, calcium channel blockers or esophageal dilation can be used.

Diagnostic testing is often begun with a roentgenographic examination in patients with suspected motor disorders. This reveals the characteristic corkscrew appearance in both diffuse esophageal spasm and presbyesophagus. An esophageal manometry confirms the presence of high-amplitude, nonperistaltic contractions within the esophageal body.

Connective Tissue Disorders

Scleroderma is the most common disease in this category that results in esophageal motor symptoms. Connective tissue disorders in this area alter the function of smooth muscle. The range of dysfunction may simply be decreased amplitude of the peristaltic waves or may progress all the way to a completely aperistaltic esophageal body. Typically, the lower esophageal sphincter and the lower two-thirds of the esophageal body are hypotonic.

These patients often have pre-existing connective tissue problems, and only later present with difficulty in swallowing. They may note problems with liquids or solids. Some variation in these symptoms is related to the stage of disease. The esophageal body is hypotonic early in the course, and problems with liquid swallowing are therefore noted. Over time, however, the lower esophageal sphincter pressure decreases and reflux esophagitis develops. The patient may progress to a peptic stricture of the lower esophagus. At this point, significant problems with solids are noted. These patients almost always have a long history of severe heartburn antedating their symptoms of dysphagia.

Esophageal manometry is the test of choice to determine the extent of dysfunction of the esophageal musculature. When patients have symptoms suggesting a mechanical obstructive process, however, upper gastrointestinal endoscopy should also be carried out to evaluate the situation further.

Various problems can result in difficulty in swallowing. A fairly complex differential can be evoked with this simple symptom. Differentiating between oropharyngeal and esophageal body sources is helpful, and further distinction between mechanical and motor processes is necessary. The investigation should be directed according to the information obtained.

REFERENCES

1. Kilman WJ, Goyal RK: Disorders of pharyngeal and upper esophageal sphincter motor function. *Arch Intern Med,* 136:592, 1976.
2. Rubin P: Cancer of the gastrointestinal tract. I. Esophagus, stomach, small intestine. JAMA, 226:1544, 1973.
3. Wynder EL, Bross IJ: A study of etiological factors in cancer of the esophagus. Cancer, 14:389, 1961.
4. Logan JS: The Plummer-Vinson stricture. Ulster Med J, 47(Suppl 2):1, 1978.
5. Schatzki R, Gary JE: Dysphagia due to a diaphragm-like localized narrowing in the lower esophagus ("lower esophageal ring"). Am J Roentgenol, 70:911, 1953.
6. Hollis JB, Costell DO: Esophageal function in elderly men. Medicine, 80:371, 1974.
7. Kekki N, Sipponen P, Sjurada M, et al: Age behavior of gastric acid secretion in males and females with a normal antral and body mucosa. Scand J Gastroenterol, 18:1009, 1983.

chapter

3

THE MANAGEMENT OF CHRONIC PEPTIC ULCER DISEASE

Kevin V. Carey

A peptic ulcer is an erosion of the intestinal mucosa resulting from destruction by acid and pepsin. The term "ulcer" is usually reserved for craters that extend into the muscle layer, and "erosion" refers to more superficial injury. Peptic ulcers occur in the duodenum, stomach, and esophagus, and in areas bordering ectopic gastric mucosa (e.g., Meckel's diverticulum).

Peptic ulcer disease is a common malady. It is estimated that about 10% of the population of the United States suffer from an ulcer in their lifetime. Peptic ulcer disease is also one of the most studied human disorders. The rapid developments in endoscopy in the last two decades have facilitated the examination of the major ulcer-bearing areas. At the same time, many new drugs to heal ulcers have been developed. These drugs required proof of their efficacy and safety, and an enormous amount of knowledge about the natural history of ulcer disease was thereby obtained. A major finding was that frequent recurrences are characteristic of peptic ulcer disease. In a study of several hundred patients with duodenal ulcer,[1] only 26% were completely symptom- and ulcer-free for 12 months following healing of their ulcer. One recurrence occurred in 33%, two recurrences in 25%, and three or more in 17% of these patients. Other studies have emphasized this, with about a 70% recurrence rate at 1 year commonly reported. The longer term recurrence rate is not known. It appears that the disease does ultimately burn out. At 10 to 15 years, about two-thirds of patients are asymptomatic. The recurrence rate seems to decrease annually.

The importance of understanding the medical treatment of peptic ulcer disease is further emphasized because it is recommended for a wide spectrum of upper abdominal complaints. Ulcer therapy is recommended for those with dyspepsia and indigestion.[2] Ulcer drugs are used to prevent stress ulcers and to treat upper intestinal bleeding. It is debatable whether the treatment is helpful in these circumstances, but, it certainly makes these drugs some of the most frequently prescribed in the world.

PATHOGENESIS

An ulcer occurs when aggressive factors overwhelm the defensive ability of the intestinal lining. Many aggressive factors can be active, and different factors are paramount in different patients.

Acid has received the greatest attention, but only a minority of ulcer patients have above-normal acid secretion. In patients with gastrinomas (Zollinger-Ellison syndrome, multiple endocrine neoplasia, type I), the high acid outputs alone seem sufficient to produce ulcers. In most patients, however, other contributing factors seem to be operative. Nonetheless, it is rare to see an ulcer in an individual with below-average acid secretion, and the adage "No acid, no ulcer" is almost always applicable.

In the past decade, great interest has arisen in a bacterium as a factor contributing to ulcer formation. Helicobacter pylori (H. pylori), formerly called Campylobacter pylori, has been found in over 90% of ulcer patients. Even before the identification of H. pylori, it was known that most patients with ulcer had active, chronic gastritis. Evidence now shows that H. pylori is the cause of this active, chronic gastritis. H. pylori is an organism uniquely adapted to its environment. It is a motile organism that moves freely in the gastric mucus, and it produces urease in large quantities. Splitting urea may help protect the bacteria from gastric acid and, in addition, may damage the gut lining, aiding in ulcer production. The question remained as to how the organism that produces a lesion in the antrum, and is found primarily in the antrum, causes ulcers mainly in the duodenum. In response, it has been suggested that islands of gastric mucosa are commonly found in the duodenum, especially in duodenal ulcer patients, and that these areas support the growth of H. pylori; therefore, ulcers may form at their borders.

H. pylori is found in over 90% of duodenal ulcer patients and in over 90% of gastric ulcer patients (when gastric ulcers related to the use of nonsteroidal anti-inflammatory drugs, or NSAIDs, are excluded). Eradication of the organism is associated with healing of the ulcer. Prevention of reinfection prevents recurrence of peptic ulcer, whereas recurrent ulcer is frequently associated with recurrent infection.

Nonetheless, H. pylori does not cause an ulcer in all those infected. Epidemic infections with H. pylori have produced gastritis, not ulcers. Subjects who intentionally drank H. pylori did not develop ulcers, but developed active, chronic gastritis. H. pylori appears to be a permissive or promoting factor.

Recognition of the importance of H. pylori has led to an examination of the relationship of this bacterium to other factors known to be related to ulcer disease. For example, an increased incidence of ulcer in certain socioeconomic groups may be a result of an increased incidence of infection. Also, the increased incidence of ulcer associated with the presence of blood group O and blood group substance nonsecretor status may be related to an increased susceptibility to infection.

Despite the fact that pepsin is part of the name "peptic ulcer," pepsin has not been as vigorously studied as acid. This is probably because drugs with antipeptic activity have not been developed. A strong correlation between acid and pepsin secretion has been noted, though, and peptic activity is greatly heightened by acid.

High levels of pepsinogen I are found in the serum of about 50% of ulcer patients. Hyperpepsinogenemia I is inherited as an autosomal dominant trait, but only about 40% of those who inherit the trait develop ulcers.

Factors that increase acid or pepsin secretion increase the incidence of ulcer. It remains to be established whether an increased incidence of H. pylori infection similarly increases ulcer incidence.

Several defensive factors are involved in the maintenance of the mucosa exposed to gastric secretions: (1) the gastric mucosal barrier to acid diffusion; (2) the mucous layer; (3) cell regeneration; (4) prostaglandin synthesis; (5) mucosal blood flow; and (6) bicarbonate secretion. A deficiency of one or more of these factors has not been convincingly shown to cause ulcers, but defensive factors probably determine the precise sites of ulcer formation. Furthermore, their importance is illustrated by the fact that patients with massive secretion of acid resulting from gastrinoma may have no ulcers but just diarrhea, whereas individuals with low-normal acid secretion may develop ulcers.

In summary, peptic ulcer disease represents an interaction between aggressive, injurious factors and defensive factors, so that the defenders are locally overwhelmed.

DIAGNOSIS

Peptic ulcer is suggested by epigastric pain, which is described as gnawing and is relieved by food or antacid. The pain usually occurs 1 to 3 hours after eating or awakens the individual from sleep in the hours just after midnight. It is unusual for ulcer pain to occur in the morning before breakfast. The ulcer may produce either an increase in appetite or anorexia and nausea.

The symptoms are neither specific nor sensitive. Symptoms of bloating, belching, or fatty food intolerance may occur in half of patients. One-third of patients with ulcers may be asymptomatic.

Although radiography can successfully diagnose peptic ulcer in most cases, endoscopy is more sensitive and provides an opportunity to biopsy suspicious lesions.

A position paper commissioned by the American College of Physicians has provided valuable guidance regarding the proper use of endoscopy in the diagnosis of peptic ulcer.[2] Endoscopy is not recommended for the evaluation of every patient with dyspepsia. A trial of ulcer therapy is suggested for the average individual, with no further diagnostic testing necessary in those who respond. It should be emphasized, however, that endoscopy is indicated in certain circumstances prior to a trial of therapy. The following groups should be endoscoped: (1) individuals with weight loss; (2) individuals who have systemic symptoms; (3) individuals with evidence of a complication (e.g., bleeding or obstruction); (4) the elderly; and (5) individuals who have recurrent symptoms (without proven diagnosis of peptic ulcer). Endoscopy is recommended for those who do not have a response to therapy in 7 to 10 days, and for those who fail to resolve their symptoms in 6 to 8 weeks.

It is instructive to consider the reasoning behind this position paper:

1. Only 20% of patients with dyspepsia actually have a duodenal ulcer, 50% have no endoscopic findings, and the rest have various findings, grouped under gastritis, duodenitis, and similar conditions.
2. The treatment is not affected by those findings. As previously noted, all dyspepsia is treated with antiulcer therapy.
3. A major concern is that a diagnosis or gastric cancer might be missed or delayed. The incidence of gastric cancer, however, is lower than 1% in most series of dyspeptic patients. Of these, about 90% have advanced lesions. Furthermore, gastric cancer patients should be found because of systemic symptoms, failure of treatment, or recurrence of symptoms.
4. Patients with a peptic ulcer should ultimately be definitively diagnosed when they develop recurrent symptoms.
5. Most ulcer patients heal on the ulcer therapy, whereas those without ulcers are seldom harmed by that treatment. The side effects of ulcer therapy have been rare and mild.

TREATMENT

Patient Education. Because peptic ulcer disease is chronic and recurrent, an important part of therapy is patient education. Patients should be informed that they are likely to develop recurrent symptoms. The patient needs to know that bleeding can occur, even in the absence of pain, and that melena is an indication of bleeding that requires urgent medical care.

Diet. Patients frequently want to discuss dietary treatment for their ulcers but, contrary to popular belief, no particular dietary regimen has been found to be of proven benefit. In particular, milk and dairy products are commonly believed to be beneficial. Indeed, there has been some interest in the possible benefit of the prostaglandin content of milk but the recommendation of milk at this time would be premature. An antacid is probably superior.

Data suggest that a high-fiber diet is helpful in reducing the incidence of ulcer and reduces recurrence.[3] In a study from India, [4] it was noted that the incidence of duodenal ulcer was much higher in the rice-eating areas than in the wheat-eating areas. A clinical trial was performed in which patients with radiographically proven duodenal ulcers were randomized to a diet of unrefined wheat or rice. The wheat diet was associated with a significantly lower ulcer recurrence rate than the rice diet.

Patients often argue that they can't have an ulcer because they can tolerate hot or spicy foods without distress. These individuals need to be assured that such foods may commonly produce indigestion, but that has little to do with their ulcer. A common sense approach is to suggest that ulcer patients avoid foods that cause discomfort. If a patient insists on a diet the high-fiber diet can be suggested, which has other benefits.

Beverages also have minor effects on ulcer disease. All beverages, including water and milk, stimulate acid production. Caffeinated and decaffeinated beverages stimulate acid secretion. No evidence has been found to indicate that these beverages are particularly harmful in ulcer disease. The one exception is alcohol. Cirrhosis is clearly associated with an increased incidence of ulcer; therefore, drinking to the point of developing cirrhosis increases the risk of ulcer. One report[5] has suggested that alcohol, even in moderate amounts, is harmful by reducing the chance of healing (in response to famotidine).

Smoking. More important than a discussion of diet is a discussion of smoking. Smoking increases the risk of ulcer and of an ulcer complication.[6] The increased risk of ulcer from smoking is dose-related, with the significant increase in risk occurring at a consumption of 10 cigarettes/day. Smoking interferes with various antiulcer drugs, reducing the speed of healing and decreasing the total response rate. Smoking increases the risk of recurrence and increases the possibility of undergoing surgical therapy because it increases the complication risk—that is, the chance of intractability to medical therapy, bleeding, obstruction, or perforation. Finally, smoking is associated with a decrease in life expectancy after ulcer surgery, not because of ulcer complications or cancer but because of the known cardiovascular complications of smoking. No matter how one looks at it, smoking is especially harmful for individuals with ulcers. This point must be strongly emphasized with patients who are smokers.

The effect of smoking on recurrence rates was clearly shown in a study reported in 1984.[7] Ulcer recurrence rates were examined in groups of patients who had healed their duodenal ulcers. A group of patients was given placebo and two other groups were given different doses of cimetidine as maintenance therapy. Smokers in all groups had an increased risk of recurrence. The smokers on placebo had a 72% recurrence rate, and smokers on either dose of cimetidine had a 34% recurrence rate. Nonsmokers on placebo had a 21% recurrence rate and nonsmokers on cimetidine had an 18% recurrence rate. The same findings were confirmed in terms of symptomatic recurrence, with a 51% rate for the smoker on placebo contrasting markedly with the 13% rate for nonsmoking subjects on placebo.

Drugs. NSAIDs clearly increase the risk of bleeding from ulcers. Also, the bleeding is often more serious when associated with NSAID use. Patients with a diagnosed ulcer should be cautioned about this risk if they decide to use NSAIDs. Patients who have bled should be strongly advised not to use these drugs at all.

It is controversial whether steroids cause ulcers or interfere with healing.

Theophyllines stimulate acid secretion and probably do increase ulcer incidence. Clearly, an increased risk of ulcer is associated with chronic obstructive pulmonary disease, independent of drug therapy for it.

Stress. Another topic that a patient often wishes to discuss is stress. The notion that certain occupations and personality types are particularly susceptible to ulcers is extremely popular. Some studies have reported findings supporting this theory, but others have found no such associations. A report from Texas considered stress and a number of different psychologic factors in relation to ulcer.[8] The authors did not find an increased incidence of stressful events in the period before the development of an ulcer, but they did find that the ulcer patients perceived stressful events as of greater import and impact than the control population. It was not the circumstances themselves but the individual's perception of those circumstances that seemed to be important. An increased incidence of various abnormalities on psychologic index testing was also noted—hypochondriasis, excessive dependency, depression-anxiety, and lower ego strength. Whether psychologic intervention has an effect on the ulcers or on their recurrence remains questionable.

PHARMACOLOGIC THERAPY

H_2 Receptor Inhibitors

The most popular drugs in the treatment of peptic ulcer disease at present are the H_2 receptor antagonists. The history of these drugs is interesting. It was known for many years that histamine stimulated acid secretion, and that, when doing a histamine stimulation test, one could block the allergy-type side effects with diphenhydramine hydrochloride (Benadryl) and other "traditional" antihistamines while maintaining the gastric secretory effect. It was speculated that the allergic symptoms (e.g., urticaria, rhinitis, flushing) were mediated by different receptors than the gastric effects. The allergic response receptors were designated H_1 receptors and the gastric secretory receptors were referred to as H_2 receptors. In 1972, Black and colleagues[9] demonstrated selective H_2 receptor blockade. Their first drug was burimamide, which had a potent antisecretory effect when administered parenterally; it was too weak, however, when given orally. The next drug developed was metiamide. This drug was given clinical trials, in which the discovery of side effects, including agranulocytosis and aplastic anemia, led to its withdrawal. Subsequently, cimetidine was developed, and this achieved extensive, widespread use. Others have followed. Four readily available H_2 inhibitors are now on the market in the United States: cimetidine (Tagamet), ranitidine (Zantac), famotidine (Pepcid), and nizatidine (Axid).

The differences between these drugs are minor and have been overemphasized. Ranitidine is predominantly cleared by the liver, whereas cimetidine, famotidine, and nizatidine are predominantly cleared by the kidney. The potency varies; famotidine is 5 to 8 times stronger than ranitidine and nizatidine, and these are in turn roughly 10 times more potent than cimetidine. This is reflected in the dosage recommendations for each drug.

All H_2 receptor antagonists share the same mode of action—by inhibiting histamine potentiation, they decrease acid secretion. They decrease nocturnal acid secretion, decrease meal-stimulated secretion, and decrease acid secretion stimulated by pentagastrin, hypoglycemia, or histamine. These drugs have been found to be particularly effective at decreasing the nighttime acid production, thereby controlling nighttime pain.

In trying to identify a "drug of choice," the side effects of the H_2 receptor antagonists have been examined in detail. Significant, but rare, complications include leukopenia, interstitial nephritis, and transaminase level elevations. Problems that have been particularly emphasized with cimetidine include gynecomastia, oligospermia (controversial), impotence (controversial), confusion in the elderly, and inhibition of the microsomal cytochrome P450 metabolism system of the liver, but clinical experience has shown that these side effects are overemphasized. It is seldom that therapy must be interrupted because of side effects. For example, in the case of cimetidine, the side effects that commonly occur are diarrhea, in about 1%, nausea and vomiting (<1%), and gynecomastia (which occurs in about 0.2% of men on long-term maintenance). The total incidence of side effects with cimetidine is between 3 and 5%.

Ranitidine has a similar incidence of side effects. The most common is headache, which occurs in about 3%. Again, with this drug, a lower than 1% incidence of a wide spectrum of side effects is noted, including malaise, dizziness, constipation, and nausea. It appears to have a lower chance of confusion and gynecomastia and approximately 10 times less impairment of the P450 enzyme system, but may have a slightly greater risk of elevation of serum transaminase levels than cimetidine.

The side effects of famotidine and nizatidine are similar to those of the other two drugs. Both famotidine and nizatidine have headache as their most frequent side effect. They appear to have insignificant effects on the P450 system. Clinical experience is not as extensive with these drugs.

The cost of these drugs to the patient is high, and cost should be a major consideration in choosing among them. According to one report,[10] cimetidine is the least expensive of the class, averaging 10 to 15% less than famotidine and ranitidine, which are similar in price. Nizatidine is intermediate in price, closer to cimetidine than to the other two.

The tremendous popularity of the H_2 receptor antagonists is well deserved. These drugs are highly effective, with a healing rate for duodenal ulcer of 75 to 85% at 4 to 6 weeks of therapy. After 8 weeks of treatment, it varies between 90 and 95% in different studies. A slight further increase is seen after 12 weeks. No significant difference in efficacy among the four drugs has been found.

Other Drugs

Sucralfate. Sucralfate (Carafate) is a major therapeutic agent that does not significantly affect acid levels. Sucralfate developed from research begun on polysaccharides in the 1960s, which showed that increasing the sulfation of some polysaccharides produced agents with increased antipeptic activity. Sucralfate is a disaccharide with multiple sulfates attached to it; the sulfates are combined with aluminum hydroxide molecules. Despite the large number of aluminum hydroxide moieties, sucralfate is an extremely weak antacid. The mechanism of action of sucralfate is still unclear. In vitro, it inactivates pepsin, binds bile salts, and protects protein membranes, to which it is bound, from peptic digestion. Binding of the drug to the mucosa, which occurs best in an acid environment, is important to its mechanism of action. Sucralfate has a "cytoprotective" effect. Pretreatment with sucralfate has been shown to limit the damage to the gastric mucosa from the subsequent administration of various caustic substances, such as concentrated acid, aspirin, and alcohol. This cytoprotective effect is associated with increased prostaglandin levels, with increased blood flow and increased gastric mucus production.

Sucralfate has an efficacy equivalent to that of the H_2 receptor antagonists in healing acute peptic ulcer. It is also equally efficacious in preventing ulcer recurrence. An advantage of sucralfate is that it is not systemically absorbed, which reduces the risk of systemic complications or significant interactions with other drugs. It can interfere with the absorption of some drugs, however, when they are bound to the sucralfate in the lumen of gut. The rate of side effects is in the same range as that of the H_2 antagonists—that is, 3 to 5%. The most frequent side effect is constipation.

The fact that sucralfate does not act through acid inhibition is a significant advantage in at least one circumstance. In the intensive care setting, in which patients are intubated for mechanical respiratory support and have nasogastric tubes in place, acid suppression has been shown not only to lead to bacterial colonization of the stomach, but to colonization of the nasopharynx and upper airway.[11] This increases the risk of pneumonia.

Omeprazole. Omeprazole (Prilosec) is the first of a new class of antisecretory drugs, the substituted benzimidazoles, to reach the market. These drugs inhibit the H^+/K^+-ATPase enzyme system at the secretory membrane of the gastric parietal cell, which is the final step in the production of acid. Omeprazole irreversibly inactivates the enzyme, and so the duration of acid inhibition lasts up to 72 hours. It is more potent than any of the H_2 receptor antagonists.

Omeprazole heals ulcers more rapidly than the other drugs but, at 4 to 6 weeks, the healing rates are similar. The major advantage has been its use in gastrinoma patients and in patients refractory to other treatment.

Omeprazole has a rate of side effects similar to that of the other drugs. The most frequent side effect is headache. A significant concern was raised by the occurrence of gastric carcinoid tumors and by hyperplasia of enterochromaffin-like cells in rats given omeprazole. Such effects have not been seen in humans, however, even though a significant rise in gastrin levels occurs with the drug. In fact, a report from the National Institutes of Health[12] has reported no significant side effects in a group of patients treated with high-dose omeprazole for Zollinger-Ellison syndrome.

At present, the drug is not FDA-approved for long-term or maintenance use. It is extremely expensive, about $3/20 mg daily dose.

Antacids. Antacid therapy is the oldest recognized therapy for peptic ulcer disease, but concepts concerning that therapy have recently begun to change. It was originally thought that antacids had to be given frequently and in high dosage to neutralize gastric acid completely to heal ulcers. The same concept was applied to the H_2 inhibitors when they were introduced. Both antacids and H_2 inhibitors were used in dosages designed to maintain a neutral or basic gastric pH throughout 24 hours. Clinical trials with H_2 inhibitors, however, have shown that excellent healing rates can be achieved when acid production is inhibited only at night. This has led to studies in which antacids were given in lower dosage and at less frequent intervals. A Scandinavian study[13] has compared a group of ulcer patients treated with antacid tablets qid (after meals and at bedtime) with a group treated with cimetidine, 800 mg, at bedtime. They found similar healing rates. About 70% of ulcers were healed in 4 weeks with this comparatively weak antacid regimen. Additionally, no difference was seen in the number of nights with pain between the group taking cimetidine and the group taking antacids.

Antacid therapy is a perfectly reasonable choice. The side effects are mainly changes in bowel habits because of the magnesium or aluminum in the antacids. Probably one of the most common reasons that they are not recommended more often is that patients don't consider antacids "real medicine," and a prescription is not required.

Antibiotics. Because H. pylori is so often associated with ulcer, and because its persistence seems critical to recurrence, therapy to eradicate H. pylori is a consideration. Eradication of H. pylori has been shown to produce healing rates comparable to those of other therapies. In addition, the relapse rates are lower, about 20% in 1 year, in contrast to more than 70% after other treatment.

In vitro, H. pylori is sensitive to a host of antibiotics: bismuth compounds, penicillins, erythromycin, tetracycline, tinidazole, metronidazole, gentamicin, and nitrofurantoins. It is resistant to sulfamethoxazole, trimethoprim, nalidixic acid, and vancomycin. The growth of H. pylori is affected only slightly by cimetidine, sucralfate, carbenoxolone, and antacids. In vivo, however, the rate of relapse and resistance has been so high that triple drug therapy is recommended.

It might be anticipated that such a regimen would be associated with a significant incidence of side effects (e.g., antibiotic-induced diarrhea, allergy). Conversely, conventional ulcer therapy has an extremely high efficacy and an enviably low rate of side effects. It seems unlikely that triple drug therapy can soon replace single-agent ulcer treatment. The challenge is to develop antimicrobial therapy that is as convenient and safe as present ulcer therapy.

Anticholinergics. Anticholinergics have long been used to treat ulcers. Anticholinergics reduce acid secretion, but the nonselective anticholinergics are not as effective as the drugs mentioned above. These drugs can be effective in combination with H_2 inhibitors and antacids.

A selective anticholinergic, pirenzipine, has been shown to be an effective single agent, with an efficacy equivalent to that of other antiulcer drugs, but it is not available in the United States.

Prostaglandins. Only one drug of this class is presently available for ulcer-related use. Misoprostil (Cytotec) has been recommended to reduce the risk of NSAID-induced gastric ulcer. In fact, it is the only drug with proven efficacy for this indication but, for ulcer unrelated to NSAID use, it is not a good choice. It carries a high risk of side effects, the most frequent of which is diarrhea. There is a risk of inducing abortion, miscarriage, or premature labor with this class of drugs.

MAINTENANCE THERAPY

The minimum effective dosage and duration of therapy have not been of major research interest. The standard duration of therapy for duodenal ulcer is 4 to 6 weeks. The healing rate at that time as found by endoscopy is 70 to 80%, but a higher percentage of patients are asymptomatic. Stopping therapy at this point does not seem to be associated with earlier recurrences or failure of ultimate healing. It would be of interest to determine the minimum required duration of therapy.

In the case of gastric ulcer, therapy must be continued until the ulcer has been documented to have healed completely. Failure of healing strongly suggests a malignant cause of the ulcer.

The appropriate use of maintenance therapy is unclear. Maintenance therapy refers to the use of drugs, usually in lower than treatment dosage, in an attempt to prevent ulcer recurrence. The rate of ulcer recurrence is high but, fortunately, most recurrences are asymptomatic.

Certainly, recurrences should be treated with standard regimens. If an endoscopic diagnosis was not previously made, an endoscopic examination is warranted.

After how many recurrences should maintenance therapy be considered? A firm consensus has not been reached. Most gastroenterologists suggest maintenance therapy if two recurrences have occurred within a year. Also, most suggest maintenance for those who have had a complicated ulcer—that is, an ulcer associated with bleeding or obstruction, or one that perforated (when a vagotomy was not performed). The length of time for continuing maintenance therapy is even more unclear. So little information is available that a recommendation can not be made.

OTHER THERAPEUTIC CONSIDERATIONS

Other considerations include refractory ulcers and nonulcer dyspepsia.

Refractory Ulcer

A refractory ulcer is one that has not healed in 6 weeks for duodenal ulcer or 8 weeks for gastric ulcer. When a patient reports symptoms for times exceeding these intervals, it is important to demonstrate first that the symptoms are caused by the ulcer. A repeat endoscopy is warranted.

If the diagnosis is confirmed, it is important to determine that the patient has taken the prescribed medication. Again, stopping smoking and NSAID use should be recommended. Sometimes, the patient is willing to reconsider at the prospect of surgery. At this point, the serum gastrin level should be measured to rule out gastrinoma.

If the patient has been reasonably compliant, and smoking and NSAID use are not relevant factors, some escalation of therapy is recommended. The addition of an anticholinergic to the drug already being given, or a change to omeprazole, are regimens most likely to be successful. Omeprazole appears particularly promising.[14] Other changes and combinations have not been found to be as useful.

After an additional 4 weeks of therapy, continuation of symptoms requires therapy according to the site of the ulcer. For gastric ulcer, surgery is recommended. Only full-thickness biopsy can exclude malignancy. For a duodenal ulcer, a trial of a different class of drug than the one previously used, and/or treatment for H. pylori, should be tried (e.g., triple drug—bismuth, metronidazole, and amoxicillin).

Failure of all these measures should lead to a recommendation of surgery. Fortunately, this is rare. The treatment of peptic ulcer disease has advanced dramatically in the last two decades. Many highly effective drugs are now available to heal ulcers that are extremely safe and have few side effects. A "cure" for the disorder, and effective therapy for its complications, however, remain challenges for the future.

Nonulcer Dyspepsia

In light of the highly successful therapy available for peptic ulcer, it has been frustrating that most patients with dyspepsia have no endoscopic lesions. No proven effective therapy is available for this nonulcer dyspepsia. Many drugs have been tried, but none is significantly superior to the high rates of symptomatic improvement seen with placebo.

For placebo-type effects, H_2 receptor antagonists, sucralfate, and omeprazole are expensive. I prefer antacids and anticholinergics. For severe cases, tricyclic antidepressants often seem to be effective.

RECOMMENDATIONS

In conclusion, some definite recommendations may be worthwhile. These are based on my own opinions and are therefore more "editorial" than scientific. For the average ulcer patient, I recommend cimetidine, because it is the least expensive choice. For long-term or maintenance therapy in a man I use nizatidine (because of the widely publicized antiandrogen effects of long-term cimetidine); for a woman, I recommend cimetidine. If the patient is taking drugs whose metabolism is likely to be significantly affected by inhibition of the P450 enzyme system, I prescribe sucralfate. Antacids can be used for symptom control, regardless of the other drug(s) used.

REFERENCES

1. Bardhan KD: Intermittent treatment of duodenal ulcer for long-term medical management. A review. Postgrad Med J, 64 (Suppl 1):40, 1988.
2. Health and Public Policy Committee, American College of Physicians: Endoscopy in the evaluation of dyspepsia. Ann Intern Med, 102:266, 1985.
3. Rydning A, Berstad A, Aadland E, Odegaard B: Prophylactic effect of dietary fibre in duodenal ulcer disease. Lancet 2:736, 1982.
4. Malhotra SL: A comparison of unrefined wheat and rice diets in the management of duodenal ulcer. Postgrad Med J, 54:6, 1978.
5. Reynolds JC: Famotidine therapy for active duodenal ulcers: A multivariate analysis of factors affecting early healing. Ann Intern Med, 111:7, 1989.
6. McCarthy DM: Smoking and ulcers—time to quit (Editorial.) N Engl J Med, 311:726, 1984.
7. Sontag S, Graham D, Belsito A, et al: Cimetidine, cigarette smoking, and recurrence of duodenal ulcer. N Engl J Med, 311:659, 1984.
8. Feldman M, Walker P, Green JL, Weingarden K: Life events, stress, and psychosocial factors in men with peptic ulcer disease. A multidimensional case-controlled study. Gastroenterology, 91:1370, 1986.
9. Wyllie JH, Hesselbo T, Black JW: The effect of burimamide on gastric secretion in man. Br J Surg, 59:902, 1972.
10. Nizatidine (Axid). Med Lett Drugs Ther, 30:78, 1988.
11. Driks MR, Craven DE, Celli BR et al: Nosocomial pneumonia in intubated patients given sucralfate as compared with antacids or histamine type 2 blockers. N Engl J Med, 317:1376, 1987.
12. Maton PN, et. al.: Long-term efficacy and safety of omeprazole in patients with Zollinger-Ellison syndrome: A prospective study. Gastroenterology, 97:827, 1989.
13. Weberg R, Aubert E, Dahlberg O, et al: Low-dose antacids or cimetidine for duodenal ulcer? Gastroenterology, 95:1465, 1988.
14. Tytgat G, et al: Omeprazole in peptic ulcers resistant to histamine H_2-receptor antagonists. Aliment Pharmacol Ther, 1:31, 1987.

chapter

4

THE APPROACH TO THE PATIENT WITH CHRONIC ABDOMINAL PAIN

Joseph T. Danzi

The management of the patient with chronic abdominal pain can be one of the most difficult clinical situations in office practice for many reasons. First, the patient is frustrated because of the inability of other physicians to diagnose the cause of their pain. Second, many of these patients have an altered personality affect, or neurotic behavior complex, that makes relating to them difficult. Finally, the physician can become frustrated because of the inability to diagnose the problem and establish a therapeutic program for relief of the patient's pain.

HISTORY AND PHYSICAL EXAMINATION

A comprehensive and detailed history and physical examination are imperative in difficult clinical situations such as this. The following should be obtained: a detailed initial history elucidating the location, characteristic, intensity, and chronology of the abdominal pain; determination of associated signs and symptoms and factors that aggravate or alleviate the pain; an evaluation of the patient's psychologic status; a history of previous gastrointestinal diseases; a history of prior abdominal or pelvic surgeries; a family history of common or unusual digestive disease, such as peptic ulcer, irritable bowel, porphyria, or cholecystitis; a complete history of prior diagnostic studies, both laboratory and radiologic; a history of prior therapies for the condition; and, a detailed physical examination. This comprehensive approach is time-consuming, but may be cost-efficient in the long-term management of the patient.

The following examples illustrate the usefulness of this approach in managing the two most common causes of chronic abdominal pain I have seen in my practice.

Case 1. If the abdominal pain is crampy in nature, located in the left lower quadrant or in both the left and right lower quadrants; is associated with a change in bowel habits, either diarrhea or constipation; is associated with mucoid material in the movements, without blood; is associated with abdominal bloating; no weight loss occurs; is associated with frequent, loose, bowel movements in the morning; is associated with a heightened gastrocolic reflex; is associated with stress or tension at work or at home; is associated with normal diagnostic laboratory studies and roentgenograms of the entire digestive tract; and is associated with a history of neurotic complaints or an altered affect, then this clinical senario is typical of a patient with the irritable bowel syndrome. It is appropriate to treat this patient with a high-fiber diet, fiber substitutes, and antispasmodics. This therapeutic trial should be continued for a period of 4 to 8 weeks, and the patient seen in follow-up. The usual clinical response is a decrease in the frequency and severity of the abdominal pain, with stabilization of the bowel habits. If the patient fails to respond to this therapeutic trial, studies to exclude a malabsorptive disease, lactose intolerance, or acute intermittent porphyria should be ordered.

Case 2. If the abdominal pain is severe enough to require frequent hospitalization and has resulted in multiple operations or exploratory laparotomies; is related to stress, menstrual cycle, or fatiguing circumstances; is brought on by the use of barbiturates, antianxiety medications, or specific antibiotics; is seen in a patient with normal diagnostic studies, including barium examinations of the complete gastrointestinal tract, (i.e., small bowel roentgenography, abdominal CT scan or ultrasound examination); is not associated with endometriosis or other ovarian causes; is observed in a patient with a normal psychologic profile; and is observed with other symptoms of autonomic neuronal dysfunction, such as hypertension or constipation, then one of the porphyrias that has neuropsychiatric symptoms and abdominal crisis secondary to its associated autonomic neuropathy is most likely. Acute intermittent or variegate porphyria, or hereditary coproporphyria, may be the cause of the patient's abdominal pain crisis. Urinary studies for D-aminolevulinic acid, porphobilinogen, and coprobilinogen, along with a blood test for uroporphyrinogen I synthetase, help establish a correct diagnosis (Table 4–1).[1] Once a correct diagnosis has been established, patient counselling regarding the

TABLE 4–1. URINARY STUDIES IN PORPHYRIA

Type	Urinary Abnormalities
Acute intermittent porphyria	↑ Porphobilinogen, ↑ D-ALA*
Variegate porphyria	↑ Porphobilinogen, ↑ D-ALA
Hereditary coproporphyria	↑ Porphobilinogen, ↑ D-ALA ↑ Coproporphyrin

*D-ALA, D-aminolevulinic acid.

medications to avoid and circumstances known to precipitate abdominal crisis should be given. The patient should be instructed to report to an emergency room with the first signs of an abdominal pain crisis, to identify themselves as a patient with a form of porphyria known to result in abdominal pain, and to request glucose infusions and pain control medication.[2]

LOCALIZATION AND CHARACTER OF THE PAIN

Much has been written of the importance of the localization of the pain within the abdominal cavity and the characteristic of the pain.[3] All sophomore or junior medical students in their clinical diagnosis classes have received lectures on the diseases that can result in pain in the epigastrium, mid-abdomen, and hypogastrium. The organs most commonly associated with epigastric pain include the esophagus, stomach, liver, pancreas, and gallbladder.[4] The small intestine is the most common source of periumbilical abdominal pain. The cause of hypogastric chronic abdominal pain includes disease of the colon, rectum, urinary bladder, uterus, and ovaries. The localization of the abdominal pain is of paramount diagnostic importance in the differential approach to patients with acute abdominal pain, but is less helpful in patients with chronic abdominal pain, except in those with an irritable bowel.

The character of the abdominal pain is helpful in the diagnostic approach to a patient with chronic abdominal pain. Is there radiation of the pain? Typically, patients with gallbladder or biliary tract disease complain of a steady pain on the right side of the epigastrium, or a midepigastrium pain. It is a misnomer that biliary pain is colicky in nature.[5] Importantly, about one-third of these patients has associated radiation of the pain to the intrascapular area or infrascapular area on the right.[6] Individuals with chronic pancreatitis have a boring, deep epigastric pain that increases with recumbency and eases with flexion of the spine. Patients with predominantly chronic inflammation of the tail of the pancreas may have radiation to the left shoulder secondary to irritation of the left diaphragm, but most patients with chronic pancreatitis complain of radiation straight through into the back.[7] Patients with the irritable bowel syndrome and associated bloating often complain of bilateral subcostal pain or costovertebral angle discomfort, which worsens as the abdominal distention increases.[8]

CLINICAL MANIFESTATIONS

Various signs and symptoms and precipitating and alleviating features are associated with chronic abdominal pain. It is a misconception in clinical practice that patients with chronic cholecystitis are often intolerant of fatty foods, but such individuals are no more intolerant of this type of food than people with a normal functioning gallbladder.[9] Importantly, fatty foods, through their release of cholecystokinin, may induce abdominal pain in a patient with the irritable bowel syndrome.[10] As mentioned, patients with chronic pancreatitis notice relief or exaggeration of their abdominal pain with certain body positions. Patients with acute intermittent or variegate porphyria, or hereditary coproporphyria, can have an abdominal crisis precipitated by certain medications or factors (Table 4–2). A high percentage of patients with the irritable bowel syndrome can correlate the start of their symptoms with stressful circumstances and a change in bowel habits.[11]

DIAGNOSTIC CONSIDERATIONS

An evaluation of the psychologic status is important in correctly diagnosing patients with the irritable bowel syndrome. These individuals frequently have associated neurotic manifestations, such as depression, chronic anxiety, or hysteria.[12] Studies have demonstrated that these patients have a lower pain threshold than healthy individuals, so they have a high incidence of associated complaints such as headaches and joint symptoms.[13] Patients with chronic pancreatitis and an associated cancer of the pancreas frequently have a sensation of impending doom. About 5 to 10% of such patients suffer from depression.[14] Individuals with one of the three porphyrias associated with abdominal pain can have associated psychiatric manifestations, such as depression or the organic brain syndrome.

Physical findings are helpful in the diagnosis of a patient with chronic abdominal pain. The most important clue to the diagnosis of a porphyria associated with abdominal pain is a normal abdominal examination when the patient is pain-free, and findings that mimic those of an acute abdomen during the abdominal crisis. Patients with an irritable bowel might demonstrate abdominal bloating, pain on palpation of the sigmoid colon, or the presence of rectal spasms on digital examination. Not infrequently, these patients demonstrate signs of anxiety, such as sweaty palms, nervousness, and labile hypertension. The presence of decreased or absent peripheral pulses in a patient with chronic abdominal pain and a normal abdominal examination should suggest a mesenteric arterial cause.

CAUSES OF THE PAIN

A number of conditions can cause chronic abdominal pain. The irritable bowel syndrome is the most frequent diagnosis in patients with an

TABLE 4–2. FACTORS PRECIPITATING AN ABDOMINAL CRISIS IN PATIENTS WITH ACUTE INTERMITTENT OR VARIEGATE PORPHYRIA AND HEREDITARY COPROPORPHYRIA

Factor	Examples
Drugs	Anticonvulsants, sulfonamides, barbiturates, chlordiazepoxide, ergot preparations
Other causes	Emotional stress, menses, fasting, infection, alcoholism

TABLE 4–3. CAUSES OF CHRONIC ABDOMINAL PAIN	
Diagnosis	**Associated Features**
Irritable bowel syndrome	Alteration of bowel habits, with mucoid material; altered affect or neurotic characteristic; association of stress or anxiety with signs and symptoms; normal gastrointestinal roentgenograms and laboratory studies
Acute intermittent or variegate porphyria, or hereditary coproporphyria	Recurrent abdominal pain crisis; association with certain medications; evidence of other autonomic neuropathy—constipation, diaphragmatic paralysis; history of multiple surgeries or laparotomies
Chronic pancreatitis	History of prior recurrent pancreatitis; history of alcoholism; compatible history and diagnostic studies
Intestinal ischemia	History of smoking; history of peripheral vascular and/or ischemic heart disease; postprandial pain that makes individual not want to eat

associated change in bowel habits. In patients with recurrent abdominal crisis, a diagnosis of acute intermittent or variegate porphyria, or hereditary coproporphyria, should be excluded. A diagnosis of chronic pancreatitis should be considered if the clinical history and diagnostic studies are compatible. Chronic abdominal pain secondary to mesenteric arterial insuffiency should be considered in a patient with a history of peripheral vascular and/or ischemic heart disease, a history of smoking, and confirmatory abdominal angiographic findings. Chronic cholecystitis without cholelithiasis can cause chronic, radiating, epigastric pain. Table 4–3 summarizes the associated features of these diagnoses.

In summary, a correct diagnosis of the cause of chronic abdominal pain requires patience, a detailed review of the history, and a complete physical examination. Although frustrating to many clinicians, a proper diagnosis often results in a satisfied patient.

REFERENCES

1. Bloomer JF: The porphyrias: Pathogenesis, manifestations, and management. Gastroenterology, 71:689, 1976.
2. Bloomer JF: The hepatic porphyrias. Viewpoints Dig Dis, 9:1, 1977.
3. Way LW: Abdominal pain. *In* Gastrointestinal Disease. Edited by MH Sleisenger and JS Fordtran. Philadelphia, WB Saunders, 1989, pp 238–250.
4. Rinaldo JA, Jr, Scheinok P, Rupe CE: Symptom diagnosis: A mathematical analysis of epigastric pain. Ann Intern Med, 59:145, 1963.

5. Way LW, Sleisenger MH: Cholelithiasis: Acute and chronic cholecystitis. *In* Gastrointestinal Disease. Edited by MH Sleisenger and JS Fordtran. Philadelphia, WB Saunders, 1989, pp 1691–1714.
6. Gunn A, Keddie N: Some clinical observations on patients with gallstones. Lancet, 2:7771, 1972.
7. Grendell JH, Cello JP: Chronic pancreatitis. *In* Gastrointestinal Disease. Edited by MH Sleisenger and JS Fordtran. Philadelphia, WB Saunders, 1989, pp 1842–1872.
8. Swarbrick ET, Hegarty JE, Bat L, et al: Site of pain from the irritable bowel. Lancet, 2:443, 1980.
9. Donaldson RM, Koch JP: A survey of food intolerances in hospitalized patients. N Engl J Med, 271:657, 1964.
10. Harvey RF, Read AE: Effect of cholecystokinin on colonic motility and symptoms in patients with irritable bowel syndrome. Lancet, 1:1, 1973.
11. Schuster MM: Irritable bowel syndrome. *In* Gastrointestinal Disease. Edited by MH Sleisenger and JS Fordtran. Philadelphia, WB Saunders, 1989, pp 1402–1418.
12. Latimer P, Sarna S, Campbell D, et al: Colonic motor and myoelectrical activity: A comparative study of normal patients, psychoneurotic patients, and patients with the irritable bowel syndrome. Gastroenterology, 80:893, 1981.
13. Whitehead WE, Winget C, Fedoravicius AS, et al: Learned illness behavior in patients with irritable bowel syndrome. Dig Dis Sci 27:202, 1982.
14. Cello JP: Carcinoma of pancreas. *In* Gastrointestinal Diseases. Edited by MH Sleisenger and JS Fordtran. Philadelphia, WB Saunders, 1989, pp 1872–1884.

chapter

5

THE APPROACH TO THE PATIENT WITH NONBLOODY DIARRHEA

Joseph A. Scopelliti

Diarrhea is defined as an increase in the number, volume, or fluidity of bowel movements from the normal, *usual* habit of an individual. The normal stool weight for an adult American is less than 150 to 200 daily. More than 200 daily is characterized by the patient as an increased number of bowel movements. In the evaluation of patients with diarrhea, it is important to try and assess objective symptoms such as the number of bowel movements, as well as subjective symptoms such as volume and fluidity.

As noted above, in Western populations, the average stool weight is 100 to 200 g daily. This varies, however, depending on patient demographics, with such factors as a rural or urban lifestyle affecting a change. Those living in rural areas in the United States have a significantly higher stool weight than those in urban areas. People in underdeveloped countries usually have a stool weight of 400 to 500 g daily, yet this is not considered diarrheal. The change from the patient's normal habit is therefore important.

ACUTE DIARRHEA

The first step in the office evaluation of patients with any diarrheal illness is to determine the duration. Acute diarrhea, by definition, is of less than 3 weeks' duration. Most typically, the patient presents to the office with a few days of changing bowel habits that are usually of sudden onset. The most common cause for this illness is a viral infection. In evaluating the history, however, several important points must be considered. First, it must be determined whether this is the first episode or is a recurrent problem. This is of critical importance, because chronic disorders such as inflammatory bowel disease can have a relapsing and remitting course. In addition, it must be determined whether blood is present with the bowel movement. If so, this points away from a viral cause and toward disorders such as inflammatory bowel disease. If the patient has no prior history of this, then bleeding with an acute diarrheal illness indicates an invasive bacterial pathogen, such as Campylobacter, Shigella, or enteroinvasive Escherichia coli. Further points to be assessed in the history include possible recent medication use, with particular attention to antibiotics and other medications that have diarrhea as a significant side effect.

The diagnosis in acute diarrhea is generally made by the history. If no repetitive episodes of similar symptoms occur, the patient has not used any medications, and no bleeding is present with the bowel movement, then the diagnosis of viral gastroenteritis is made by exclusion. At this point, no further diagnostic work-up need be undertaken.

Treatment at this point is supportive. The patient should be placed on a clear liquid diet for 48 hours. This significantly decreases the duration of illness. Avoidance of milk products later on may also be important, because the brush border of the small bowel could be damaged. Rehydration formulas (e.g., the World Health Organization formula) are particularly useful in children and the elderly, two groups that are at significant risk for dehydration. Bismuth subsalicylate is helpful in relieving traveler's diarrhea and may be of considerable use for all types of acute diarrhea. Finally, antidiarrheal medications, such as Lomotil or Imodium, are generally not necessary. They may be used, in extreme cases, but should be reserved for patients with persistent symptoms beyond 5 to 7 days. If the patient has continued symptoms, an evaluation for chronic diarrhea should be undertaken (see below).

CHRONIC DIARRHEA

Chronicity in the case of a diarrheal illness is indicated by repetitive bouts of diarrhea or diarrhea of continued duration, longer than 3 weeks. The first point in the history should be a determination of the anatomic source of the diarrhea. Generally, colonic sources are characterized by small volume and by frequent and urgent bowel movements. The sensation of tenesmus or rectal pressure is a prominent feature. In inflammatory bowel disease, gross bleeding is often noticed (discussed elsewhere in this text). In contradistinction, diseases of the small bowel are characterized by large- or normal-volume bowel movements that are increased in frequency and number from the usual. The patient does not have blood with the bowel movements, and, most importantly, has a considerable degree of weight loss.

The symptom of weight loss in diarrheal illness is important to evaluate for several reasons. First, it indicates a probable organic source of the patient's diarrhea. Second, it can identify a small bowel source. Weight loss indicates that a malabsorptive process is active. A note of caution here: patients with colonic sources of diarrhea often recognize a pattern of postprandial bowel movements. They avoid eating and, as a result, lose weight. It is crucial to question patients as to their dietary intake and to determine whether they believe that their dietary intake has been sufficient to maintain their weight. Typically, patients with small bowel processes note that their dietary intake is actually greater than normal, despite their illness.

Age is a serious consideration in the evaluation of this process. Of clear importance is the patient older than 50 years. In this population, all changes in bowel habits must be considered indicative of a colonic neoplasm until proven otherwise. The initial work-up should be aimed directly at this, regardless of the other findings. This may cause some patients to have testing that may not prove to be helpful, but it is such a necessary evaluation that it cannot be disregarded.

More recently, the sexual history of the patient has become increasingly important. In the situation of the diarrheal illness, the patient's risk factors for the development of acquired immunodeficiency syndrome (AIDS) must be evaluated. The frequency of diarrhea in this particular patient population is extraordinarily high, and has been reported to be as high as 30 to 80%,[1,2] (this is discussed further below).

Other points to be evaluated include a history of any abdominal surgeries, which may have predisposed the patient to diarrhea. Medication use, especially antibiotics, is important to ascertain. Travel history or exposure to parasitic infestations must be considered. Finally, the pattern of alternating constipation and diarrhea may indicate a functional disorder, such as irritable bowel syndrome (Chap. 12).

Physical examination of the patient with chronic diarrhea is generally directed toward identifying signs of malnutrition. The skin should be examined for any rashes, in particular looking for the bullous rash of dermatitis herpetiformis. This can be seen on the extensor surfaces of the elbows and knees. The patient should be examined for signs of muscle wasting, particularly temporal atrophy, and mucous membranes should be examined for evidence of dehydration, which again indicates an organic process.

The abdominal examination should be carried out, paying close attention to the presence of any palpable masses. Also, the patient should be examined for ascites and peripheral edema, because these indicate a hypoproteinemia state. Rectal examination with hemoccult testing is necessary. The patient should also be evaluated for any perianal diseases, such as a fistula, which might indicate the presence of inflammatory bowel disease. The last two areas of investigation are determination of the presence of lymph adenopathy, which could indicate an AIDS-related disorder, and the neurologic examination, which looks for peripheral neuropathies; these could indicate a chronic malabsorptive state that results in vitamin deficiencies.

BASELINE STUDIES

The work-up of chronic diarrhea should begin once an adequate history and physical examination have been performed. At this point, baseline studies are needed, including a complete blood count to evaluate the patient for an anemia. Specifically, the type of anemia needs to be identified. A hypochromic microcytic anemia indicates chronic blood loss, but may also represent malabsorption of iron, such as in celiac sprue. Megaloblastic anemias are often associated with small bowel pathology. The presence of an elevated white blood count is a nonspecific finding, but indicates inflammatory bowel disease as a possibility. Serum electrolyte levels are determined. The major findings here are a low potassium level and the presence of a metabolic acidosis, indicating a severe diarrhea. The possibility of secretory diarrheas is more likely under these circumstances. The measurement of serum cholesterol and protein levels provides information on the patient's nutritional status and on the severity of the diarrhea. A low serum calcium level indicates malabsorption, particularly of fat-soluble vitamins. This can be confirmed further by measuring the prothrombin time.

Finally, proctosigmoidoscopy and stool collection should be performed initially in the work-up of all patients with chronic diarrhea. The stool should be examined with Wright's stain to demonstrate fecal leukocytes, which indicates a breach of the intestinal mucosa. Inflammatory bowel disease and an infectious diarrhea are the two most likely diagnoses here. Examination for ova and parasites, as well as stool culture, should be performed routinely. Use of a Sudan stain is also helpful, because this provides a qualitative assessment of fat malabsorption. Note that use of a Sudan stain often yields positive results, but that a negative result does not rule out fat malabsorption. Sigmoidoscopy should be done, preferably without a preparation, because this could distort the mucosal pattern (Chap. 10). Biopsies should be performed, as needed.

At this point, a decision must be made as to the likely origin of the diarrhea. The work-up from this point on is distinctly different, depending on whether it is a midgut diarrhea or has a colonic source. Again, a review of the history would indicate large, voluminous stools, with extremely rapid weight loss, indicative of a midgut diarrhea. Colonic diarrhea is characterized by frequent, small stools and urgency; tenesmus and hematochezia are also common features.

Midgut Diarrhea

Midgut diarrhea can be broken down further into maldigestion and malabsorption; these refer to the various stages of the intestinal process. Digestion is a luminal process that requires the presence of bile salts, pancreatic enzymes, and appropriate intestinal transit so that the food can be prepared properly for mucosal absorption. This is in contrast to malabsorption, which assumes that the luminal digestive phase has proceeded normally. Absorption requires an intact mucosal surface and appropriate transport mechanisms for absorbed nutrients. The product of malabsorption and maldigestion is steatorrhea.

Therefore, the first step in the evaluation of suspected midgut diarrhea is an evaluation for steatorrhea. As noted above, a simple stool examination with Sudan stain is sometimes helpful but, more often, the investigation requires some quantitative measurement of stool fat. This is best done with a 72-hour fecal fat collection. Fat absorption is 93% efficient; thus, a stool fat greater than 7 grams while on a 100-g fat diet, indicates malabsorption. Another method for determining fat malabsorption is to use the triolein breath test. In this, a carbon-14 labeled triglyceride is ingested. If not absorbed (steatorrhea), then no carbon-14 is excreted in the breath during the examination. Although not as widely available, this is an accurate measurement of fat absorption.

Once fat malabsorption has been confirmed, a decision must be made as to whether this represents maldigestion or malabsorption. This can be done using the D-xylose test, which involves giving the patient an oral solution of xylose that can be passively absorbed through the small bowel mucosa. It is absorbed primarily in the proximal small bowel. When the D-xylose test result is abnormal, malabsorption is the diagnosis. Further investigation is necessary to determine the mucosal pattern of the small intestine and to characterize the problem further. Diseases that cause malabsorption generally have a specific mucosal pattern that can be identified roentgenographically. For example, the dilated small bowel and thickened folds seen in celiac sprue are almost always characteristic of this disease. If the site of malabsorption is suspected to be the distal small bowel, a Schilling test can be performed. Although not as specific a test of mucosal function as the D-xylose test, it is helpful in assessing ileal absorptive capabilities.

If the D-xylose test is normal, the diagnosis of maldigestion is suggested. Maldigestion requires a normally functioning liver and pancreas, as well as appropriate intestinal transit. Patients with cirrhosis have diminished bile salt production and therefore may malabsorb fats because of poor luminal mixing between the bile salts and ingested fats. This represents one type of maldigestion. A second type of maldigestion occurs when insufficient pancreatic enzymes are present to digest fat to an absorbable state. Pancreatic insufficiency can occur because of damage to the pancreas or an obstruction to the pancreatic duct, both of which produce functional disruptions to the pancreas. Visualization of the pancreas is generally the first step in the evaluation; CT scanning or endoscopic retrograde cholangiopancreatography (ERCP) is generally used.

If further work-up is necessary, a secretin stimulation test can be carried out. Secretin is given intravenously and pancreatic secretion is collected through a duodenal catheter. This is measured for the bicarbonate and amylase concentrations in response to secretin.

The third type of maldigestion that can occur is inappropriate luminal transport. In patients with diseases of the smooth muscle or anatomic variations such as the blind loop syndrome, bacterial overgrowth occurs. This syndrome results in luminal maldigestion and diarrhea. The diagnosis is usually confirmed by small bowel roentgenographic studies. The typical patient with bacterial overgrowth is someone who has scleroderma. Postoperative changes are usually identified quickly by history. Small bowel sampling for culture is generally not done in patients with bacterial overgrowth, because this is difficult to carry out and the results are not always reliable.

Colonic Diarrhea

In contrast to patients suspected of midgut diarrhea, colonic diarrheas are generally easy to evaluate. These almost always occur because of mucosal inflammatory changes or an obstructive process in the colon. When colonic diarrhea is suspected, flexible sigmoidoscopy, barium enema, and colonoscopy are the diagnostic tests of choice. The one that is specifically used depends on the physician in charge.

Flexible sigmoidoscopy is helpful for the evaluation of inflammatory bowel disease, because ulcerative colitis rarely spares the rectum. Crohn's disease may, however, not be identified by the sigmoidoscopic examination. Neoplastic diseases, if considered, require a more thorough investigation of the lower intestine.

A barium enema is useful in identifying inflammatory bowel disease when an air contrast study is performed. Single-contrast studies are nonspecific, however, and often miss the diagnosis of inflammatory bowel disease. Both single- and double-contrast barium enemas are highly diagnostic in evaluating neoplastic causes of diarrhea.

Colonoscopy is the most sophisticated of the examination techniques available for the lower intestine. It is the most sensitive and specific test for diagnosing inflammatory bowel disease, and offers the capability of colonic biopsy if a neoplastic process is suspected. It is the preferred test for determining a colonic source of diarrhea.

Secretory Diarrhea

The last type of diarrhea to be considered is that of secretory diarrhea, which is defined as a stool weight of greater than 250 g daily while the patient is NPO. Secretory diarrhea is caused by an active secretory process within the bowel. It can be the result of infections such as Vibrio cholera, or it can be hormonally mediated. The hormone source may be a primary gut tumor, such as a carcinoid, or the hormone may be related to a paraneoplastic process from an extraintestinal neoplasm.

If secretory diarrhea is suspected, a clue can be obtained from the history. Patients note that their diarrhea does not change, even if they avoid eating for long periods. If this is present, the patient should be brought into the hospital and fasted while stool samples are collected and weighed. If secretory diarrhea is confirmed, an investigation for infectious sources should be undertaken. If negative, hormone studies should be performed. The main hormones to look for include gastrin, vasoactive intestinal peptide, calcitonin, glucagon, and 5-hydroxyindoleacetic acid. If one of these is found, its source must be ascertained. The likely sources are specific, depending on the hormone.

SPECIAL CONSIDERATIONS

In the evaluation of patients with chronic diarrhea, several special situations need to be addressed.

Suspicion of Colonic Carcinoma

Any patient with a change in their bowel habit who is over 50 years old needs an evaluation to rule out the presence of a colonic carcinoma. This should be carried out regardless of the patient's hemoccult status. The false-positive rate for hemoccult testing is 30 to 60%.[3,4] The investigation should be intensified if the patient has any family history of colonic neoplasms, including adenomatous polyps.

Immunocompromised Patients

The second special situation is that of the homosexual or immunocompromised patient. In recent years, it has become clear that this group is at particular risk for the development of intestinal infections. At first, it simply seemed to be a matter of sexually transmitted disease, but it is now clear that many diarrheal illnesses are associated with an immunocompromised state. Viral infections of the gastrointestinal tract are common in patients with AIDS. The viral infections are not self-limited, however, and are usually profoundly severe. Herpes simplex virus types I and II have been identified as a common cause of nonbacterial proctitis. These viruses are typically found in sexually active male homosexuals. The characteristics of this infection include a severe anorectal pain, fever, sacral paresthesias, and perianal ulcerations. With this pattern of symptoms, sigmoidoscopic examination is the diagnostic test of choice. It reveals typically aphthous-like ulcers involving the rectum, but generally not extending higher up into the colon. The intervening rectal mucosa may be completely normal.

Cytomegalovirus (CMV) infection has also been reported as a cause of colitis in this population. It has been shown to produce a syndrome similar to that of herpes proctitis, but the main differentiating point is that CMV results in a pancolitis with severe diarrhea. This is a premorbid finding, and patients usually die within 6 months of onset of this disease.[5] It is the harbinger of an acceleration in the immunodeficiency state. Diagnosis is again established by sigmoidoscopic biopsy, with typical histologic findings of intranuclear inclusions, and can be confirmed by culture of the biopsy specimen.

Bacterial causes for diarrhea in this population include Neisseria gonorrhoeae. This was initially believed to represent a sexually transmitted disease, but this has been questioned. It is often identified in conjunction with other sexually transmitted organisms, such as syphilis and Chlamydia trachomatis. Salmonella and Shigella are also notable colonic pathogens, as are Campylobacter-like organisms. These can present with a proctitis or pancolitis.

Parasitic disease runs a wide spectrum in this population. The most common organisms are Giardia lamblia and Entamoeba histolytica. Their presentation is exactly the same as in the nonimmunocompromised host, but their numbers are significantly increased.

The most devastating infections of the gastrointestinal tract in the AIDS population are Cryptosporidium and Mycobacterium avium intracellulare. Cryptosporidium is a small protozoan with the potential for producing a severe infection in AIDS patients. It causes a profound diarrhea, with extraordinary fluid losses. Specialized culture techniques using sugar flotation to separate the oocysts have been useful in making the diagnosis. Treatment is limited. Spriamycin was thought to have some promise, but this has not held true.[6] More recently, courses of somatostatin have met with some success.[7]

Mycobacterium avium intracellulare is a known pulmonary pathogen. Both small and large bowel infections with this organism have been described.[8] It is usually part of a disseminated disease that results in a malabsorptive process, with profound weight loss. Biopsy of the intestinal region involved using an acid-fast stain is generally diagnostic. Treatment can be directed according to susceptibility testing; some response is expected.

In AIDS patients, a nonspecific enteropathy pattern has been described.[9] This is characterized by malabsorption findings with abnormal small and large bowel mucosa. Its exact pathogenesis is unclear, but it appears to be a slowly progressive disease that does not respond to a wide variety of antibiotic regimens. It is invariably part of a continuous, progressive deterioration in the patient's health.

The evaluation of a patient with AIDS-related diarrhea focuses on infectious organisms, with sigmoidoscopy as the first step. Stool should be collected at the time of sigmoidoscopy to demonstrate ova, parasites, and/or bacterial infections. Mucosal specimens can be obtained for viral studies. Mycobacterium avium intracellulare can be identified by stool examination for acid-fast bacilli. Pending the results, a full colonoscopy might be warranted to look for other evidence of mucosal disease. If a complete examination of the colon is unremarkable, further investigation into the small bowel may be necessary. Giardia can be particularly difficult to identify on stool examination, with a recovery rate of 50% being common.[10] Small bowel biopsy to diagnose Giardia is the test of choice if this is suspected. Small bowel roentgenography may be helpful if enteropathy is suspected. Thus, AIDS patients have a nonspecific enteropathy that is not infectious in origin, but this has not been well classified as yet.

This chapter has addressed the work-up of organically caused diarrheal illnesses. Treatment has not discussed, because this depends on the specific diagnosis. Other causes of diarrheal complaints are functional disorders, which are discussed elsewhere in this text.

REFERENCES

1. Anthony MA, Brandt LJ, Klein RS, et al: Infectious diarrhea in patients with AIDS. Dig Dis Sci, 33:1141, 1988.
2. Bartelsman IF, Sars PR, Tytgat GN, et al: Gastrointestinal complications in patients with acquired immunodeficiency. Scand J Gastroenterol, 24:112, 1989.
3. Winawer SJ, Andrews M, Miller CH, et al: Review of screening for colorectal cancer using fecal occult blood testing. *In* Progress in Cancer Research and Therapy, Vol 13: Colorectal Cancer, Prevention, Epidemiology, and Screening. Edited by SJ Winawer, D Schottenfeld, and P Sherlock. New York, Raven Press, 1980, pp 249–259.
4. Winawer SJ, Andrews M, Flehinger B, et al: Progress report on controlled trial of fecal occult blood testing for the detection of colorectal neoplasia. Cancer, 45:2959, 1980.
5. Frager DH, Frager JD, Wolf EL, et al: Cytomegalovirus colitis in acquired immunodeficiency syndrome: Radiologic spectrum. Gastrointest Radiol, 11:241, 1986.
6. Soave R, Johnson WD: Cryptosporidium and Isospora belli infections. J Infect Dis, 157:225, 1988.
7. Cook DJ, Kelton JG, Stanisz AM, et al: Somatostatin treatment for cryptosporidial diarrhea in a patient with AIDS. Ann Intern Med, 108:708, 1988.
8. Wolke A, Meyers S, Adelsberg BR, et al: Mycobacterium avium intracellulare-associated colitis in a patient with the acquired immunodeficiency syndrome. J Clin Gastroenterol, 6:225, 1984.
9. Kotler DP, Gaetz HP, Lange M, et al: Enteropathy associated with the acquired immunodeficiency syndrome. Ann Intern Med, 101:421, 1984.
10. Ament ME, Rubin CE: Relation of giardiasis to abnormal intestinal structure and function in gastrointestinal immunodeficiency syndrome. Gastroenterology 62:216, 1972.

chapter

6

THE APPROACH TO THE PATIENT WITH BLOODY DIARRHEA

Joseph T. Danzi

The diagnostic approach to patients with bloody diarrhea can be subdivided into five major findings:

1. The distinction between hematochezia or lower gastrointestinal hemorrhage and bloody diarrhea
2. Bloody diarrhea resulting from a colonic infection
3. Bloody diarrhea resulting from a flare-up of existing conditions, such as inflammatory bowel disease
4. Bloody diarrhea as a consequence of prior therapy resulting in conditions such as radiation proctocolitis or pseudomembranous colitis
5. Bloody diarrhea resulting from colonic neoplasia (Table 6–1).

The distinction between hematochezia and bloody diarrhea is usually not clinically difficult. An individual with lower gastrointestinal hemor-

TABLE 6–1. DIAGNOSTIC CONSIDERATIONS IN A PATIENT WITH BLOODY DIARRHEA
Distinction between bloody diarrhea and rectal bleeding
Exclusion of an infectious cause (parasitic; bacterial, including C. difficile)
Diagnosis of initial flare-up or an exacerbation of known ulcerative or Crohn's colitis
Consequence of prior radiation or antibiotic therapy
Result of a colonic neoplasia (adenoma or adenocarcinoma)

rhage typically presents with the passage of blood clots or unclotted blood rectally, and usually develops signs and symptoms of hypovolemia, such as hypotension, postural blood pressure changes, and tachycardia. Evidence of acute blood loss is noted, with a decreasing hemoglobin and hematocrit, and often the source of the hemorrhage is angiodysplasia of the colon or acute diverticular arterial bleeding.[1,2] A patient with bloody diarrhea only has blood-tinged diarrheal movements or fresh blood mixed with a loose stool, uncommonly develops signs or symptoms of hypovolemia, and may have a slow decrease in the hematocrit. The blood in their diarrheal movements does not originate from either colonic angiodysplasia or acute diverticular bleeding. If an individual with the irritable bowel syndrome develops a diverticular hemorrhage, it is not difficult to distinguish between hematochezia and bloody diarrhea (Table 6–2).

The three most common causes of bloody diarrhea are infectious colitis, inflammatory bowel disease, and colonic neoplasia.[3] It is more common for a colonic cancer to bleed than a colonic polyp, and it is more common for a patient with an obstructing colonic cancer to have bloody diarrhea because of the fermentation diarrhea that results. It is of paramount importance to exclude an infectious cause for bloody diarrhea in patients in remission with known inflammatory bowel disease, rather than to assume a relapse. It is equally important to exclude an infectious cause in patients newly diagnosed with inflammatory bowel disease before initiating steroid therapy.

The exclusion of an infectious colitis as the cause of bloody diarrhea is usually accomplished easily by submitting from all patients two or more fresh stool specimens for ova and parasite evaluation and stool culture. In addition, the stool should be analyzed by Wright's stain to detect the presence or absence of neutrophils. Conditions other than an infectious colitis that could produce a positive result with Wright's stain are inflammatory bowel disease and radiation enterocolitis. These diseases have a negative bacterial and parasitic stool evaluation, a history compatible with either disease, and specific sigmoidoscopic findings (see

TABLE 6–2. DISTINCTION BETWEEN BLOODY DIARRHEA AND HEMATOCHEZIA

Feature	Bloody Diarrhea	Hematochezia
Signs of Hypovolemia (hypotension, tachycardia)	Not common	Usual
Evidence of acute blood loss (hemoglobin; hematocrit)	Usual evidence of chronic blood loss	Usual
Bowel movement characteristic	Rare—usually blood mixed with stool	Usually only blood without stools
Cause	Infectious; inflammatory bowel disease; chronic radiation therapy; colonic neoplasia	40%; diverticular bleeding; 40%; vascular anomalies

Chap. 11). I routinely order a stool analysis for Clostridium difficile antitoxin assay in patients with bloody diarrhea. This is especially important if the patient has a history of prior antibiotic use before the onset of the bloody diarrhea, and if individuals have known inflammatory colitis. A small percentage of patients with ulcerative or Crohn's colitis have bloody diarrhea secondary to this bacterial infestation without a prior history of antibiotic use.[4]

Three guidelines must be remembered when collecting a stool specimen for bacterial or parasitic evaluation. First, the stool specimen should be submitted to the laboratory within 1 hour of collection. Second, the laboratory needs to exclude such bacterial diseases as Campylobacter jejuni and Yersinia enterocolitica in the stool culture analysis. Third, prior barium studies can produce a false-negative parasitic evaluation for Entamoeba histolytica. I recommend obtaining a serologic E. histolytica titer in a patient having a barium enema done before excluding this colonic infestation, especially if the sigmoidoscopic features are compatible with a diagnosis of E. histolytica (see Chap. 11). A titer between 1:200 and 1:2000 dilution is diagnostic of a concurrent E. histolytica infection.[5]

The most common cause of an infectious colitis in the United States is still C. jejuni, subspecies fetalis. Infection with Yersinia, Salmonella, or Shigella organisms are still frequent in this country, and all cases of bloody diarrhea require bacteriologic culture exclusion.[6] With the present sushi "craze" in this country, various organisms can result in an infestation that produces an enterocolitis that may mimic either type of idiopathic inflammatory bowel disease, as determined clinically or sigmoidoscopically.[7,8] An infection with C. jejuni, Y. enterocolitis, Salmonella, or Shigella can result in a colitis that produces radiographic or sigmoidoscopic features that can be confused with those of ulcerative or Crohn's colitis (see Chap. 10).

The emergence of E. coli 0157:H7 as a significant gastrointestinal pathogen has now been recognized. This enteric organism causes a hemorrhagic colitis that may be associated with hemolytic uremic syndrome or thrombotic thrombocytopenia purpura. One study[9] has demonstrated four important findings: (1) E. coli 0157:H7 is second to C. jejuni in the incidence of enteric infestation, ahead of Salmonella and Shigella; (2) this organism is associated with a 96% incidence of bloody diarrhea, whereas bloody diarrhea with C. jejuni, Salmonella, and Shigella infestation has an incidence of 46, 41, and 40%, respectively; and (3) ground beef and raw milk are the most common vehicles for transmitting the infection. I recommend screening for E. coli 0157:H7 in bacteriologic stool analysis for all patients with a history of bloody diarrhea.

A patient with ulcerative or Crohn's colitis usually presents with bloody diarrhea during an exacerbation of the disease. The diarrhea typically has a daytime and a nocturnal component. Associated signs and symptoms include crampy abdominal pain, tenesmus, malaise, fatigue, and a low-grade fever. Laboratory studies commonly demonstrate an increase in the erythrocyte sedimentation rate, a slight leukocytosis, thrombocytosis, variable degrees of anemia, and hypokalemia and hypoalbuminemia if protein-calorie malnutrition is associated. The sigmoidoscopic features of the mild to severe form of both types of inflammatory bowel disease are described in Chapter 10. As stated, it is important to exclude an infectious cause for the bloody diarrhea in patients with known ulcerative colitis or Crohn's disease before initiating steroid therapy. The patient with amebic colitis who is placed on high-dose steroid therapy has a high risk of resultant disseminated amebiasis, with a high rate of morbidity and mortality.

The pattern of response to therapy of severe ulcerative or Crohn's colitis is the resolution of the nocturnal diarrhea, followed first by the disappearance of the blood in the stool and then by the resumption of normal bowel movements. Any patient with severe colitis who suddenly has no bowel movements should have toxic megacolon excluded through serial radiography of the abdomen.[10] Only an ileus, such as that associated with a megacolon, produces a rapid cessation of bloody diarrhea in patients with severe colitis. The time required for the medical therapy of severe ulcerative or Crohn's colitis to normalize bowel movements is usually 7 to 21 days.

A past medical history of radiation therapy to the pelvis for prostate or uterine cancer is an important part of the evaluation of a patient with bloody diarrhea. Typically, patients with chronic radiation colitis develop their symptoms 4 to 6 months after the completion of therapy.[11] Bloody diarrhea is a common presenting symptom in patients with chronic radiation proctocolitis. The blood in the stool results from the atrophic mucosa and mucosal telangiectasia observed in the colonic mucosa during sigmoidoscopy (Chap. 10).[11] These mucosal abnormalities are a result of the radiation-induced obliterative arteritis. A mucosal biopsy usually confirms the observed endoscopic features of mucosal atrophy, radiation-related arteritis, and telangiectasia.

It is especially important to know the history of prior radiation therapy before proceeding with diagnostic colonoscopy. Colonic stricture and pelvic adhesions are consequences of chronic radiation arterial injury. This, in combination with mucosal atrophy, can result in colonic perforation during colonoscopy if excessive instrument pressure is applied to the sigmoid or left colon.

Typically, the features of chronic radiation proctocolitis are identified within the sigmoid colon in patients receiving radiation therapy for uterine or prostatic cancer.[12] With the identification of distal colonic chronic radiation injury, it is not mandatory to perform a total colonoscopy in a patient with a stricture or pelvic adhesions. A barium enema examination can exclude any concomitant colonic lesion, such as colonic polyps or colonic cancer. It is prudent in this clinical situation to limit the colonoscopic procedure to the distal colon.

The therapeutic approach to a patient with bloody diarrhea secondary to chronic radiation proctocolitis is as follows:

1. Place the individual on a strict, low-residue diet.
2. Use steroid suppositories or enemas, as determined by the extent of colonic involvement.

3. Add oral steroids in patients failing local (enema) steroid therapy or with extensive colonic injury.
4. Institute transfusions, as required.
5. Consider a proximal colostomy if all the preceding therapeutic measures fail.[13]

In my experience, chronic, low-dose oral steroid therapy in the range of 10 to 20 mg of prednisone daily is highly successful in most patients with extensive or medically resistant chronic radiation colitis.

In individuals presenting initially with bloody diarrhea secondary to chronic radiation proctocolitis who have resolution of the rectal bleeding but persistent diarrhea with medical therapy, it is important to exclude an enteric radiation injury as the cause. Small bowel radiography can demonstrate enteric strictures, delayed transit time, and enteric dilation.[14] These features can predispose the patient to a bacterial overgrowth syndrome, with its associated megaloblastic anemia and steatorrhea. The steatorrhea results from the bacterial deconjugation of the bile acids and the resultant decreased micellar formation. The anemia is secondary to the bacterial uptake of vitamin B_{12}. Treatment of a bacterial overgrowth syndrome includes the use of a broad-spectrum antibiotic, such as tetracycline, usually tid for 3 of the 4 weeks during a month. If a patient fails single antibiotic therapy, metronidazole can be added in conjunction with the original antibiotic.[15]

If small bowel radiography demonstrates only enteric wall thickening, without strictures or dilation, the patient's diarrhea is probably secondary to a malabsorptive state related to the radiation mucosal injury. Medical therapy varies if the radiation injury is predominantly in the proximal or distal small bowel. With proximal chronic radiation enteritis, the use of elemental dietary supplements alone or in conjunction with oral steroid therapy may be successful.[11] Unfortunately, some of these patients require long-term total parenteral nutrition at home. With distal chronic radiation enteritis, the use of medium-chain triglyceride supplements may decrease the diarrhea and prevent the development of fat malabsorption. In addition, monthly injections are indicated to prevent a vitamin B_{12} deficiency.

The widespread use of broad-spectrum antibiotics requires that any patient with bloody diarrhea have a thorough review of medication use. Many individuals take antibiotics fairly regularly for chronic sinus problems, chronic bronchitis, acne, urinary tract infections, and upper respiratory viral infections. This pattern of antibiotic use is directly associated with the increased recognition of C. difficile-associated pseudomembranous colitis. The colitis results from the effect of the bacterial cytotoxin on the colonic mucosa.[16] The cytotoxic mucosal injury results in mucosal inflammation with superficial ulcerations, bloody diarrhea, pseudomembranes on the mucosa (Chap. 10), the presence of fecal leukocytes as demonstrated by the Wright's stain of the stool, and the clinical signs associated with a colitis.[17] A confirmed diagnosis of C. difficile-related colitis can be established by obtaining a positive antitoxin assay result on a stool specimen.

Unfortunately, about 10% of patients with C. difficile-related pseudomembranous colitis do not have a history of antibiotic use prior to the onset of their colitis.[16] In addition, a small percentage of apparent flare-ups of ulcerative or Crohn's colitis results from a C. difficile infestation that is not associated with antibiotic use. The exact reservoir for this type of C. difficile infection is unknown. Finally, a small percentage of individuals have a positive bacterial stool culture for C. difficile with a negative antitoxin assay result.[17] These individuals are only carriers of the organism.

The mucosal features evident in the rectosigmoid colon are typical of the patient with C. difficile-related pseudomembranous colitis. One-third of such patients, however, may have the findings limited to the right colon only.[18] A total colonoscopy and positive antitoxin assay confirm the diagnosis in this subgroup of patients.

The therapy of C. difficile-related pseudomembranous colitis consists of the eradication of the bacteria with metronidazole or vancomycin treatment. The primary advantage of metronidazole is its low cost as compared to that of vancomycin, and their equal efficacy. After the completion of a 2-week course of antibiotic therapy, most patients have complete resolution of their symptoms. In addition, the resin-binding agent cholestyramine may be used in conjunction with the antibiotic to bind and inactivate the bacterial cytotoxin, and to decrease the severity and frequency of the diarrhea.

A significant percentage of patients, however, experiences a relapse after the initial course of therapy.[19] In these patients, a change in antibiotic is indicated, along with a prolonged, second course of antibiotic treatment. It is usually at this time that the patient realizes that a month's treatment with vancomycin costs about 350 to 500 dollars. The sequence of its use in the treatment of a C. difficile-associated pseudomembranous colitis relapse is qid for 2 weeks, tid for the third week, bid for the fourth week, and then one tablet daily for the final week of treatment.[17]

The final diagnostic consideration in a patient with bloody diarrhea is the exclusion of a colonic tumor. As stated, a colonic adenoma or nonobstructing colonic cancer most commonly presents with hematochezia rather than bloody diarrhea. An obstructing colonic adenocarcinoma could result in bloody diarrhea because of concomitant bleeding from the neoplasia, and the fermentation diarrhea that results from the colonic obstruction. In addition, a distal villous adenocarcinoma of the colon could produce a bloody diarrhea secondary to its high mucoid output and the bleeding associated with the cancer. Each patient who presents with bloody diarrhea requires a total colonoscopy to exclude a colonic neoplasia as its cause. The approach to the management of a patient with a colonic adenoma is discussed in detail in Chapter 9.

In summary, the diagnostic approach to a patient with bloody diarrhea includes the following: (1) a complete history and physical examination to differentiate bloody diarrhea from rectal bleeding, and to obtain a past history of inflammatory bowel disease, radiation therapy, and antibiotic usage; (2) fresh stool analysis to exclude a parasitic or bacterial cause, a Wright's stain to confirm the presence of an exudative process within

TABLE 6–3. DIAGNOSTIC APPROACH TO A PATIENT WITH BLOODY DIARRHEA

Approach	Aim
Thorough history and physical examination	Distinguish bloody diarrhea from hematochezia; obtain history of inflammatory bowel disease, radiation therapy and antibiotic use
Stool analysis, ova and parasites, culture and sensitivity, Wright's stain, C. difficile antitoxin assay	Exclusion of parasitic and bacterial colonic infestation, including C. difficile
Total colonoscopy	Exclusion of colonic neoplasia and confirmation of disease-specific endoscopic features

the colon (either infectious or inflammatory), and a C. difficile antitoxin assay; and (3) a complete colonoscopy to define the endoscopic features of the colon. With this approach, it is possible to distinguish among inflammatory, infectious, post-therapeutic, and neoplastic considerations (Table 6–3).

REFERENCES

1. Nath RL, Sequeira JC, Weitzman AF, et al: Lower gastrointestinal bleeding. Am J Surg, 141:478, 1981.
2. Welch CE, Athanasoulis CA, Galdabini JJ: Hemorrhage from the large bowel with special reference to angiodysplasia and diverticular disease. World J Surg, 2:73, 1978.
3. Peterson WL: Gastrointestinal bleeding. *In* Gastrointestinal Disease. Edited by MH Sleisenger and JS Fordtran. Philadelphia, WB Saunders, 1988, pp 397–427.
4. Trnka YM, LaMont JT: Association of Clostridium difficile toxin with symptomatic relapse of chronic inflammatory bowel disease. Gastroenterology, 80:693, 1981.
5. Owen RL: Parasitic diseases. *In* Gastrointestinal Disease. Edited by MH Sleisenger and JS Fordtran. Philadelphia, WB Saunders, 1989, pp 1153–1191.
6. Gorbach SL (ed): Infectious Diarrhea. Boston, Blackwell Scientific Publications, 1986, pp 1–328.
7. Valdiserri RQ: Intestinal anisakiasis. Report of a case. Am J Clin Pathol, 76:329, 1981.
8. Hsiu J, Gamsey AJ, Ives CE, et al: Gastric anisakiasis. Am J Gastroenterol, 81:1185, 1986.
9. MacDonald KL, O'Leary MJ, Cohon ML, et al: E. coli 0157:H7, An emerging gastrointestinal pathogen. JAMA, 259:3567, 1988.
10. Cello JP, Schneiderman DJ: Ulcerative colitis. *In* Gastrointestinal Disease. Edited by MH Sleisenger and JS Fordtran. Philadelphia, WB Saunders, 1988, pp 1435–1477.
11. Earnest DL, Trier JS: Radiation enteritis and colitis. *In* Gastrointestinal Disease. Edited by MH Sleisenger and JS Fordtran. Philadelphia, WB Saunders, 1988, pp 1369–1382.
12. Den Hartog JFC, van Haastert M, Balterman J, et al: The endoscopic spectrum of late radiation damage of the rectosigmoid colon. Endoscopy, 17:214, 1985.
13. Loiudice TA, Lang JA: Treatment of radiation enterocolitis: A comparison study. Am J Gastroenterol, 78:841, 1983.
14. Mendelson RM, Nolan DJ. The radiological features of chronic radiation enteritis. Clin Radiol, 36:141, 1985.

15. Toskes PP, Donaldson RM: The blind loop syndrome. *In* Gastrointestinal Disease. Edited by MH Sleisenger and JS Fordtran. Philadelphia, WB Saunders, 1988, pp 1289–1297.
16. Lyerly DM, Krivan HC, Wilkins TD: Clostridium difficile: Its disease and its toxins. Clin Microbiol Rev, 1:1, 1988.
17. Bartlett JG: The pseudomembranous enterocolitides. *In* Gastrointestinal Disease. Edited by MH Sleisenger and JS Fordtran. Philadelphia, WB Saunders, 1988, pp 1307–1320.
18. Tedesco FJ, Corless JK, Brownstein RF: Rectal sparing in antibiotic-associated pseudomembranous colitis: A prospective study. Gastroenterology, 83:1259, 1982.
19. Bartlett JG: Treatment of Clostridium difficile colitis. Gastroenterology, 89:1192, 1985.

chapter

7

DIVERTICULAR DISEASE OF THE COLON

Joseph T. Danzi
Richard J. Fastiggi

Diverticular disease of the colon is characterized by the presence of pseudodiverticula within the large intestine and their associated complications. The pathognomonic feature of diverticulosis is the herniation of colonic mucosa through the colonic muscular wall, whereas that of diverticulitis is a microperforation of a diverticulum, with its attendant inflammatory reaction. It is estimated that one-third to one-half of all Americans over the age of 60 years have diverticulosis, that 10 to 25% of them develop diverticulitis, and that 1 to 2% of patients with diverticulosis require surgery for a complication of it.[1,2]

Diverticulosis can involve any part of the colon, but colonic diverticula are more common in the distal left and sigmoid colons. Right colonic diverticula can occur as an isolated finding or in conjunction with total colonic diverticulosis. Diverticular disease of the right colon is associated with the same complications as diverticula of the distal colon.[3]

The complications of diverticulosis include diverticulitis and diverticular bleeding. The secondary complications of diverticulitis are fistula, colonic stricture, and intraabdominal abscess. Hemorrhage from a diverticular bleed is the most common cause of severe, lower gastrointestinal bleeding in the elderly in this country.[4]

The medical literature contains many articles about the controversy over the exact cause of diverticular disease of the colon. One main theory states that the pseudodiverticula of the colon are a result of abnormal colonic motility, with its subsequent high intracolonic pressure and herniation of the colonic mucosa through a weakness in the muscular wall adjacent to the penetration from the serosa of the nutrient artery. The incidence of diverticular disease of the colon is high in patients with the irritable bowel syndrome.[5] The presence of the diverticula in the sigmoid colon correlates with the area of the colon having the highest pressure gradient. Another theory suggests that a primary muscular defect permits the subsequent hernia of the colonic mucosa. This hypothesis is partially substantiated by the known association of diverticulosis of the colon in patients with scleroderma and conditions such as Marfan's syndrome.[6]

The role of dietary fiber in the subsequent development of colonic diverticula seems to have been clarified. A number of epidemiologic studies have supported an inverse relationship between dietary fiber intake and the occurrence of diverticulosis. The initial observations of Burkitt and colleagues[7] regarding the association of high-fiber diet in underdeveloped countries and the low incidence of diverticular disease of the colon in their inhabitants can now be abstracted to individuals worldwide.[7] The most important concept related to dietary intake is the fact that a high-fiber diet must be maintained from early childhood throughout life to help prevent the subsequent development of diverticulosis. Many Americans begin their high-fiber intake later in life in an attempt to protect themselves from colonic cancer and diverticular disease. Whether this latter approach is successful is unknown.

How does dietary fiber prevent the subsequent development of diverticulosis? This question presently remains unanswered. It appears, however, that the amount of dietary fiber is the important factor, rather than the type of fiber ingested. Bingham has demonstrated that a total daily fiber intake of 100 g seems to be protective against the subsequent development of diverticulosis.[8] That same study illustrated that most individuals in developed countries have a total daily fiber intake of only 10 to 25 g. Dietary fiber does not seem to alter the abnormal colonic motility seen in patients with diverticulosis, but it seems to disperse the intracolonic pressure throughout the colon, rendering it less susceptible to herniation of the mucosa.[9]

Considerable debate has arisen in the medical literature regarding the best way to supply 100 g of fiber daily. Clearly, the most cost-efficient method is the consumption of a high-fiber diet, rather than relying on the use of a fiber supplement.[10] Vegetable fiber seems to exert a more protective effect on the colon than animal fiber. Some patients require both a high-fiber diet and fiber supplementation to have regular bowel movements and to reduce the associated abdominal pain.

Most people with diverticulosis have no associated signs or symptoms related to their colonic mucosal outpouching. A Scandinavian study has demonstrated that individuals with asymptomatic diverticulosis have manometric studies similar to those of normal individuals, whereas people with diverticulosis and complaints of abdominal bloating, pain, and irregular bowel habits have sigmoid motility studies indistinguishable from those of patients with the irritable bowel syndrome.[11] It is not uncommon for a patient to be diagnosed with both diverticulosis and irritable bowel syndrome.

Two studies have demonstrated that no symptoms can be considered characteristic of uncomplicated diverticular disease.[12,13] Indeed, the data seem to support the idea that when bowel symptoms occur in patients with colonic diverticulosis, the symptoms are usually a result of a coexistent irritable bowel syndrome.

The management of uncomplicated diverticular disease usually involves only reassurance, because most patients are asymptomatic. In those individuals with diverticulosis coli and symptoms compatible with an irritable bowel, the use of a high-fiber diet seems justified. No evidence from the literature has shown that a high-fiber diet in individuals with uncomplicated diverticulosis prevents the development of the complications of the diverticular disease.[7]

Diverticular hemorrhage occurs in about 15% of individuals with diverticulosis coli.[1] The characteristics of diverticular hemorrhage include its occurrence in an elderly patient who might have a diagnosis of diverticulosis coli, massive rectal bleeding associated with symptoms of hypovolemia, and the tendency to stop bleeding spontaneously or in association with the symptoms of hypovolemia. Most commonly, the hemorrhage occurs in a segment of uncomplicated diverticulosis and is rarely associated with inflammation of the diverticula. It is more common for hemorrhage to occur from a sigmoid diverticula, but most severe diverticular bleeding episodes occur in the right colon.[14]

It is uncommon for diverticular bleeding to present as the passage of blood mixed with stools in the daily bowel movement. This clinical presentation requires the exclusion of a colonic neoplasia in a patient with known diverticulosis coli.

Diverticular hemorrhage and colonic bleeding associated with angiodysplasia of the colon are the two most frequent causes of colonic hemorrhage in individuals over the age of 70 years.[15] The correct diagnosis can be established by colonoscopy. Indeed, many patients in this age group may have both diseases concomittantly.

Approximately 25% of patients have recurrent bleeding after their first diverticular hemorrhage. A patient who has had a second episode of bleeding from a diverticular source has a 50% chance of further episodes of diverticular hemorrhage.[16] These findings are important in the management of patients with recurrent diverticular hemorrhage. It should be strongly recommended to an individual with two episodes of bleeding from a diverticular source that they have a subtotal colectomy if their condition dictates that they can withstand the surgery.

It is difficult to know with certainty the actual percentage of those with diverticulosis coli who go on to develop acute diverticulitis. Many sources have estimated, however, that between 20 and 25% of such individuals are diagnosed with an acute inflammatory complication of their diverticular disease. Typically, the signs and symptoms of acute diverticulitis include the presence of severe, left-sided lower abdominal pain, the association of chills and fever, and the presence of anorexia. The physical examination usually reveals left lower quadrant tenderness, guarding, and signs of local peritoneal inflammation. Laboratory findings included a leukocytosis, an elevated erythrocyte sedimentation rate, and possibly the presence of microscopic hematuria secondary to ureteral inflammation. This clinical picture in a patient with known diverticulosis coli is strongly suggestive of acute diverticulitis.

A mild episode of acute peridiverticulitis can be managed at home with bed rest, clear liquids, oral antibiotics such as ampicillin, 500 mg qid, and close contact with the patient by telephone. If no clinical improvement is noted within 48 hours, it is best to hospitalize the patient for intravenous fluid and antibiotic therapy and the exclusion of a secondary inflammatory complication.

It has been estimated that 20% of those admitted for a diagnosis of acute diverticulitis require surgery during that admission, and that 50% have a second acute inflammatory complication of their diverticular disease within the year.[1] All patients with a history of a resolved episode of acute diverticulitis require a flexible sigmoidoscopy to exclude a colonic neoplasia as the cause of their inflammatory episode. It is rarely necessary to perform a sigmoidoscopy during the acute episode, except to exclude a secondary complication or to confirm the diagnosis in a patient not responding to therapy.

Associated complications of acute diverticulitis include pericolonic abscess, fistula, and bowel obstruction. When the pericolonic inflammation extends beyond the mesentery and pericolonic fat, an abscess can result. Clinically, the association of an abdominal or pelvic mass, spiky fever and chills, and signs of toxicity in a patient with acute diverticulitis should raise the suspicion of a pericolonic abcess. The management of these patients requires hospitalization with intravenous antibiotic therapy and a surgical consultation.

Fistula can result from the association of the pericolonic inflammation with contiguous organs. Colovesical and colovaginal fistula are not uncommon, but colocutaneous fistula can also result from an episode of severe, acute diverticulitis.[17] The incidence of fistula formation in patients with acute diverticulitis has varied from 12 to 25% in different studies.[18] Clinical symptoms associated with a colovesical fistula include recurrent urinary tract infections, fecaluria, and pneumaturia. Clinical findings associated with a colovaginal fistula include recurrent vaginal infections and a fecal vaginal discharge.

Bowel obstruction of both the small and large intestines can result as a consequence of acute diverticulitis. Small bowel obstruction occurs more commonly than large bowel obstruction because the small intestinal loops lying within the pelvis become involved with the adhesions associated with the acute pericolonic inflammation.[18] Large bowel obstruction occurs after a severe episode or repeated episodes of acute diverticulitis and the resultant pericolonic fibrosis.

Any patient with symptoms of colonic obstruction requires an endoscopy of the involved colonic segment to exclude a colonic neoplasia as the cause of the obstruction.

REFERENCES

1. Almy TP, Howell DA: Diverticular disease of the colon. N Engl J Med, 302:324, 1980.
2. Mendeloff AI: Thoughts on the epidemiology of diverticular disease. Clin Gastroenterol, 15:855, 1986.
3. Peck DA, Labat R, Waite VC: Diverticular disease of the right colon. Dis Col. Rectum, 11:49, 1968.
4. Behringer GE, Albright NL: Diverticular disease of the colon: A frequent cause of massive rectal bleeding. Am J Surg, 125:419, 1973.
5. Ritchie J: Similarity of bowel distension characteristics in the irritable bowel syndrome and diverticulosis (abstract). Gut, 18:990, 1977.
6. Smith AN: Colonic muscle in diverticular disease. Clin Gastroenterol, 4:917, 1986.
7. Burkitt DP, Clements JL, Eaton SB: Prevalence of diverticular disease, hiatal hernia, and pelvic phleboliths in black and white Americans. Lancet, 2:880, 1985.
8. Bingham S: Dietary fibers intake: Intake studies, problems, methods, and results. In Dietary Fibre, Fibre-Depleted Foods, and Diseases. Edited by H Trowell, DP Burkitt, and K Heaton. London, Academic Press, 1985, pp. 77–104.
9. Painter NS, Truelove SC: The intraluminal pressure patterns in diverticulosis of the colon. Gut, 5:201, 1964.
10. Hull C, Greco RS, Brooks DL: Alleviation of constipation in the elderly by dietary fiber supplementation. Geriatr Soc, 28:410, 1980.
11. Weinreich J, Anderson D: Intraluminal pressure in the sigmoid colon. II: Patients with sigmoid diverticula and related condition. Scand J Gastroenterol, 11:581, 1976.
12. Thompson WG, Heaton KW: Functional bowel disorders in apparently healthy people. Gastroenterology, 79:283, 1980.
13. Drossman DA, Sandler RS, McKee DC, et al: Bowel symptoms among subjects not seeking health care. Gastroenterology, 83:529, 1982.
14. Casarella WJ, Kanter IE, Seaman WB: Right-sided colonic diverticula as a cause of acute rectal hemorrhage. N Engl J Med, 286:450, 1972.
15. Boley SJ, Dibiase A, Brandt LJ, et al: Lower intestinal bleeding in the elderly. Am J Surg, 137:57, 1979.
16. McQuire HH, Jr, Haynes BW, Jr: Massive hemorrhage from diverticulosis of the colon. Ann Surg, 175:847, 1972.
17. Small WP, Smith AN: Fistula and conditions associated with diverticular disease of the colon. Clin Gastroenterol, 4:171, 1975.
18. Whiteway J, Morrison BC: Pathology of the aging—diverticular disease. Clin Gastroenterol, 4:829, 1985.

c h a p t e r

8

CANCER IN INFLAMMATORY BOWEL DISEASE

Richard G. Farmer

Cancer of the colon and rectum as a complication of ulcerative colitis has been recognized since the description by Bargen[1] over 60 years ago. Although the clinical characteristics have been known since then, the incidence, risk factors involved, and detection, and possible prevention of the development of colorectal cancer in patients with ulcerative colitis have remained significant problems. An obvious deterrent to the recommendation of prophylactic colectomy has been the magnitude and risk of the operation itself, coupled with the need for a permanent ileostomy. Because it could not be determined with accuracy which patient might be at highest risk for developing cancer, or whether cancer had actually developed, insignificant progress was made until the recognition of the histologic lesion now called dysplasia and the ability to perform colonoscopy with the surveillance biopsy technique. Because of these significant improvements in the understanding of precancerous lesions in patients with inflammatory bowel disease (IBD), the question of which patient should be screened for cancer and how this should be done is of great concern, both from the clinical perspective and in regard to the cost-benefit relationship of procedures for accomplishing this.

In recent years a number of significant breakthroughs have been made, with steady improvements in understanding the morphologic significance of histologic dysplasia or precancerous lesions and in the development of fiberoptic colonoscopy, which has enabled multiple biopsy surveillance techniques to be carried out. This understanding has developed over about 15 to 20 years, but has been greatly clarified in the past 5 years, with increasing recognition occurring to date. The clinical situation represents a rapidly evolving area. It is important because the vast majority of patients undergoing surveillance for cancer are much younger than typical patients with colorectal cancer, and early cancer detection appears to be the key for long-term survival. Furthermore, the development of pull-through ileal pouch procedures for patients with ulcerative colitis, which obviates the need for a permanent ileostomy, has significantly improved patient compliance for such procedures and has stimulated the interest of physicians and surgeons in assessing which patients might gain greatest benefit from these procedures.

RISK FACTORS

The assessment of risk factors in IBD for the subsequent development of intestinal cancer has been largely related to patients with ulcerative colitis. It is only recently that patients with Crohn's disease have been observed to be at higher risk than the general population for the development of intestinal cancer. The actual number of patients with inflammatory bowel disease who develop intestinal cancer remains small, particularly in any one institution. Therefore, the necessity for uniformity in the determination of risk assessment, data collection, interpretation, and analysis is obvious. Although excellent cooperation on an international basis has been noted, progress in this area continues to be slow.

CANCER AND ULCERATIVE COLITIS

Patients with ulcerative colitis involving the entire colon and present for 10 years or longer are known to have a higher risk for the development of large bowel cancer than the general population, and this has been known for many years.[2] Predicting the patient who might develop large bowel cancer has, however, been difficult. Colonoscopy has been performed frequently in most centers for about the past 15 years and, subsequently, the use of surveillance biopsy techniques has further improved the situation.[3] In addition, the definition of dysplasia morphologically has been clarified,[4] although its exact clinical correlation has not yet been delineated. A number of methodologic problems are involved in the current assessment of the risk of colon cancer in those with ulcerative colitis.[5] These include the use of referral center populations, patients already known to have cancer, the duration of the study, and projections of risk using small numbers of patients. High cumulative risk factors have been reported, which has created confusion for the physician or surgeon who encounters such cases infrequently. The question of the prevention of cancer by prophylactic colectomy has similarly been raised, and concerns have been expressed regarding the cost-benefit of such action and about the quality of life of the patient.

A cooperative review article from the American Gastroenterological Association and the American Society for Gastrointestinal Endoscopy[6] has

TABLE 8–1. CUMULATIVE RISK OF COLORECTAL CANCER IN ULCERATIVE COLITIS*

Source	Reference Number	Year of Report	Patients with Ulcerative Colitis	Cancer Risk (%)
Lennard-Jones, et al.	13	1977	229	10.3
Maratka, et al.	14	1985	305	5.0
Hendriksen, et al.	15	1985	124	1.3
Brostrom, et al.	11	1987	1274	5.0
Gilat, et al.	12	1988	147	13.8

*Extensive (total) colitis, with 20 years' duration of disease.

Data from Desaint D, Legendre C, Florant C: Dysplasia and cancer in ulcerative colitis. Hepatogastroenterology, 36:219, 1989.

emphasized that 145,000 new cases of colorectal cancer occur in the United States annually, of which ulcerative colitis represents only a small percentage of such lesions. Because of the factors mentioned, however, cancer screening in IBD is considered part of an overall spectrum of colonoscopy surveillance generally. This is an important consideration, because fecal occult blood testing does not have a place in the assessment of patients with IBD (because of their propensity for bleeding to occur as a result of the inflammatory process, thus creating confusion), but patients with ulcerative colitis should be placed in a high-risk group for colorectal cancer screening.

The risk for and frequency of cancer in patients with ulcerative colitis has been extensively studied, with some important information coming from western Europe, particularly Scandinavia and Great Britain.[7,8] A cohort study from Birmingham and Oxford in Great Britain and from Stockholm has shown that the predicted risk at 20 years from onset of disease for patients with extensive ulcerative colitis is only 7%, although previous data assessed by these authors indicated the risk as 20 to 25%.[8] In a review article by Desaint and colleagues,[9] studies regarding the cumulative cancer incidence in patients with ulcerative colitis were summarized. These data are presented in Table 8–1, with estimates of cancer risk in patients with extensive (total) colitis ranging from 1.3 to 13.8% at 20 years. Prior and associates[10] expressed their data in actuarial terms, with a cumulative probability of developing colorectal cancer as 8% at 25 years after the diagnosis of ulcerative colitis. Brostrom and co-workers[11] and Gilat and colleagues[12] calculated ratios for the observed number of cases of colorectal cancer in patients with ulcerative colitis above those expected in a similar group of the general population, ranging from 3:1 to 6.5:1 in the studies noted. Lennard-Jones and associates[13] described the risk as cancer incidence per patient-year, with the risk in the second decade of disease being approximately 1 in 200 patient-years, and 1 in 60 patient-years in the third decade. A lower incidence was found in the studies reported from Czechoslovakia[14] and Denmark.[15] Ransohoff[16] has estimated that the risk

TABLE 8–2. COLORECTAL CANCER IN PATIENTS WITH ULCERATIVE COLITIS (UC)

Total patients followed	1248*
Patients with extensive (total) colitis	562
Patients with colorectal cancer	82
Mean age (years) of diagnosis of cancer	43
Duration from colitis diagnosis to cancer diagnosis (years)	
Extensive colitis	18
Left-sided colitis	22.4
Cumulative risk of colorectal cancer in UC (% at 20 years' duration)	
Extensive colitis	11.9
Left-sided colitis	1.8

*Mean follow-up, 14.4 years.

Data from Mir-Madjlessi SH, Farmer RG, Easley KA, Beck GJ: Colorectal and extracolonic malignancy in ulcerative colitis. Cancer 58:1569, 1986.

of cancer among patients with extensive (total) colitis is approximately 0.5 to 1% per person annually.

In 1986, we reported the Cleveland Clinic experience[17] with colorectal and extracolonic malignancy in ulcerative colitis patients. Based on a review of 1248 cases of ulcerative colitis seen at the Cleveland Clinic and followed through 1984, we reported our experience with 82 patients with colorectal cancer and 48 patients with extracolonic malignancy. The mean follow-up for all patients was 14.4 years. The clinical data for these patients are presented in Table 8–2. Among the patients with colorectal cancer, men outnumbered women 2:1, and 90% of the patients had extensive colitis; only 10% had inflammatory changes that were confined distal to the splenic flexure. The duration of disease was 10 years or more in 93% of cases, and the mean duration of disease was 18 years from diagnosis to the development of cancer. Desaint and colleagues[9] have reported a compilation of 11 different series of patients who had developed cancer in ulcerative colitis, and found that the mean duration from the diagnosis of ulcerative colitis to the diagnosis of cancer is 18 ± 1 years, which is exactly what we have found.[17]

For patients with left-sided colitis only who developed colonic cancer, we found a mean duration of disease of 22.4 years.[17] Cancer of the large bowel developed in 11% of patients with extensive colitis and in 1.6% of those with left-sided colitis. The colitis had been inactive before the diagnosis of cancer in 48% of all cases. The onset of the colitis had been acute in 7% and insidious in 93% of patients, and was continuously active in 8% and remittent in 92%. The mean age at diagnosis of cancer was 43 years.

Grundfest and associates[18] have studied the development of cancer of the retained rectum after colectomy with ileorectal anastomosis. They found the risk of cancer per patient-year to be 1 in 206 in the second decade and 1 in 116 in the third decade. Desaint and colleagues[9] reviewed four

TABLE 8–3. CANCER IN PATIENTS WITH ULCERATIVE COLITIS

Pathologic Features	Occurrence (%)
Multifocal	13.5
Poorly differentiated	34
Proximal to splenic flexure	44
	No. of Patients
Extraintestinal cancer (most common neoplasms: bile duct, leukemia, bone tumor, endometrial)	48
Concurrent colorectal cancer	6

Data from Mir-Madjlessi SH, Farmer RG, Easley KA, Beck GJ: Colorectal and extracolonic malignancy in ulcerative colitis. Cancer, 58:1569, 1986.

similar studies and observed that the cumulative risk of developing cancer in the rectal stump was 6% at 20 years and 15% at 30 years of disease.

We have found[17] that the cumulative risk of colorectal cancer is significantly higher in patients with extensive colitis than in those with left-sided disease ($p = 0.0001$): 1.9 versus 1.8% at 20 years and 25.3 versus 3.7% at 30 years). With regard to the clinical features of cancer, 25% of patients presented with obstructive bowel symptoms and 39% experienced reappearance of bowel symptoms when the colitis had been inactive. At the time the cancer was detected, 19% of the patients were asymptomatic.

The prognosis for colorectal cancer in patients with ulcerative colitis, based on our experience,[17] appears to be similar to that of colorectal cancer in the general population, with a cumulative 5-year survival rate of 54%. In their survey, Desaint and co-workers,[9] demonstrated a mean 5-year survival rate of 36.9 ± 4.4%, ranging from a low of 17 to 22% to a high of 55 to 65%. Thus, our experience[17] concurs favorably with that of others.

In our experience,[17] 48 patients had extracolonic malignancy, and 6 of them had associated colorectal cancer. The most common lesions found were bile duct carcinoma, leukemia, bone tumors, and endometrial cancer, the probability of which were significantly greater than expected ($p = 0.01$), whereas that of lung cancer was lower than expected ($p = 0.01$).

Table 8–3 lists the pathologic features found in the patients with colorectal cancer; of these 48 patients, 6 had concurrent colorectal cancer in conjunction with extraintestinal malignancies. Thus, cancer associated with ulcerative colitis is characterized by a tendency for a higher percentage of poorly differentiated lesions and a higher percentage of multifocal lesions than are typically seen in patients with colorectal cancer unassociated with ulcerative colitis.[6] In the review by Desaint and colleagues,[9] the location of cancer was compared in five studies with more than 20 cases of cancer each (ranging to a high of 74 separate cancers found in patients in the Cleveland Clinic experience). Four other studies found fewer than 10 cancers; these are summarized and extrapolated in Table 8–4. In the past, cancer associated with ulcerative colitis was thought to be of a higher degree of malignancy and situated more proximally than in

TABLE 8–4. LOCATION OF CANCER IN ULCERATIVE COLITIS

			Location						
Source	Reference Number	No. of Cancers	Multifocal Sites	Rectum	Sigmoid Colon	Descending Colon	Transverse Colon	Ascending Colon	Cecum
Mir-Madjlessi, et al.	17	74	10	24	17	7	17	10	11
Prior, et al.	10	35	4	14	5	2	6	3	2
Gilat, et al.	12	26	0	9	0	13	4	0	0
Brostrom, et al.	11	25	5	17	8	4	8	1	3
Ransohoff	16	22	6	4	5	0	3	5	0
Cases reviewed by Desaint, et al.	19	209	27	69 (33%)	40 (19%)	27 (13%)	42 (20)%	23 (11%)	18 (9%)

Data from Desaint B, Legendre C, Florent C: Dysplasia and cancer in ulcerative colitis. Hepatogastroenterology, 36:219, 1989.

patients whose lesions occur without ulcerative colitis.[2] The same increased percentage of proximal tumors noted in colorectal cancer patients without ulcerative colitis, however, has been found in patients with or without ulcerative colitis.[19]

Dysplasia in Ulcerative Colitis

Dysplasia, the presumed precancerous epithelial change, has been recognized in colonic mucosal specimens adjacent to and distant from colitis-associated carcinomas. In fact, circumstantial evidence has suggested that dysplasia may not only be a marker for carcinoma, but may itself be the carcinoma in an early preinvasive phase.[4]

Dysplastic changes can occur in grossly flat mucosa, in mucosa with a villous configuration, or in a nodular growth resembling an adenoma. Dysplasia is recognized by histologic examination of biopsy specimens using well-defined cytologic criteria, including nuclear enlargement with hyperchromasia, increased mitotic figures, and decreased intracellular mucin. Most colitis-associated dysplasias resemble adenomas similar to those seen in the noncolitic patient. Pathologists currently use the term "dysplasia" only as a synonym for intraepithelial neoplasia, and it should not be used to refer to the reactive or reparative changes seen with active inflammation.[20]

The Inflammatory Bowel Disease–Dysplasia Morphology Study Group[4] has proposed a three-tiered classification for biopsy interpretation in inflammatory bowel disease: positive, negative, and indefinite for dysplasia (Figs. 8–1 to 8–3). We have found this classification to be useful and reasonably reproducible.[3,20] Desaint and colleagues[9] have found interobserver variations in the assessment of dysplasia to be 4 to 8% among experienced pathologists, and probably higher among those with less experience in dysplasia assessment. Biopsy specimens negative for dysplasia include normal colon and those showing changes of active or quiescent colitis. Positive biopsy specimens are reported as showing either high-grade or low-grade dysplasia, with the distinction based on the cytologic atypia present. At the cytologic level, dysplasia is characterized by increased nuclear size with nuclear crowding, stratification of nuclei, and abnormal cellular proliferation.[9,16]

Biopsy specimens are classified as showing changes indefinite for dysplasia when unusual cytologic abnormalities are seen, but these are of insufficient degree to warrant a diagnosis of true dysplasia. Indefinite changes are usually encountered in a background of active inflammation, in which atypical epithelial changes may represent repair or regeneration following healing of the inflammation, rather than actual dysplasia. The category of indefinite dysplasia is a legitimate diagnosis, alerting the treating physician that worrisome cytologic changes are present that could place a patient in a higher risk category, thus requiring more frequent surveillance.[20]

Management recommendations for patients with low-grade dysplasia are difficult to make because of the paucity of information available concerning long-term follow-up in this group. It seems safe to continue

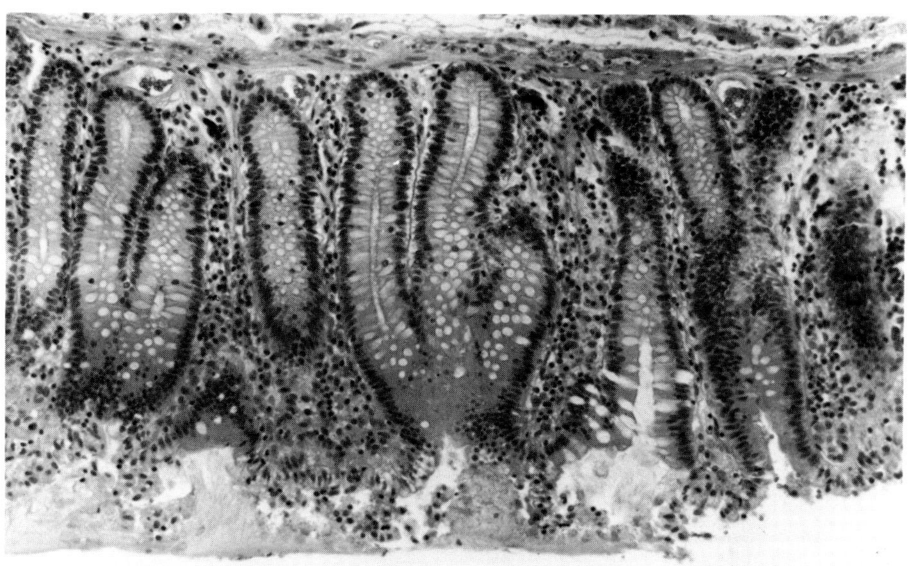

FIG. 8–1. Colonic mucosa showing changes of an inactive (quiescent) colitis, negative for dysplasia. The colonic crypts have lost their parallel arrangement and many crypts are branching. The nuclei are small, regular in shape, and not hyperchromatic. The cells maintain a low nuclear to cytoplasmic size ratio.

short-term follow-up (e.g., 6 months) for patients with low-grade dysplasia but, if dysplasia persists or is associated with any suspicious gross lesion or stricture, colectomy should be strongly considered. In our experience,[3] 38 patients with low-grade dysplasia were followed for a mean of 5 years without clinical evidence of the development of cancer. If high-grade dysplasia is encountered, it should be confirmed, and colectomy should be recommended. Our experience with surveillance biopsy interpretation[3] has shown that true negatives are rarely interpreted as dysplasia, and dysplasia, especially high-grade dysplasia, is rarely missed. Variations in interpretation do occur, however, and confirmation of a biopsy diagnosis is usually desirable before colectomy.[20] One or more of the following may be considered as adequate confirmation: (1) finding dysplasia in repeat biopsy from the same site; (2) finding dysplasia in one or more additional sites during the same endoscopic examination; and (3) review and confirmation of the dysplasia interpretation by another pathologist experienced with the classification system advocated by Riddell and associates.[4]

Surveillance endoscopy with biopsy has a number of limitations. Dysplasia is not commonly encountered, it is difficult for any one pathologist to acquire extensive experience, and interobserver variability can occur.[20] In addition, dysplasia can be focal, with considerable sampling error. If dysplasia is considered a neoplastic change, however, complete resolution is unlikely, and continued surveillance is important. Furthermore, although we have found that dysplasia is universally located

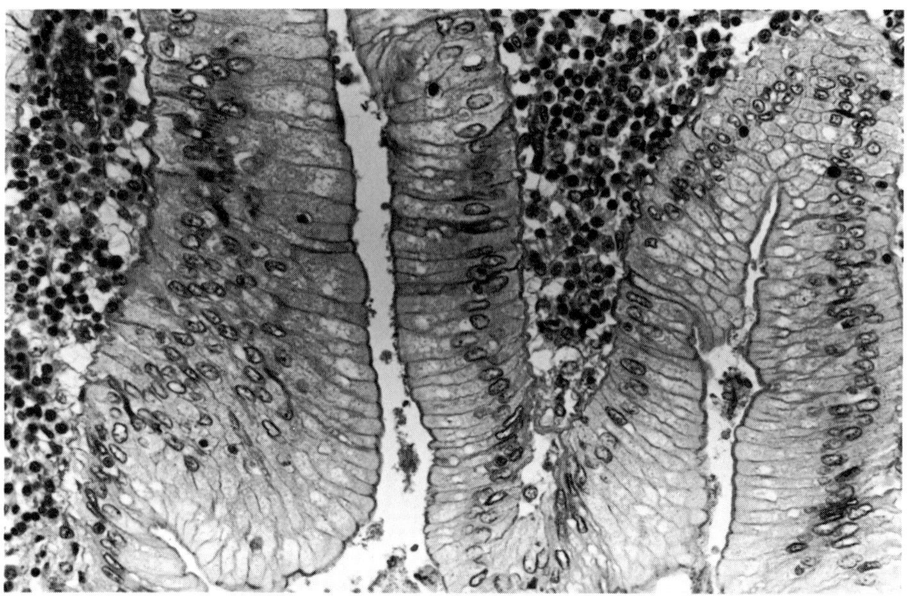

FIG. 8–2. Colonic mucosal segment considered indefinite for dysplasia. The luminal aspect of each cell contains small mucin droplets and the epithelial cells resemble those seen in gastric foveolar epithelium. This type of mucous cell is often seen in areas of dysplasia, but in this field the crypt epithelium lacks diagnostic criteria for dysplasia. The nuclei are only minimally enlarged, nuclei are not hyperchromatic, and the cells maintain a low nuclear to cytoplasmic size ratio.

adjacent to any lesion that has been found to be malignant histologically, in only half of patients was dysplasia distant to the lesion or throughout the large bowel.[3,20] Thus, surveillance rectal biopsies have no value (unless, of course, positive), because a negative rectal biopsy can occur in at least half of patients who have either proximal dysplasia or carcinoma. Dysplasia often occurs at a distance from the cancer itself, even though not universally spread throughout the colon and rectum. In the study that is generally considered to be the one that stimulated the current interest and understanding in dysplasia as a histologic lesion, Morson and Pang[21] found dysplasia distant from the cancer in all 23 of the patients they studied. Desaint and co-workers[9] have assessed this study, and found that 88% of the specimens at a distance from the cancer were positive. Of the 137 specimens assessed, 121 had dysplasia distant from the cancer, although this was only in the rectum in about 50%.[9]

In our study of patients undergoing a surveillance program,[3] no cases were found in which a patient subsequently had surgery performed for cancer if their biopsies had been negative for dysplasia on surveillance. More simply stated, the absence of dysplasia correlated with the absence of cancer. Patients with high-grade dysplasia who undergo colectomy, however, have an approximately 45% chance that cancer will be found somewhere in the resected specimen.[9,13,21] Desaint and colleagues[9] have

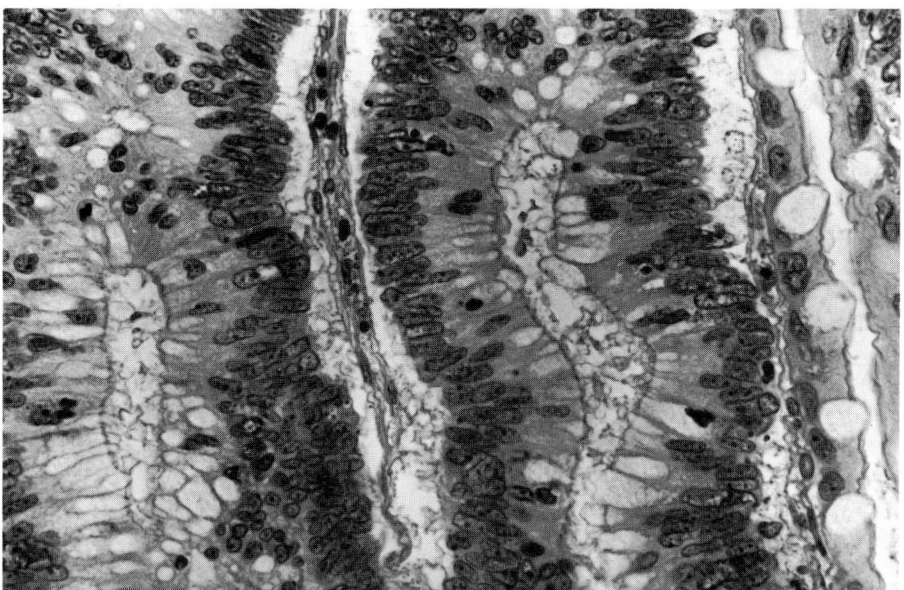

FIG. 8–3. Colonic mucosa positive for high-grade epithelial dysplasia. In contrast to epithelium negative for dysplasia (Fig. 8–1), the dysplastic epithelium demonstrates larger hyperchromatic nuclei, with nuclear crowding and stratification. Intracellular mucin is decreased, and the cells demonstrate a relatively high nuclear to cytoplasmic size ratio. In general, the changes present resemble those seen in colonic adenoma.

reviewed the results of five of the largest surveillance studies in patients with ulcerative colitis and assessed the results of 1211 patients entered in these programs. Among these, dysplasia was present before colectomy in 84% and cancer was found at colectomy in 42% of patients with dysplasia. Ransohoff[16] has observed that high-grade dysplasia is found in only 50% of patients found to have colon cancer. Furthermore, the mean interval between the development of low-grade and high-grade dysplasia-cancer is approximately 3 years,[9] so that even though a strong correlation is found between dysplasia and cancer, it is not absolute.

"Adenoma" in the Colitic Patient

Because most inflammatory bowel disease-associated dysplasias represent adenomas, it can be difficult to distinguish among them, but generally a diagnosis of "adenoma" in a patient with IBD must be viewed with skepticism, and probably represents IBD-associated dysplasia. It has been increasingly recognized, though, that adenomas can be found in patients with ulcerative colitis, but only if the following criteria are met: (1) the patient is in an adenoma age group (i.e., over 40 years); (2) the dysplasia lesion is pedunculated; (3) the excision is complete; (4) the mucosa of the stalk lacks dysplasia; and (5) it occurs in an area not affected by inflammatory bowel disease (e.g., cecal adenoma in a patient with left-sided colitis). Pseudopolyps, common in patients with ulcerative colitis, do not have a higher risk of dysplastic change than flat mucosa.[20]

DYSPLASIA AND CARCINOMA IN CROHN'S DISEASE

Increasing clinical and pathologic evidence have suggested that patients with Crohn's disease are also at increased risk for the development of intestinal carcinoma.[22] The small bowel carcinomas found in our experience in patients with Crohn's disease have occurred (on average) 20 years after the onset of Crohn's disease. Most involve the ileum and almost always occur in areas actively involved by Crohn's disease. The carcinomas are clinically and grossly subtle, and often occur in strictured areas that resemble the inflammatory strictures of Crohn's disease. Small intestinal carcinomas in Crohn's disease tend to be of poor differentiation and are associated with a poor prognosis. Approximately 25% of cases have occurred in bypassed or out-of-circuit segments.[22]

Colonic carcinomas found in patients with Crohn's disease have generally been found also to occur after many years of disease. That this lesion is increasingly being recognized is illustrated by our report,[22] in which we found dysplasia in epithelium adjacent to the lesions. Thus, these features may indicate that a dysplasia-carcinoma sequence similar to that proposed for ulcerative colitis also occurs in Crohn's disease, but not enough information is available as yet to make this statement definitely.

Based on our experience,[22] endoscopic surveillance would be of limited value in small bowel (ileal) Crohn's disease. Because of the general inaccessibility to endoscopic examination and the focal nature of dysplasia, few studies on dysplasia occurring in small intestine cancer in patients with Crohn's disease have been reported. Because only approximately 80 cases of Crohn's disease associated small bowel carcinoma have been reported, with approximately 25% of these occurring in out-of-circuit segments, the expected cancer or dysplasia yield of a surveillance program would be expected to be small. Endoscopic surveillance in colonic Crohn's disease might be of value, however, and our experience indicates that dysplasia occasionally occurs, but technical difficulties might be encountered in some patients with colonic Crohn's disease because of stricturing and skip lesions generally. In addition, the absolute number of cases of colonic carcinoma in Crohn's disease probably would not warrant that such a program be undertaken at present.

Our experience[20,22] has shown that a patient with recrudescence of colitis-like symptoms and a background of long-standing, inactive Crohn's disease should be thoroughly investigated for colonic carcinoma, including colonoscopy. Annual surveillance of an out-of-circuit rectum seems reasonable, considering that approximately 20% of reported cases of cancer in Crohn's disease have occurred in such segments.[20] It may, however, be better to advise removal of a defunctionalized rectum, especially if reanastomosis is not planned, is not possible, or is contraindicated. The presence of dysplasia in a biopsy specimen from a patient with Crohn's disease must alert the physician to the possibility of a coexistent invasive malignancy; in this situation we recommend colectomy, as for ulcerative colitis. Clinicians should also recognize that chronic fistula or anal strictures in Crohn's disease may be complicated by squamous cell carcinoma or adenocarcinoma.

CURRENT DEVELOPMENTS IN THE DETECTION OF DYSPLASIA

Current approaches to the assessment of precancerous lesions in inflammatory bowel disease have moved somewhat away from morphologic histologic features and more into flow cytometry.[23–25] Flow cytometry can be used to detect deoxyribonucleic acid (DNA) aneuploidy. Data from one study have suggested that "neoplastic progression in ulcerative colitis is associated with production of abnormal clonal populations of cells."[24] This phenomenon is called aneuploidy and, in the study mentioned, aneuploid populations were not detected in biopsy specimens of normal controls or in patients with ulcerative colitis without dysplasia. Melville and colleagues[23] have used flow cytometry to analyze 353 specimens from 58 patients with extensive ulcerative colitis, 22 of whom had developed carcinoma. DNA aneuploidy was easier to recognize than dysplasia and was found to be associated with patients who had developed colonic carcinoma.[9,23] A significant correlation was found between dysplasia and the incidence of DNA aneuploidy.[23]

The biologic significance of DNA aneuploidy in ulcerative colitis as a predictor of impending malignant transformation continues to be evaluated. Studies of aneuploidy assessed by flow cytometry have shown that aneuploidy is associated with ulcerative colitis, even in the absence of dysplasia, but rarely if ever in patients with Crohn's disease or in controls.[25] Thus, flow cytometry with detection of DNA aneuploidy may be an important future adjunct, or even the primary detection modality, for patients with long-standing ulcerative colitis suspected of being at risk for the development of colorectal cancer.

PATIENT MANAGEMENT RECOMMENDATIONS

As a result of the experience at the Cleveland Clinic Foundation,[2,3,17,20] patient management recommendations based on colonic surveillance with biopsy for patients with ulcerative colitis are presented in Table 8–5. Experience from the perspective of physicians, surgeons, and pathologists appears to indicate that surveillance programs of this type are beneficial to patients and are cost-effective. Patients with extensive colitis who have had disease for more than 7 to 10 years, and whose biopsy specimens remain negative for dysplasia, can probably safely continue regular surveillance with total colonoscopy every 1 to 2 years. Patients with changes indefinite

TABLE 8–5. INFLAMMATORY BOWEL DISEASE AND CANCER: PATIENT MANAGEMENT RECOMMENDATIONS, COLONOSCOPY SURVEILLANCE

Biopsy Interpretation	Recommendation
Negative	Regular follow-up, 2 years
Indefinite	Short-term follow-up, 6 months–1 year
Positive low-grade dysplasia	Short-term follow-up, 6 months; consider colectomy if associated with suspicious gross lesion
Positive high-grade dysplasia	Colectomy

for dysplasia require shorter term follow-up, 6 months to 1 year, and management recommendations for patients with low-grade dysplasia are the same. For patients whose disease is less than total colon cancer, risk is higher than in the general population, but much lower than in patients with total colon ulcerative colitis.[9,17,26] Critical factors continue to be the assessment of patients with low-grade dysplasia and the obvious need for compliance by patients for the surveillance biopsy program. In a program of surveillance colonoscopy biopsies are obtained from flat mucosa approximately every 10 cm, and strictures and "suspicious" or mass lesions are biopsied. Our experience, however, is that pseudopolyps are not associated with the development of cancer.[20] For patients with high-grade dysplasia in the colonic epithelium, colectomy is recommended.

The usefulness of cancer surveillance programs in patients with Crohn's disease appears to be of limited value, and are probably of no value in those with small intestine Crohn's disease. Although cases of large bowel dysplasia have occurred in Crohn's disease, colonoscopy may be technically difficult and the absolute number of cases is small. The expected yield of positive cases in a surveillance program would also be small, and it would be difficult to assess the clinical significance and cost-effectiveness.

SUMMARY AND CONCLUSIONS

1. Intestinal cancer associated with inflammatory bowel disease is more common in patients with ulcerative colitis than in those with Crohn's disease. In our experience,[17] the duration of the disease prior to the diagnosis of cancer was almost always greater than 10 years, with a mean of 18 years.
2. Extensive total colon disease occurs in 90% of patients who develop colonic cancer.[17]
3. The age of onset is not significant as a risk factor, but the duration of disease is significant.[17]
4. The severity of the episodes of colitis or the course of disease is not related to the subsequent development of colonic carcinoma.

Similarly, no relationship to any form of therapy or lack of same has been found,[17] and no relationship to the development of sclerosing cholangitis has been noted.[27]

5. Patients with proctitis alone probably do not have a greater risk of developing colonic cancer than the general population.[28]
6. Patients with left-sided colitis (i.e., inflammatory changes extending to the splenic flexure) have a higher risk for the development of colonic cancer than the general population, but a lower risk than those with total colon ulcerative colitis.[17,26] The duration of disease is longer for cancer to develop than for those with extensive colitis, with a mean age in our experience of 22 years after diagnosis.[17]
7. Almost all patients with extensive ulcerative colitis who develop colonic cancer have dysplasia, and almost all have high-grade dysplasia and/or a mass lesion.[3]
8. Not all patients with high-grade dysplasia have cancer (although may develop it in the future); about half are found to have cancer if colectomy is performed.[3]
9. Dysplasia is found adjacent to the carcinoma in almost all cases. Only half have widespread (i.e., rectal) dysplasia, although dysplasia distant to the lesion is common.[3]
10. Low-grade dysplasia appears not to progress to cancer frequently, although this is a subject for further study.[3]
11. Patients without dysplasia who undergo surgery for symptoms have a low risk of having cancer found unexpectedly.[3]
12. For patients with Crohn's disease, although dysplasia has been found in occasional cases of colonic carcinoma, surveillance programs do not appear to be warranted at this time.[22]

REFERENCES

1. Bargen JA: Chronic ulcerative colitis associated with malignant disease. Arch Surg, 17:561, 1928.
2. Farmer RG, Hawk WA, Turnbull RB: Carcinoma associated with mucosal ulcerative colitis and with transmural ulcerative colitis and enteritis (Crohn's disease). Cancer, 28:289, 1971.
3. Rosenstock E, Farmer RG, Petras R, et al: Surveillance for colonic carcinoma in ulcerative colitis. Gastroenterology, 89:1342, 1985.
4. Riddell RH, Goldman H, Ransohoff DF, et al: Dysplasia and inflammatory bowel disease: Standardized classification with provisional clinical application. Hum Pathol, 14:951, 1983.
5. Collins RH, Feldman M, Fordtran JS: Colon cancer, dysplasia, and surveillance in patients with ulcerative colitis. A critical review. N Engl J Med, 316:1654, 1987.
6. Fleischer ED, Goldberg SB, Browning TH, et al: Detection and surveillance of colorectal cancer. JAMA, 261:580, 1989.
7. Brostrom O, Lofberg R, Nordenvall B, et al: The risk of colorectal cancer in ulcerative colitis. An epidemiologic study. Scand J Gastroenterol, 22:1193, 1987.
8. Gyde SN, Prior P, Allan RN, et al: Colorectal cancer in ulcerative colitis: A cohort study of primary referrals from three centers. Gut, 29:206, 1988.
9. Desaint B, Legendre C, Florent C: Dysplasia and cancer in ulcerative colitis. Hepatogastroenterology, 36:219, 1989.

10. Prior P, Gyde SN, Macartney JC, et al: Cancer morbidity in ulcerative colitis. Gut, 23:490, 1982.
11. Brostrom O, Lofberg B, Ost A, Reichard H: Cancer surveillance of patients with long-standing ulcerative colitis: A clinical, endoscopic, and histological study. Gut, 27:1193, 1987.
12. Gilat T, Fireman Z, Grossman A: Colorectal cancer in patients with ulcerative colitis. A population study in central Israel. Gastroenterology, 94:870, 1988.
13. Lennard-Jones JE, Morson BC, Ritchie JK, et al: Cancer in colitis: Assessment of the individual risk by clinical and histological criteria. Gastroenterology, 73:1280, 1977.
14. Maratka Z, Nedbal J, Kocianova J, et al: Incidence of colorectal cancer in proctocolitis: A retrospective study of 959 cases over 40 years. Gut, 26:43, 1985.
15. Hendriksen C, Kreiner S, Binder V: Long-term prognosis in ulcerative colitis based on results from a regional patient group from the county of Copenhagen. Gut, 26:158, 1985.
16. Ransohoff DF: Colon cancer in ulcerative colitis. Gastroenterology, 94:1089, 1988.
17. Mir-Madjlessi SH, Farmer RG, Easley KA, Beck GJ: Colorectal and extracolonic malignancy in ulcerative colitis. Cancer, 58:1569, 1986.
18. Grundfest SF, Fazio V, Weiss RA, et al: The risk of cancer following colectomy and ileo-rectal anastomosis for extensive mucosal ulcerative colitis. Ann Surg, 193:9, 1981.
19. Slater G, Greenstein AJ, Gelernt I, et al: Distribution of colorectal cancer in patients with and without ulcerative colitis. Am J Surg, 149:780, 1985.
20. Petras RE: Inflammatory bowel disease, dysplasia, and carcinoma. Guthrie J, 58:15, 1989.
21. Morson BC, Pang LSC: Rectal biopsy as an aid to cancer control in ulcerative colitis. Gut, 8:423, 1967.
22. Petras RE, Mir-Madjlessi SH, Farmer RG: Crohn's disease and intestinal carcinoma. A report of 11 cases with emphasis on associated epithelial dysplasia. Gastroenterology, 93:1307, 1987.
23. Melville DM, Jass JR, Shepherd JF, et al: Dysplasia and deoxyribonucleic acid aneuploidy in the assessment of precancerous changes in chronic ulcerative colitis. Observer variation and correlations. Gastroenterology, 95:668, 1988.
24. Levine DS, Reid BJ, Hagitt RC, et al: Frequency and distribution of aneuploid cell populations in chronic ulcerative colitis. Gastroenterology, 94 (Part II):A260, 1988.
25. Porschen R, Robin U, Schumacher A, et al: Detection of DNA aneuploidy by flow cytometry reflects the epidemiological difference in colorectal cancer risk between Crohn's disease (CD) and ulcerative colitis (UC). Gastroenterology, 96 (Part II):A152, 1989.
26. Greenstein AJ, Sachar DB, Smith H, et al: Cancer in universal and left-sided ulcerative colitis: Factors determining risk. Gastroenterology, 77:290, 1979.
27. Farmer RG, Winkelman EI, McGonagle B: Ulcerative colitis and high-grade mucosal dysplasia and sclerosing cholangitis occurring simultaneously; evaluation and management. Gastroenterol Hepat J, 4:11, 1989.
28. Farmer RG: Nonspecific ulcerative proctitis. Gastroenterol Clin North Am, 16:157, 1987.

chapter

9

THE SCREENING AND MANAGEMENT OF COLONIC NEOPLASIA

Joseph T. Danzi

Colonic neoplasia includes adenomatous polyps and adenocarcinoma. Both types of colonic neoplasia are frequent in Americans over the age of 40 years. Colorectal cancer ranks as the second most common internal malignancy in both sexes in this country, and one study has suggested that at least two-thirds of Americans over the age of 65 have at least one colonic polyp.[1] It is now generally accepted that colonic cancers arise in benign adenomatous polyps that have undergone malignant degeneration. This dysplastic change is referred to as the colonic adenoma-cancer sequence.

Two factors affect the colonic adenoma-cancer sequence. The first is the histologic type of the colonic adenoma. The three types of adenoma are tubular adenoma, tubulovillous adenoma, and villous adenomas. It is generally accepted that a villous adenoma has a greater premalignant potential than a tubular adenoma of the colon; The second factor is the size of the adenomatous polyp. For all histologic types of adenoma, a polyp under 1 cm in size has approximately a 1% chance of harboring an invasive cancer. An adenoma between 1 and 2 cm in size has about a 10% chance of having an invasive cancer, and an adenoma of more than 2 cm in size has a more than 40% chance of containing an invasive cancer. It is generally agreed in the gastroenterology literature that the normal doubling time, the time it takes for a polyp to double in size, is about 2½ to 3 years. This time sequence affects the subsequent management of patients with known colonic adenomas and influences their follow-up.

Another important factor in the colonic adenoma-cancer sequence is the incidence of synchronous and metachronous colonic neoplasia. Literature reports have estimated that about 30 to 50% of patients with a distal colonic

TABLE 9–1. FACTORS INFLUENCING THE COLON ADENOMA-CANCER SEQUENCE

Factor	
Histologic type of adenoma	Villous adenoma has a greater malignant potential than tubular adenoma
Size of polyp	For all types of adenomas: <1.0 cm ≈ 1% risk of invasive cancer 1–2 cm ≈ 10–12% risk of invasive cancer >2 cm ≈ 40% risk of invasive cancer
Doubling time of adenoma size	$2\frac{1}{2}$–3 years
Incidence of synchronous adenoma more proximal in colon	30–50%
Incidence of metachronous adenoma	30%
National Polyp Study time analysis	10 years from a "clean" colon to presence of a colon cancer; 5 years from a "clean" colon to presence of a colonic adenoma

adenoma are found to have synchronous adenoma or adenocarcinoma when total colonoscopy is performed.[2] The significant incidence of synchronous colonic lesions is the main reason a total colonoscopic examination is required for all patients in whom adenomas are detected on sigmoidoscopic examination. In addition, a patient with an adenoma in the distal colon has about a 30% chance of developing a subsequent colonic adenoma.[3,4] This makes it clinically important to follow a patient with a known history of colonic neoplasia.

The National Polyp Study has been providing important clinical data regarding the colonic adenoma-cancer sequence:[3]

1. Statistics show that, histologically, 68% of colonic polyps are adenomas, 15% are hyperplastic, and the remainder are various non-neoplastic polyps.
2. An average of 10 years exists between a colon having no polyps and the subsequent presence of a colon cancer, with a mean interval of 5 years between a "clean" colon and the subsequent detection of a colonic adenoma (Table 9–1).

Information from the National Polyp Study has resulted in the new recommendations of the American Cancer Society's colorectal screening program. This program aims to detect and remove colonic adenomas before their conversion to colon cancer. The American Cancer Society has suggested that all patients over the age of 40 years have an annual digital examination and fecal hemoccult testing, that all patients over 50 should have a screening sigmoidoscopy, in addition to the above testing, that a follow-up screening sigmoidoscopy be performed in 1 year if the initial evaluation was normal, and that a subsequent examination of the

TABLE 9–2. AMERICAN CANCER SOCIETY'S SCREENING RECOMMENDATIONS FOR ASYMPTOMATIC, LOW-RISK PATIENTS

Age (years)	Recommendation
Over 40	Annual digital examination; annual fecal occult blood test (FOBT)
Over 50	Annual digital examination; annual FOBT; flexible sigmoidoscopy at age 50: repeat in 1 year if normal; if two successive sigmoidoscopic examinations normal, then every 3 years

rectosigmoid be performed every 3 to 5 years (Table 9–2).[5] These screening recommendations are for those individuals with no increased risk of colonic neoplasia—that is, no patient history of known colonic neoplasia, no known family history of colonic cancer or colonic polyposis syndrome, no patient history of gynecologic or breast cancer, and no patient history of ulcerative colitis of more than 7 years' duration.

Such screening programs for asymptomatic individuals at no increased risk for the development of colorectal cancer appear to be effective. One randomized, controlled study of patients in the Kaiser-Permanente Health Plan, aged 35 to 59 years, has demonstrated a significantly lower mortality from colorectal cancer in the study group (receiving regular sigmoidoscopic examinations) as compared to that of the control group.[6] A more recent study on the same patient population has indicated that the study group had a significantly higher incidence of early colorectal cancers (Child's classifications A and B) when compared to that of the control group.[7] It is estimated that screening flexible sigmoidoscopy in asymptomatic patients can detect colonic adenoma in about 10 percent of cases and colonic cancer in less than 0.5% of cases.[8] Finally, two significant studies have illustrated the value of a digital examination and rigid sigmoidoscopy in the detection of rectal cancer.[9,10] Therefore, all patients in this age group and category should be made aware of the screening recommendations of the American Cancer Society and should be encouraged to follow them.

Information regarding compliance by asymptomatic individuals for such screening programs is more difficult to ascertain. It is well known that the use of flexible sigmoidoscopy has increased patient acceptance of the procedure when compared to the use of rigid sigmoidoscopy.[11] In addition, the availability of flexible sigmoidoscopy seems to have increased physician compliance in regard to the performance of screening sigmoid examinations.[12] Despite both patient and physician willingness to participate, one report has suggested that only about one-third of such patients have a screening sigmoidoscopy examination.[13] Therefore, it requires a combination of patient education and encouragement, along with physician enthusiasm about the program, to achieve a successful sigmoidoscopic screening program in asymptomatic patients.

Many studies have verified the increased diagnostic yield of the flexible sigmoidoscopic evaluation when compared to that of the rigid sigmoidoscopic examination.[14,15] In addition, evidence has been found to support

TABLE 9–3. JUSTIFICATIONS FOR FLEXIBLE SIGMOIDOSCOPIC SCREENING
Increased diagnostic yield of colonic neoplasia when compared to rigid sigmoidoscopy
Data supporting hypothesis of colonic neoplasia moving more proximal in colon away from distal rectosigmoid area
Increased patient and physician compliance with performing flexible sigmoidoscopy

the hypothesis that both types of colonic neoplasia (polyps and cancer) are shifting to the right side of the colon, away from the distal rectosigmoid area.[16,17] This suggests that longer sigmoidoscopic examinations are needed. Clearly, the 35- or 60-cm flexible sigmoidoscope is preferred to the rigid sigmoidoscope for screening purposes. It is also apparent that the longer flexible instrument has a higher detection rate for colonic neoplasia and is tolerated as well as the shorter flexible instrument by patients (Table 9–3).[18,19] The specific flexible sigmoidoscope used depends on the physician's training and background.

Once a polyp has been detected on screening flexible sigmoidoscopy in an asymptomatic individual, the following steps are critical.

Histologic Confirmation. The type of distal colonic polyp needs to be confirmed by biopsy. If the polyp is adenomatous, total colonoscopy needs to be performed to exclude a synchronous colonic lesion. I believe that failure to recommend and confirm the performance of such a procedure constitutes clinical negligence because of the medical evidence supporting its usefulness in detecting early cancers in these patients. The determination of when a polyp is shown to be hyperplastic remains a subject of debate. The National Polyp Study has suggested a weakly positive association with synchronous adenoma, but their data do not support the fact that a distal rectosigmoid hyperplastic polyp is predictive of colonic neoplasia more proximally in the colon.[3] An article from the Cleveland Clinic experience, however, has suggested that a rectosigmoid hyperplastic polyp is predictive of distal colonic neoplasia.[20] Importantly, all polyps, regardless of their size, should be biopsied to confirm their histologic type. Much has been written about the small or diminutive polyp, a polyp of less than 5 mm in diameter, that does not require biopsy or follow-up because of the belief that most of these polyps are hyperplastic.[13] All colonic polyps require biopsy and endoscopic removal, if adenomatous, to decrease the subsequent development of colonic cancer.[21] Sessile polyps can be removed by the hot biopsy technique or the sequential polypectomy technique (Table 9–4).

Fecal Occult Blood Testing. It has been estimated that, of all patients having a fecal occult blood test (FOBT), 2 to 6% test positive and, of those, colonic cancer is found in 5 to 10% and colonic adenomas in 20%.[22] This means that a high false-positive rate is inherent in this type of testing, most commonly because of the patient's dietary intake of beef, certain fruits and vegetables with a high peroxidase content, or the intake of iron in vitamin preparations.[23,24] I recommend that any patient found to have a positive

TABLE 9–4. SEQUENCE AFTER DETECTING A COLONIC POLYP IN AN ASYMPTOMATIC PATIENT WITH FLEXIBLE SIGMOIDOSCOPY
1. Biopsy to define histologic type of polyp a. If adenoma: total colonoscopy to exclude synchronous colonic neoplasia b. If hyperplastic: controversy presently exists about predictive value of a rectosigmoid hyperplastic polyp and synchronous proximal colonic neoplasia
2. Therapeutic colonoscopy of all diagnosed colonic adenoma in an attempt to produce a "clean" colon

FOBT result on routine digital examination also have a confirmatory home hemoccult 3-day slide collection before starting a diagnostic evaluation. For the 2 days preceding and the 3 days of the collection, the patient is instructed to avoid all the known factors that can result in a false-positive test result. If one of the six slides is FOBT-positive with a properly collected sample, a diagnostic evaluation is mandatory.

Unfortunately, the false-negative rate of fecal occult blood testing in patients with known colonic neoplasia is alarmingly high. In patients with known colon cancer, it is from 13 to 50%, for patients with known colonic adenoma it can be as high as 75%, and in asymptomatic patients with colonic adenoma it can be as high as 90%.[25–28]

One survey has estimated that only half of the practicing physicians in the United States comply with the recommended guidelines for fecal occult blood testing.[29] Patient compliance varies from about 33% to about 95 to 98%, depending on physician motivation of the patient group.[30] Improvement in patient compliance appears to be related to an older age, knowledge of a friend with colon cancer, and an interest in preventative health care.[31]

In summary, fecal occult blood testing is not a perfect solution for the detection of colonic neoplasia, but it is the best we have to offer presently in conjunction with the other guidelines suggested by the American Cancer Society.

Specific recommendations can be made for patients at high risk of developing colonic cancer. It is first important to identify the patient who is at a higher risk for the development of colonic cancer. A family history of familial polyposis coli or Gardner's syndrome is associated with a 100% risk for the development of colon cancer by the age of 40 years. Patients with a history of cancer family syndrome have a 50% chance of developing colon cancer.[13] The incidence of colorectal cancer increases up to three times that of other groups in patients with one or two first-degree relatives who have developed the disease.[32] A history of universal ulcerative colitis of greater than 7 years' duration is associated with an increasing risk over the course of the disease. A history of prior colonic neoplasia is associated with an increased risk of developing colon cancer. Metachronous colonic adenoma recurs in about 30% of patients with a prior history of colonic adenoma. Colon cancer recurs in 3% of patients.[8] Finally, the risk of developing colorectal cancer doubles in patients with a history of endometrial, ovarian, or breast cancer (Table 9–5).[33]

TABLE 9–5. HIGH-RISK PATIENTS FOR THE DEVELOPMENT OF COLON CANCER

Factor	Risk (%)
Family history	
Familial polyposis coli or Gardner's syndrome	100 (by age 40)
Cancer family syndrome	50 (by age 40)
One or two first-degree relatives with colon cancer	Up to three times increased risk
Personal history	
Universal ulcerative colitis of greater than 7 years' duration	Increases annually
Ovarian, breast, or endometrial cancer	Twice increased risk
Prior colon cancer	3%

Changes in screening recommendations vary among different groups of high-risk patients. For those patients with a history of familial polyposis coli or Gardner's syndrome, flexible sigmoidoscopy is recommended twice annually from the age of 10 to the age of 40 years. Once multiple adenomas are found, total colectomy is indicated. For those patients with a cancer family syndrome, a colonoscopy is recommended beginning at the age of 20 years and every 2 to 3 years thereafter. For patients with a family history of colon cancer (one or two first-degree relatives), it is recommended that annual fecal occult blood testing begin 10 years before the age of the index case, with flexible sigmoidoscopy being performed at the same time and as determined by the positivity of the FOBT, or every 3 years thereafter. For patients with a greater than 7-year history of ulcerative colitis, annual to biannual colonoscopy with biopsy for the exclusion of mucosal dysplasia, beginning in the eighth year of the disease, is recommended. For a patient with a prior colon cancer, a colonoscopy should be done 6 and 18 months postoperatively, and every 3 years thereafter as long as the results are normal. For the patient with a history of colonic adenoma, a follow-up colonoscopy is required 1 year after the initial therapeutic colonoscopy to verify a "clean" colon, and then every 3 years. A history of endometrial, ovarian, or breast cancer makes it mandatory that the patient adhere strictly to the American Cancer Society guidelines.[8]

In addition to colonoscopy, the colorectal screening program provides guidelines for ordering specific laboratory studies, such as chorioembryonic antigen blood tests, liver function tests, and chest roentgenograms in patients who have had recent surgery for colon cancer. Basically, the patient needs to be examined every 3 to 6 months for the first 2 years, every 6 to 12 months for the next 2 years, and annually thereafter. A blood sample and chest roentgenogram should be obtained every 6 months for 2 years, and annually thereafter. Rigorous follow-up is necessary for early detection of a recurrence or of a metastatic disease.

It is hoped that increased physician and patient compliance with all these recommendations, including asymptomatic individuals or individuals with a positive family or personal history, can be equated with a decrease in the incidence of colon cancer and with an improved survival for those patients diagnosed with it in the future. To answer these important questions large, controlled studies are presently underway in the United States, Sweden, Great Britain, and Denmark.

REFERENCES

1. Rickert RR, Auerbach O, Garfinkel L, et al: Adenomatous lesions of the large bowel: An autopsy survey. Cancer, 43:1847, 1981.
2. ASGE Position Paper: The role of colonoscopy in the management of patients with colonic polyps. Gastrointest Endosc, 34:6, 1988.
3. Winawer SJ, Zauber A, Diaz B, et al: The National Polyp Study: Overview of program and preliminary report of patient and polyp characteristics. *In* Basic and Clinical Perspectives of Colorectal Polyps and Cancer. Edited by Glen Steele. New York, Alan R Liss, 1988, pp 35–49.
4. Winawer SJ: The natural history of colorectal cancer: opportunities for intervention. New Dev Med, 2:55, 1988.
5. American Cancer Society: Cancer of the colon and rectum. CA, 30:208, 1980.
6. Friedman GD, Collins MF, Fireman BH: Multiphasic health check-up evaluation: A sixteen-year follow-up. J Chron Dis 39:453, 1986.
7. Shelby JV, Friedman GD: Sigmoidoscopy and mortality from colorectal cancer: The Kaiser-Permanente Multiphasic Evaluation Study. J Clin Epidemiol 41:427, 1988.
8. Fleischer DE, Goldberg SB, Browning TH, et al: Detection and surveillance of colorectal cancer. JAMA, 261:580, 1989.
9. Gilbertsen VA: Proctosigmoidoscopy and polypectomy in reducing the incidence of rectal cancer. Cancer 34:936, 1974.
10. Hertz REL, Deddish MR, Day E: Value of periodic examinations in detecting cancer of the colon and rectum. Postgrad Med, 27:290, 1960.
11. Winawer SJ, Miller C, Lightdale C, et al: Patient response to sigmoidoscopy: A randomized controlled trial of rigid and flexible sigmoidoscopy. Cancer, 60:1905, 1987.
12. Rodney WM, Beaker RJ, Johnson RA, et al: Physician compliance with colorectal cancer screening (1978–1983): The impact of flexible sigmoidoscopy on protocol. J Fam Pract, 20:265, 1985.
13. Selby JV, Friedman GD: Sigmoidoscopy in the periodic health examination of asymptomatic adults. JAMA, 261:595, 1989.
14. Bohlman TW, Katon RM, Lipshutz GR, et al: Fiberoptic pansigmoidoscopy: An evaluation and comparison to rigid sigmoidoscopy. Gastroenterology, 72:644, 1977.
15. Winawer SJ, Leidner SD, Boyle C, et al: Comparison of flexible sigmoidoscopy with other diagnostic techniques in the diagnosis of rectocolon neoplasia. Dig Dis Sci 24:277, 1979.
16. Greene FL: Distribution of colorectal neoplasms: A left-to-right shift of polyps and cancer. Am Surg, 49:62, 1983.
17. Gillespie PE, Chambers TJ, Chan KW, et al: Colonic adenoma—a colonoscopy survey. Gut 20:240, 1979.
18. Lehman GA, Buchner DM, Lappas JC, et al: Anatomical extent of fiberoptic sigmoidoscopy. Gastroenterology, 84:803, 1983.
19. Dubow RA, Katon RM, Benner KG, et al: Short versus long flexible sigmoidoscopy: A comparison of findings and tolerance in asymptomatic patients screened for colorectal neoplasia. Gastrointest Endosc, 31:305, 1985.
20. Achkar E, Carey WD: Small polyps found during fiberoptic sigmoidoscopy in asymptomatic patients. Ann Intern Med 109:880, 1988.

21. Lambert R, Sabin LH, Waye JD: The management of patients with colorectal adenomas. CA, 34:167, 1984.
22. Knight KK, Fielding JE, Battista RN: Occult blood testing for colorectal cancer. JAMA, 261:587, 1989.
23. Macrae FA, St John DJB, Caligore P, et al: Optimal dietary conditions for hemoccult testing. Gastroenterology, 82:899, 1982.
24. Lifton LJ, Kreiser J: False-positive stool occult blood tests caused by iron preparations: A controlled study and review of the literature. Gastroenterology, 83:860, 1982.
25. Crowley ML, Freeman LD, Mohet MD, et al: Sensitivity of guaiac-impregnated cards for the detection of colorectal neoplasia. J Clin Gastroenterol, 5:127, 1983.
26. Macrae FA, St John DJB: Relationships between patterns of bleeding and hemoccult sensitivity in patients with colorectal cancers or adenomas. Gastroenterology, 82:891, 1982.
27. Ribet A, Frexinos J, Escourrou J, et al: Occult blood tests and colorectal tumors. Lancet 1:417, 1980.
28. Demers RY, Stawick LE, Demers P: Relative sensitivity of the fecal occult blood test and flexible sigmoidoscopy in detecting polyps. Prev Med 14:55, 1985.
29. Survey of physician's attitudes and practices in early cancer detection. CA, 35:197, 1984.
30. Gilson BS, Michnich ME, Thompson RS, et al: Physician effectiveness in preventive care: Final report. National Center for Health Services Research, US Dept of Health and Human Services, Rockville, Md., 1987.
31. Blalock SJ, DeVellis BM, Sandler RS: Participation in fecal occult blood testing: A critical review. Prev Med, 16:9, 1987.
32. Rozen P, Fireman Z, Figer A, et al: Family history of colorectal cancer as a marker of potential malignancy in a screening program. Cancer, 60:248, 1987.
33. Howell MA: The association between colorectal cancer and breast cancer. J Chron Dis, 29:243, 1976.

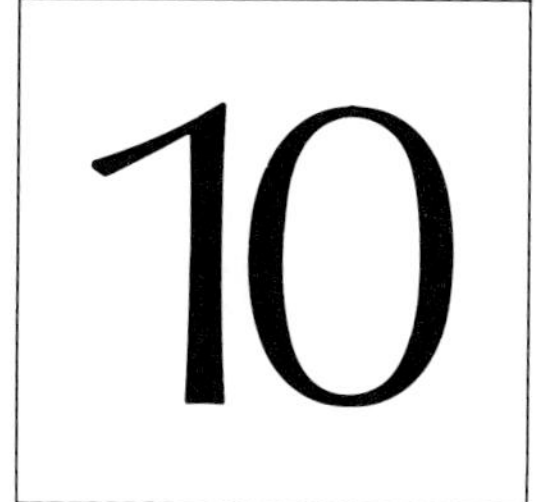

FLEXIBLE SIGMOIDOSCOPY

Joseph T. Danzi

The American public's awareness of diseases of the sigmoid colon has never been as astute as it is now, mainly because of the health-related television programs on satellite channels and the American Cancer Society's colorectal health program. This awareness can be equated to the primary care physician's need to perform screening sigmoidoscopies and to be conversant in diseases of the sigmoid colon, from diverticulosis to colorectal cancer.

The advent of flexible sigmoidoscopy has done much to increase the patient population's acceptance of routine sigmoid examinations. It is well known that patients prefer flexible over rigid sigmoidoscopy. This important consideration supplements the fact that screening with the flexible instrument increases the yield of positive sigmoidoscopic findings when compared to that of rigid examinations.[1]

The debate over whether it is best to screen patients with the 35- or 60-cm instrument continues.[2] Conflicting reports have been published regarding diagnostic yields with either flexible sigmoidoscope. I believe that all primary care physicians should become proficient with one of these instruments, and it is easier to learn the technique required for the 35-cm sigmoidoscope than for the 60-cm sigmoidoscope. Once the physician's proficiency has met patients' requirements, the average depth of inspection is greater than 25 cm, and the technique of retroflexion in the rectum is mastered, the switch from the 35- to 60-cm sigmoidoscope is easily accomplished.

It is important that physicians meet the requirements of competency for the performance of flexible sigmoidoscopy, as outlined either by the American College of Physicians or the American Board of Family Practice,

TABLE 10–1. INDICATIONS FOR ANOSCOPY
Suspected anal or perianal disease
Rectal biopsy for suspected amyloidosis
Diagnosis of infectious proctitis
History of rectal bleeding with a normal colonoscopy and sigmoidoscopy

before performing screening examinations. The two societies differ somewhat in the prerequisites needed to establish clinical competency with the flexible sigmoidoscope, so I recommend that physicians contact the appropriate society regarding their training requirements.

It is important to remember that the flexible sigmoidoscope has not entirely replaced the rigid instrument. What are the indications for the use of the rigid sigmoidoscope? First, the suspected presence of anal disease is justification for the performance of a rigid examination. Often, a rigid inspection is done initially and followed immediately with a flexible examination in this patient population. My experience is that the rigid instrument is superior to the flexible scope for the diagnosis of anal fissures, fistulae, anal papillitis, and infectious proctitis. Second, the biopsy specimens obtained with the rigid instrument are larger than those obtained with the biopsy forceps from the flexible sigmoidoscope. This is of clinical importance in establishing the diagnosis of rectal involvement with amyloidosis. Third, the diagnosis of infectious proctitis is made easier with the rigid sigmoidoscope because its large examination channel makes it easier to obtain cytologic, histologic, and bacteriologic specimens. Fourth, a rigid sigmoidoscopic examination is indicated in a patient with rectal bleeding and a normal flexible sigmoidoscopy and colonoscopic examination should be done before carrying out other diagnostic procedures (Table 10–1).

PATIENT PREPARATION

Preparation of the patient is important before performing flexible sigmoidoscopy. Usually, two disposable Fleet enemas can adequately prepare most patients. If, on initial inspection of the rectum, it is found that the sigmoid colon has been inadequately prepped, it is best to give the patient another enema to help ensure that no lesions have been missed. This is sometimes a difficult decision with a busy office practice, but it is most important in guaranteeing an adequate sigmoidoscopic examination.

It is important to determine the following before performing flexible sigmoidoscopy: a prior history of acute diverticulitis, with or without complications; previous radiotherapy for prostate, bladder, or uterine cancer; whether a hysterectomy has been performed; and previous sigmoid colon surgery. These conditions can result in a limited sigmoidoscopic examination because of adhesions. It is especially important that excessive insertion pressure be restricted in patients with chronic radiation proctocolitis because of the increased risk of perforation.

TABLE 10–2. "TIPS OF THE TRADE" IN FLEXIBLE SIGMOIDOSCOPY
Be properly prepared.
Obtain a history of prior diverticulitis or pelvic surgery and of previous radiation therapy to the pelvis.
Talk to the patient during the procedure.
Use adequate inflation pressure.
Be prudent of time.

It is imperative to explain to the patient during the procedure what they are experiencing to help relieve some of their anxiety. The patient should be reminded to tell the physician of any discomfort, because this can frequently be eased by reducing the inflation pressure. I have found the teaching attachment accepted by sophisticated patients in visualizing sigmoid abnormalities such as polyps or diverticular orifices.

It is important to use adequate inflation pressure to visualize the sigmoid colon and to facilitate passage of the sigmoidoscope. The sigmoid colon can be rapidly decompressed with the suction capabilities of the instrument. Inadequate visualization caused by underinflation of the bowel, however, is a frequent reason for an incomplete examination.

It is advisable to complete the procedure as quickly as possible. A prolonged initial examination does little to increase patient compliance for follow-up examinations (Table 10–2).

INDICATIONS AND CONTRAINDICATIONS

INDICATIONS FOR FLEXIBLE SIGMOIDOSCOPY

The primary reason for the use of this diagnostic procedure in primary care practice is screening for colorectal neoplasia (Table 10–3). The American Cancer Society has recommended that all patients over the age of 50 years, without a family history of colorectal cancer or polyps, have two normal sequential sigmoidoscopic examinations (1 year apart) and a follow-up examination every 3 to 5 years.[3] The changes made in this screening recommendation based on a positive family or patient history have been reviewed in Chapter 9.

The next most common indication is a history of or current rectal bleeding. Every patient with this history merits a flexible sigmoidoscopic

TABLE 10–3. INDICATIONS FOR FLEXIBLE SIGMOIDOSCOPY
Screening for colorectal neoplasia
History of or current rectal bleeding
Evaluation of distal colonic diseases
Assessment of rectosigmoid area in patient with abnormal barium enema

examination. If an anal cause of the bleeding is suspected, a rigid sigmoidoscopic examination can be done immediately after a normal flexible sigmoidoscopy.

Patients with distal colonic diseases, such as ulcerative colitis, Crohn's disease, complicated diverticular disease, or a rectosigmoid stricture, require sigmoidoscopic examinations to assess their response to medical therapy and changes in symptoms, and to evaluate a change in bowel habits.

A flexible sigmoidoscopy is indicated to assess the rectosigmoid colon in a patient with an abnormal barium enema study. It is important to confirm the radiologic finding and to exclude a false-positive radiologic interpretation.

CONTRAINDICATIONS FOR FLEXIBLE SIGMOIDOSCOPY

The clinical suspicion of a colonic perforation is an absolute reason *not* to perform a flexible sigmoid examination. In patients with acute diverticulitis and peritoneal signs, it is prudent to delay the sigmoidoscopic examination until the acute inflammation has resolved. All patients with an episode of acute diverticulitis who have not had a recent sigmoidoscopy, however, merit an examination during their convalescence to exclude colorectal neoplasia as the cause of the acute attack.

A flexible sigmoid examination should not be performed when a total colonoscopy is indicated.

Finally, if anal or perianal disease is suspected, and the patient has had a recent sigmoidoscopic evaluation, a rigid anoscopic or sigmoidoscopic examination should be performed (Table 10–4).

INDICATIONS FOR TOTAL COLONOSCOPY

A proximal colon abnormality demonstrated on a barium enema examination requires colonoscopy for its confirmation. Patients with unexplained gastrointestinal bleeding, whether it is hematochezia, melena of unknown cause, a positive fecal occult blood test, or an iron deficiency anemia, require a total colonoscopy to exclude a colonic cause. Patients needing colon cancer surveillance require total colonoscopy. A past history of a colon cancer resection, or individuals with a history of colonic adenoma, need regular follow-up, as outlined in Chapter 9. Individuals with a family history of colon cancer or a history of polyposis syndrome require surveillance by colonoscopy to exclude a change from colonic adenoma to colonic cancer.[4] A history of universal ulcerative colitis for longer than 7 years or indeterminate inflammatory bowel disease of the

TABLE 10–4. CONTRAINDICATIONS TO FLEXIBLE SIGMOIDOSCOPY
Clinical suspicion of a colonic perforation
Patient has an indication for total colonoscopy
Suspicion of anal or perianal disease

TABLE 10–5. INDICATIONS FOR TOTAL COLONOSCOPY
Evaluation of a proximal colon abnormality seen on barium enema
Unexplained rectal bleeding, either occult or overt
Colon cancer surveillance in appropriate patients
Exclusion of synchronous or metachronous colonic adenoma
Evaluation of colonic strictures
Colonic decompression in intestinal pseudo-obstruction

colon for longer than 10 years requires colon surveillance for evidence of dysplasia.[5] Colonoscopy is indicated for the evaluation of colonic strictures and for colonic decompression in patients with intestinal pseudo-obstruction. Total colonoscopy is indicated for the exclusion of synchronous or metachronous colonic adenoma in patients with hyperplastic or adenomatous polyps on flexible or rigid sigmoidoscopy (Table 10–5).

SIGMOIDOSCOPIC FINDINGS

Flexible sigmoidoscopy can be used to verify the normal sigmoid colon and to find evidence of specific disease.

NORMAL FINDINGS

The normal appearance of the sigmoid colon is characterized by the physician's ability to see through the normal mucosa and to visualize the submucosal vascularity. This easily recognized feature is the most important endoscopic characteristic of the sigmoid colon (Fig. 10–1). Whenever edema or inflammation of the mucosa is present, the sigmoidoscopist cannot visualize the submucosal vessels.

Diverticular orifices in the sigmoid colon are a common finding in patients over the age of 50. In uncomplicated diverticulosis, these diverticular openings can be visualized among the normally seen submucosal vessels. Not infrequently, fecoliths are seen in the diverticular orifices, but are of no clinical consequence (Figs. 10–2 and 10–3).

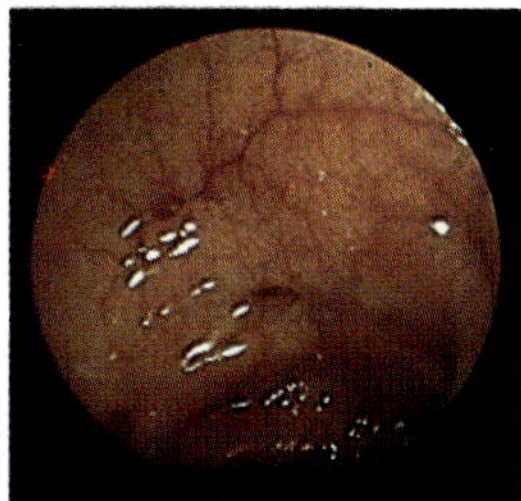

FIG. 10–1. Normal sigmoid colon.

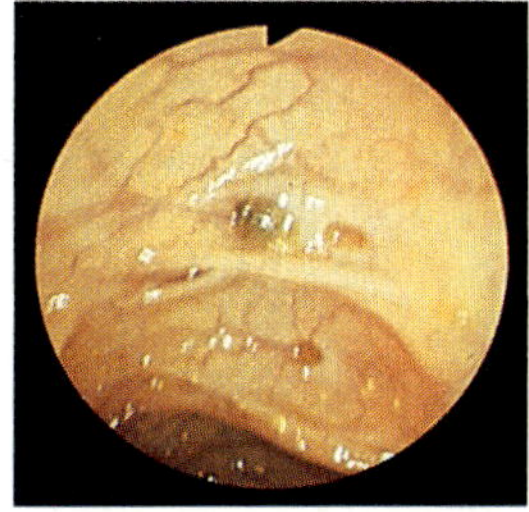

FIG. 10–2. Sigmoid diverticulosis.

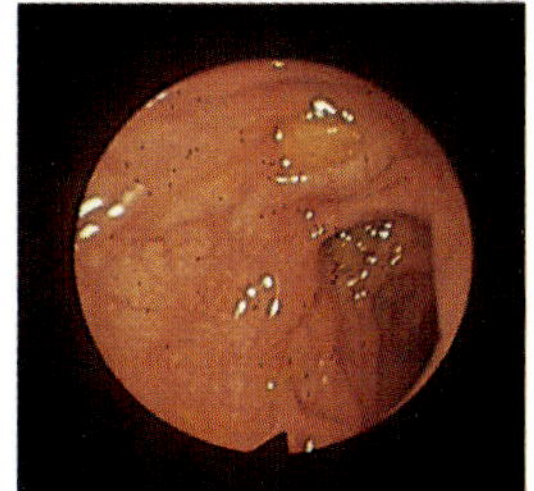

FIG. 10–3. Sigmoid diverticulosis with fecolith.

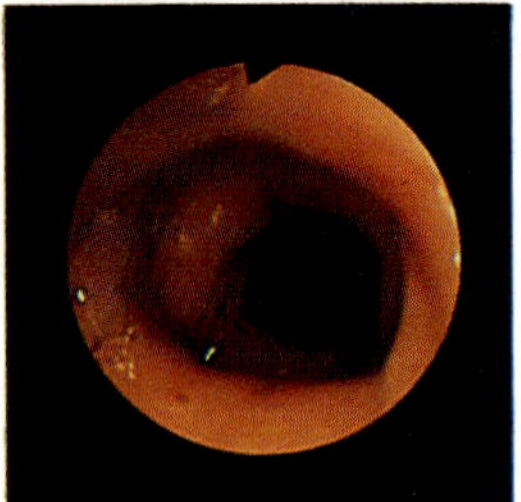
FIG. 10–4. Oval configuration of left colon.

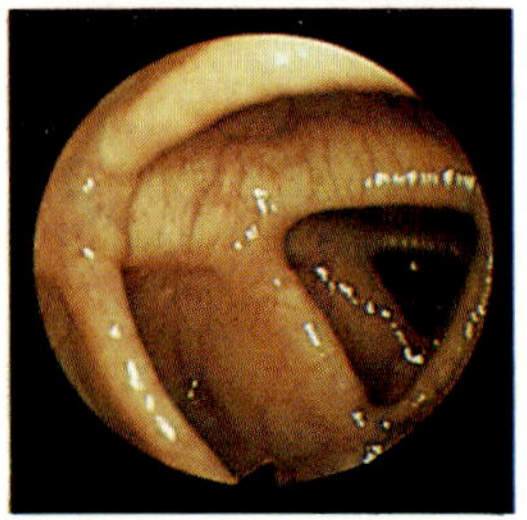
FIG. 10–5. Triangular configuration of transverse colon.

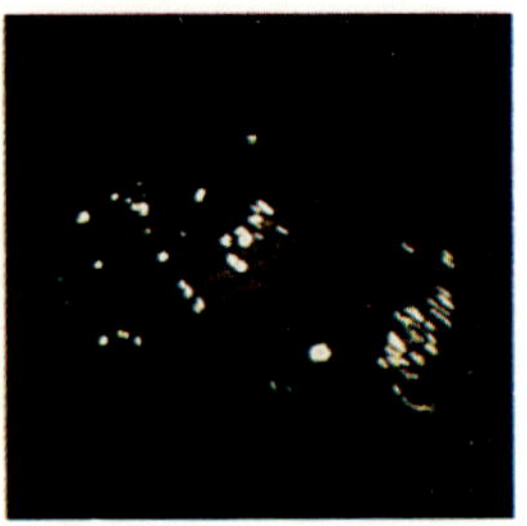
FIG. 10–6. Melanosis coli.

Occasionally, the sigmoidoscopist using the 65-instrument passes through the splenic flexure and enters the transverse colon. The configuration of the transverse colon is triangular, in contrast to the oval shape of the sigmoid and left colons (Figs. 10–4 and 10–5).

Many patients abuse laxatives. If the cathartic contains anthracene-derived chemicals, the sigmoid colon may appear blackish in color as a result of the deposition of these compounds in the submucosa of the bowel.[6] This sigmoidoscopic appearance is known as melanosis coli, but has no relationship to any abnormality of melanin synthesis or metabolism (Fig. 10–6).

SPECIFIC DISEASES

A number of diseases can be characterized by their appearance using flexible sigmoidoscopy.

Inflammatory Bowel Disease

The most common sigmoidoscopic finding with either mild ulcerative colitis or Crohn's disease of the colon is the presence of edema or inflammation of the mucosa, with a loss of the normally seen submucosal vascularity. Edema of the mucosa may cause it to reflect light or give it a granular appearance. Another important sigmoidoscopic feature of the mild forms of either type of inflammatory bowel disease is the friability of colonic mucosa when touched by the sigmoidoscope. The inflamed mucosa bleeds easily, and can have an erythematous appearance (Fig. 10–7).

Small aphthoid ulcerations are extremely rare in the mucosa of patients with mild ulcerative colitis, but are common in the colonic lining of patients with mild Crohn's colitis (Figs. 10–8 and 10–9).

When these diseases become moderately severe, their sigmoidoscopic features change. In moderately severe ulcerative colitis, the mucosa becomes more granular in appearance, with a definite erythematous hue. Touch friability is accentuated, and small aphthoid ulcerations are seen among the granular mucosa (Fig. 10–10).

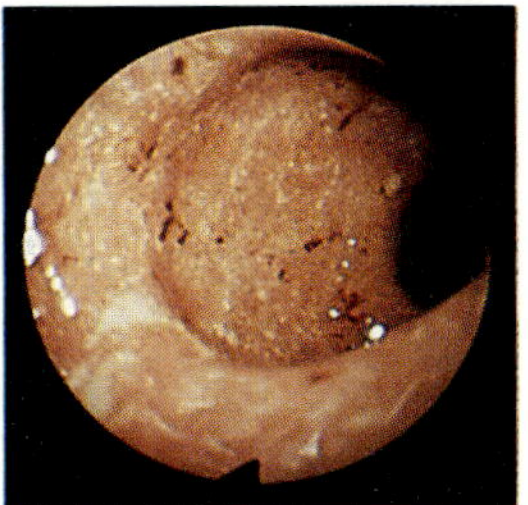

FIG. 10–7. Mild ulcerative colitis.

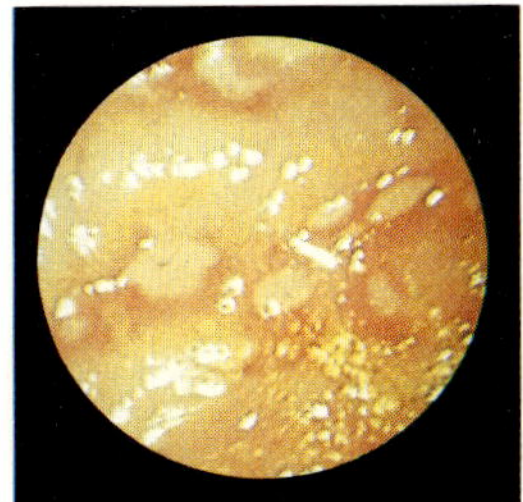

FIG. 10–8. Mild Crohn's colitis.

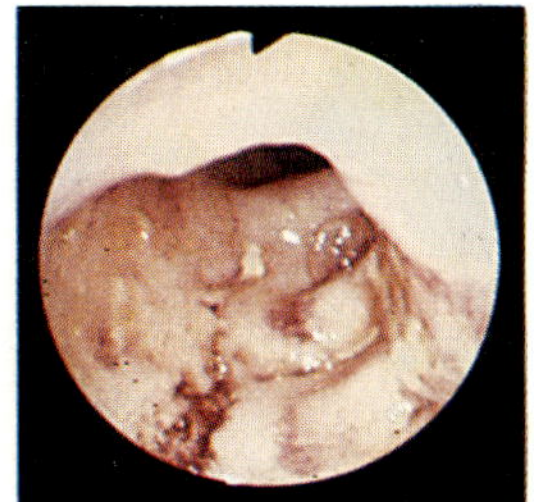

FIG. 10–9. Mild Crohn's colitis with aphthoid ulcerations.

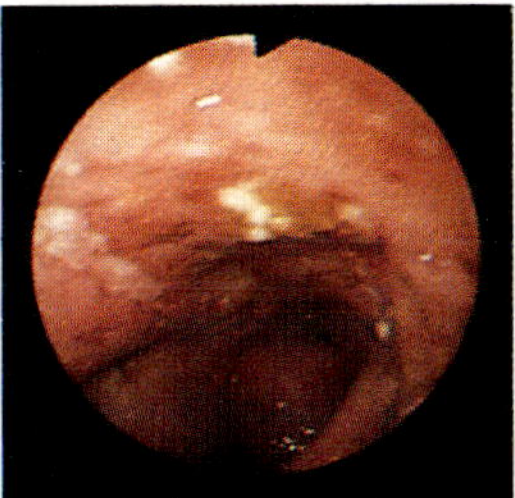

FIG. 10–10. Moderately severe ulcerative colitis.

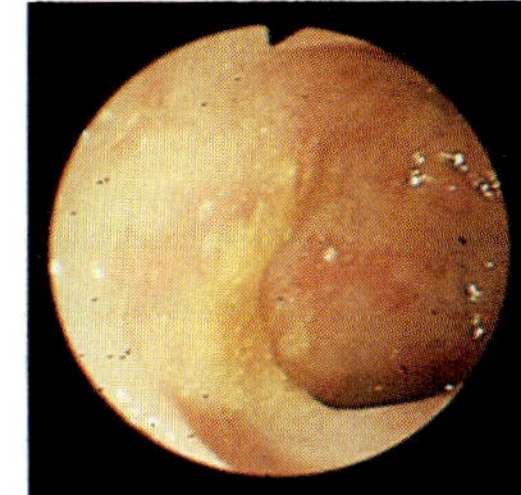

FIG. 10–11. Moderately severe Crohn's colitis with oval ulcerations.

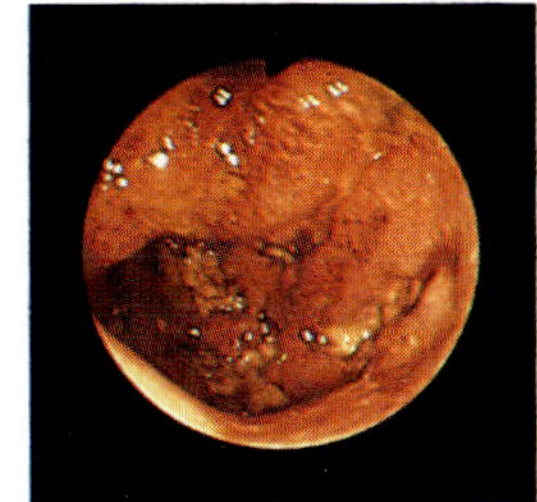

FIG. 10–12. Moderately severe Crohn's colitis with linear ulcerations and cobblestoned mucosa.

In patients with moderately severe Crohn's disease of the sigmoid colon, the sigmoidoscopist is likely to see large ulcerations that vary in configuration from ovoid to stellate to linear. These ulcerations are seen in a thickened, swollen mucosa, producing a cobblestoned appearance of the sigmoid colon (Figs. 10–11 and 10–12).[7]

In moderately severe forms of either type of inflammatory bowel disease, pseudopolyps can be seen on sigmoidoscopic examination. Pseudopolyps appear as irregular, polypoid projections off the mucosal lining. These are not true colonic polyps but represent a polypoid collection of normal mucosa that has not been ulcerated or denuded by a prior, severe attack of the inflammatory bowel disease (Fig. 10–13).

The clinician should never make a diagnosis of ulcerative or Crohn's colitis until the analyses of two sets of fresh stool have excluded an infectious cause of the sigmoidoscopic features. An infestation with Amoeba histolytica, Salmonella, Yersinia, or Campylobacter jejuni can produce the same sigmoidoscopic features. It should never be assumed that a patient with either type of inflammatory bowel disease is having a flare-up until an infectious cause has been excluded. It is especially important that no patient with presumed severe ulcerative colitis or

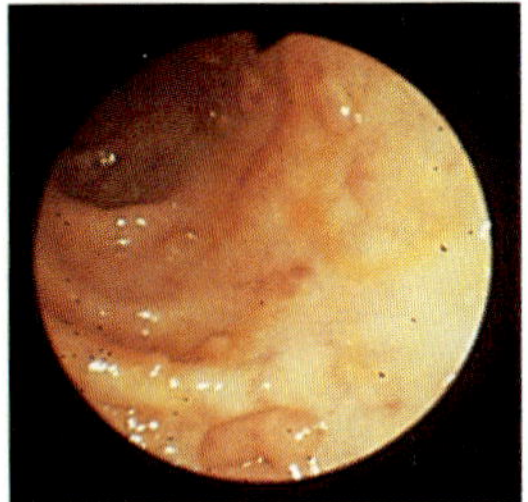

FIG. 10–13. Pseudopolyps in chronic ulcerative colitis.

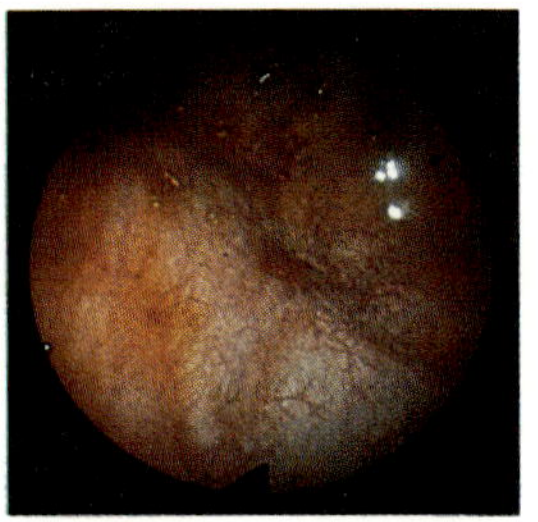

FIG. 10–14. Colonic arteriovenous malformation.

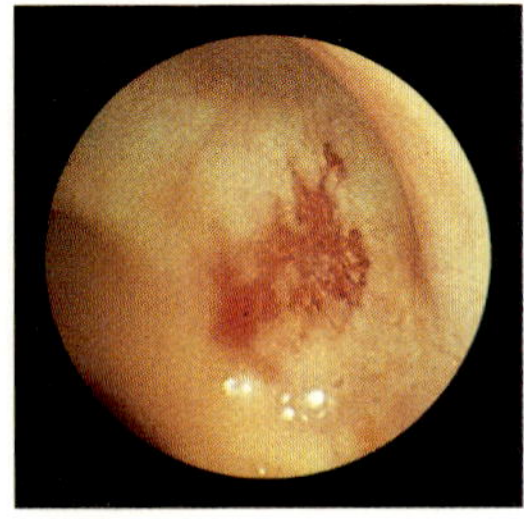

FIG. 10–15. Colonic telangiectasia.

Crohn's colitis be placed on steroid therapy until an amebic infestation has been ruled out.

Arteriovenous Malformations and Telangiectasia

Arteriovenous malformations of the colon are an important cause of colonic bleeding in patients over the age of 55. These vascular abnormalities can be found in any part of the large or small intestine, and tend to be multiple in occurrence. Arteriovenous malformations can be found in the absence of other disease or they may be seen in association with cardiovascular diseases, mainly aortic stenosis.[8]

These vascular abnormalities can be identified by endoscopic inspection of the colon in about 50% of cases. If they are located in the submucosa, the sigmoidoscopist cannot visualize them. If the arteriovenous malformations are located in the mucosa or submucosa, however, they appear as irregular, erythematous, macular defects. The size of these vascular malformations can vary, but they are usually less than 10 mm in diameter. The vascular origin of these mucosal defects can be confirmed by histologic review, but I rarely biopsy a presumed vascular abnormality because of the risk of bleeding. I recommend that primary care physicians refer these patients for a total colonoscopy, with possible therapeutic endoscopy if active bleeding is found (Fig. 10–14).

The presence of telangiectasia in the colonic mucosa is most commonly observed in patients with chronic renal failure or in individuals with hereditary telangiectasia. These vascular abnormalities are found in an otherwise normal colonic mucosa. They vary in size, are usually multiple, have an intense red color, and typically have an irregular, sawtoothed border.

Telangiectasia of the colon can result in occult or overt bleeding. Their presence should be considered in individuals with chronic renal failure and gastrointestinal bleeding or in patients with a history of epistaxis, mucosal telangiectasia of the oral or nasal cavity, and a history of gastrointestinal blood loss.[9] These mucosal vascular lesions respond well to electrocoagulative or photocoagulative endoscopic therapy (Fig. 10–15).

Chronic radiation proctocolitis can result after radiation therapy for

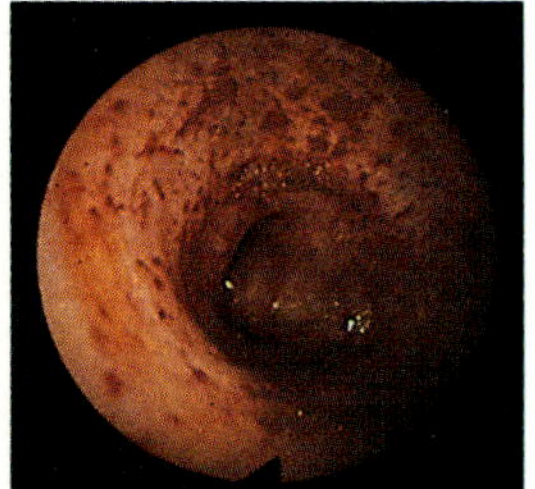

FIG. 10–16. Chronic radiation colitis.

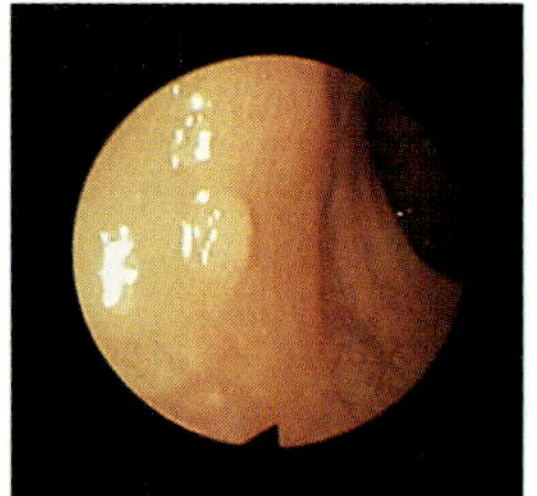

FIG. 10–17. Hyperplastic polyps.

bladder, prostate, or uterine cancer. It most commonly presents as painless rectal bleeding. The patient might have diarrhea. Typically, these symptoms occur 6 months after completion of the radiation therapy.

The important sigmoidoscopic features of chronic radiation colitis include numerous small telangiectasia among an atrophic or pale colonic mucosa. The mucosa is friable, and a biopsy specimen demonstrates an atrophic mucosa and proliferative vascular changes (Fig. 10–16).

Colon Polyps

Neoplastic and non-neoplastic polyps can be observed sigmoidoscopically.

Non-Neoplastic Polyps. The most common type of polyp in this category is the "suction artifact polyp," which is most frequently observed by the clinician during the initial experience with the instrument. This polypoid mucosal collection results from the tenting of the mucosa in the suction channel of the endoscope. The use of adequate inflation pressure through the sigmoidoscope eliminates these false polyps.

The most common type of non-neoplastic colon polyp is the hyperplastic polyp. Typically, hyperplastic polyps are the same color as the normal colonic mucosa and are usually less than 1 cm in diameter. This type of colonic polyp tends to be multiple in occurrence. As the name implies, it has no premalignant potential. The significance of this type of polyp as a predictor of synchronous colonic adenomatous polyps and its importance as an indication for total colonoscopy are uncertain.[10,11] Presently, it is the recommendation of the Section of Gastroenterology of the Guthrie Clinic that patients found to have sigmoid hyperplastic polyps have a total colon examination to exclude synchronous neoplastic polyps (Fig. 10–17).

The pseudopolyp found in patients with Crohn's colitis or ulcerative colitis is also listed in the non-neoplastic category.

Juvenile polyps are non-neoplastic, most commonly found in the rectum, usually pedunculated, single in occurrence, and typically found in patients under the age of 10 years. They are cherry-colored, with milky cystic areas, in a predominantly round, pedunculated polyp. Usually, a parent notices intermittent rectal bleeding or prolapsing of the polyp in the child. This type of polyp may slough or regress spontaneously but, if

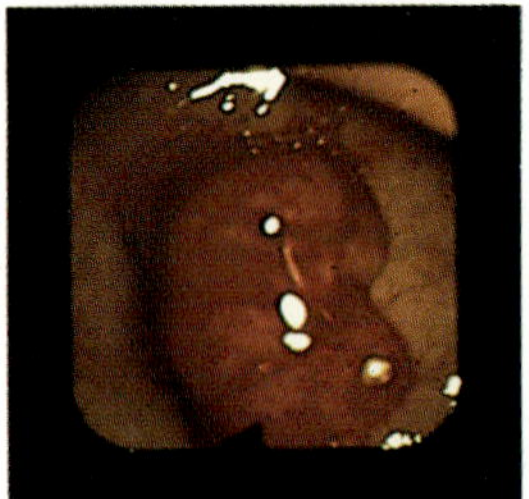

FIG. 10–18. Colonic tubular adenoma.

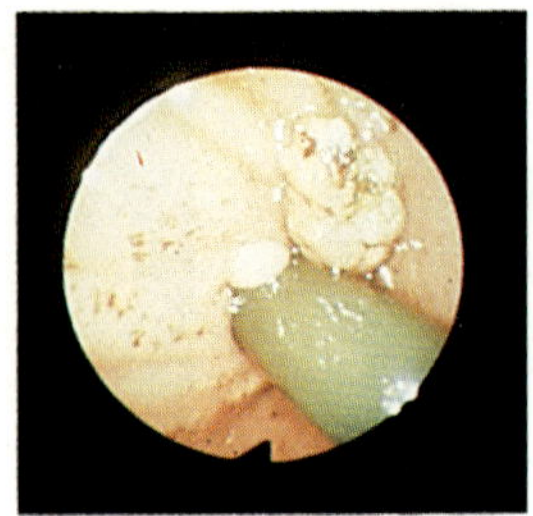

FIG. 10–19. Colonic villous adenoma.

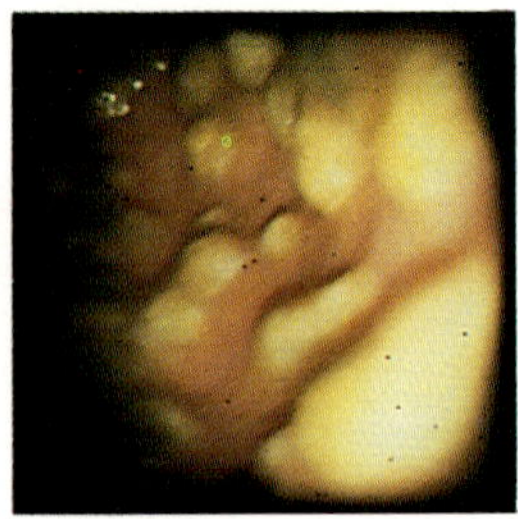

FIG. 10–20. Pseudomembranous colitis.

detected during sigmoidoscopy, it is recommended that it be removed.

Neoplastic Polyps. Colonic adenomas have a variable sigmoidoscopic appearance, depending on their histologic classification. Tubular adenomas are typically round, have variable hues of red coloration, may be sessile or pedunculated in configuration, and have a smooth surface that is disrupted by cleft-like furrows, which create lobules on the polyp's surface. Villous adenomas of the rectosigmoid colon are usually sessile, larger in size than tubular adenomas, and have the same color characteristics as tubular adenomas, but with an irregular surface resembling a head of cauliflower. Tubulovillous adenomas are variable in size, have the same color as tubular adenomas, may be sessile or pedunculated in configuration, and have polyp surfaces characteristic of both tubular and villous adenomas.

The size of the adenoma is an important indicator of malignancy within the polyp. When all histologic types of colonic adenomas are grouped together according to polyp size, the risk of detecting invasive cancer is the following: under 1 cm, approximately 1%; 1 to 2 cm, about 10%; and over 2 cm, over 40% (Figs. 10–18 and 10–19).[12]

Infectious Diarrheas

Clostridium difficile-Related Diarrheas. C. difficile is the most common bacterial cause of an antibiotic-related diarrheal illness in this country. Clinical features that suggest C. difficile are severe diarrhea, a recurrent diarrheal illness, and the associated signs of colitis, such as fever, an elevated white blood cell count, and the presence of fecal leukocytes. A stool analysis for C. difficile antitoxin assay and sigmoidoscopy are indicated in every patient who develops diarrhea after antibiotic use, in conjunction with the clinical features outlined above.

The sigmoidoscopic features of C. difficile-related diarrhea can vary from that of mucosal edema, friability, and erythema to a pseudomembranous colitis. The endoscopic features of a pseudomembranous colitis are the presence of plaque-like, yellowish-white collections that adhere to the mucosa, increased amounts of mucous, intervening mucosa that is edematous and erythematous, and the presence of mucosal ulcerations that result from sloughing of the pseudomembranous plaques (Fig. 10–20).

Two-thirds of patients with a pseudomembranous colitis have sigmoid colon involvement, but one-third of patients have only proximal (right colon) colonic involvement, with a normal sigmoid colon.[13] If the history and clinical features suggest a C. difficile-related colitis and the flexible sigmoidoscopic examination is normal, total colonoscopy is indicated to exclude right colonic pseudomembranous colitis.

Bacterial Diarrheas. Campylobacter jejuni is the primary cause of infectious diarrhea in this country.[14] The animal reservoir of this pathogen includes cattle, fowl, and house pets, and the transmission of a C. jejuni infection most commonly occurs through contaminated milk, eggs, and exposure to an infected house pet. A nonbloody diarrhea is typical of this type of infestation, but bloody diarrhea can result if an enterocolitis develops. The clinical, radiographic, and endoscopic features of C. jejuni enterocolitis mimic those of Crohn's disease (see Figs. 10–8 and 10–12).

Yersinia enterocolitica is a bacterial pathogen that can cause a simple diarrhea or result in an enterocolitis that is often indistinguishable from Crohn's disease. The common animal reservoirs of this organism are cattle and house pets. Most epidemics caused by Y. enterocolitica are associated with infected milk or ice cream. Children commonly present with enterocolitis and adults with simple gastroenteritis.[15] It is important to remember this organism as a cause of ileitis with associated mesenteric adenitis in children. The sigmoidoscopic features of a Yersinia-associated colitis are similar to those of a mild to moderately severe Crohn's disease. Fresh stool analysis should be done in all patients presumed to have inflammatory bowel disease.

Nontyphoidal Salmonella strains can cause gastroenteritis of variable severity. Usually, these strains of Salmonella are associated with mild diarrhea that lasts for 4 to 5 days and is not associated with bloody diarrheal movements. Occasionally, these bacterial infestations can result in colitis with bloody diarrhea and the sigmoidoscopic features of mild ulcerative colitis (see Figs. 10–7 and 10–10). Antibiotic therapy is appropriate in a Salmonella colitis, but it is usually not necessary in patients with mild gastroenteritis.

All strains of Shigella can cause a bacterial dysentery that results in colitis of variable severity. A Shigella-related colitis is associated with nonbloody or bloody diarrhea, fever, abdominal pain, and tenesmus. Because of the associated colonic ulcerations, toxic megacolon and colonic perforation have been reported. A diagnosis is established by a positive stool culture and by the sigmoidoscopic feature of colonic ulcerations of variable depth with piled up margins. Important therapeutic considerations include adequate hydration, the avoidance of antidiarrheal medications, and appropriate antibiotic therapy.

Parasite-Related Diarrheas. In this country, the two most important parasitic causes of diarrheal illness are Giardia lamblia and Entamoeba histolytica. Many other parasitic organisms can cause colitis or diarrhea, but these are usually diagnosed in immune-compromised patients, such as those with AIDS.

Entamoeba histolytica is the only species of ameba that is pathogenic in

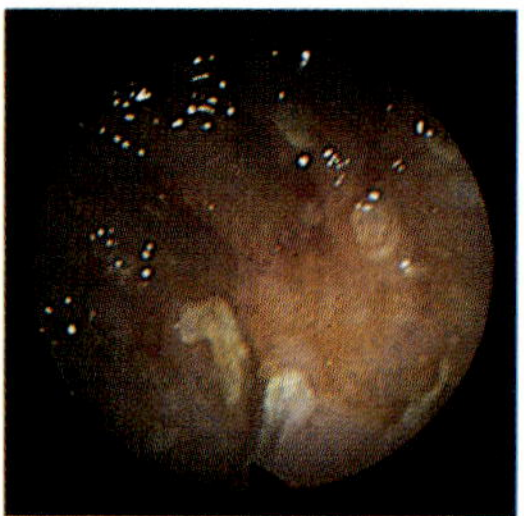

FIG. 10–21. Amebic colitis.

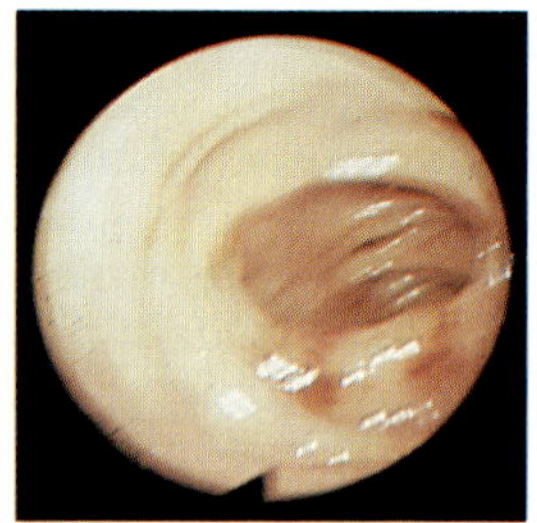

FIG. 10–22. Acute diverticulitis.

humans. It is transmitted by the fecal-oral route and is common in Americans without a travel history. This parasite can result in diarrhea or colitis of varying severity. Bloody mucoid movements, fever, and combined rectal and abdominal pain indicate the presence of colitis. The sigmoidoscopic features of amebic colitis usually (75%) demonstrate oval ulcerations with undermined edges that are seen among normal mucosa, whereas 25% of patients have the mucosal characteristics of moderately severe ulcerative colitis.[16] The colonic ulcerations seen with amebic colitis vary in size, but can approach 1 cm in diameter (Fig. 10–21).

Giardia lamblia is an important cause of diarrhea in Americans, but it does not cause colitis in normal individuals. The infestation results from drinking water that is contaminated with the parasite. It is common in campers who drink untreated water from mountain streams and can be epidemic in communities whose water purification systems fail to remove the cysts of the parasite. Giardia cysts can be killed by boiling the water or by adding 12 ml of a saturated iodine solution to 1 liter of clear, untreated water. Because this parasite does not cause colitis, the sigmoid colon examination in these individuals is normal.

Acute and Chronic Diverticulitis

The sigmoidoscopic features of diverticulosis have been described above (see Normal Findings; Figs. 10–2 and 10–3).

It has been estimated that 10 to 25% of individuals with diverticular disease develop clinically apparent diverticulitis. The exact cause of the acute inflammation is uncertain, but it does not appear to be related to a high-fiber diet.

If a patient with known diverticulosis develops clinical features compatible with a diagnosis of acute diverticulitis, it is not necessary to perform sigmoidoscopy during the acute stage. In fact, the performance of flexible sigmoidoscopy in patients with peritoneal signs is contraindicated in this clinical situation because this could exacerbate pericolonic inflammation.

Sigmoidoscopic examination of a resolving acute diverticulitis reveals mucosal edema around the diverticular orifices, with frequent obliteration of the diverticular orifice (Fig. 10–22). Pus drainage from a diverticulum in a patient with resolving acute diverticulitis is uncommon.

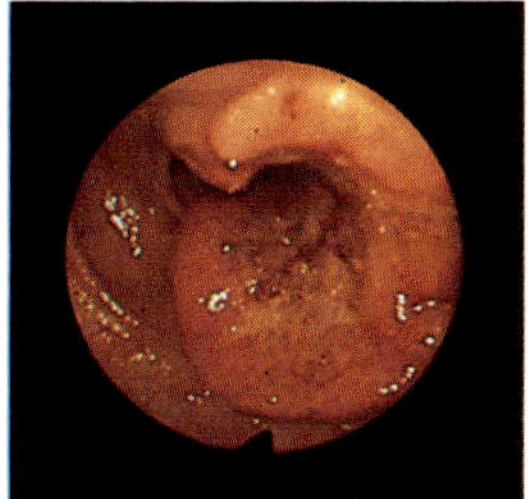

FIG. 10–23. Colonic adenocarcinoma.

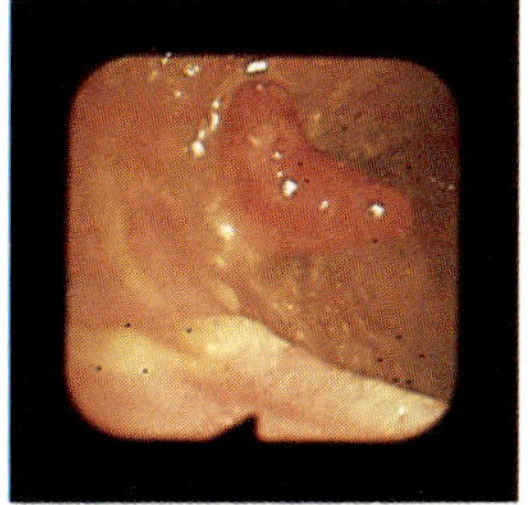

FIG. 10–24. Ulcerating tubular adenocarcinoma.

A flexible sigmoidoscopic examination after the resolution of the acute symptoms is indicated to exclude a neoplastic lesion as the cause of the acute diverticulitis. This inspection also excludes any complication of acute diverticulitis, such as a fistula or a pericolonic abscess.

The most common feature of chronic diverticulitis is the presence of a colonic stricture after an episode of acute diverticulitis. This stricture results from the pericolonic fibrosis associated with a severe episode of acute diverticulitis. Constipation is the most common symptom of colonic stricture following acute diverticulitis. A colonic stricture resulting from chronic diverticulitis has the same endoscopic and radiographic features as one resulting from an ischemic colonic episode. Because ischemic colonic strictures most often occur in the flexures of the colon, they might also occur in the sigmoid colon of patients with known diverticulosis. The clinical history allows an episode of acute diverticulitis to be differentiated from an acute ischemic colonic event.

Colon Cancer

The colonic adenoma-carcinoma sequence and the guidelines for screening flexible sigmoidoscopy in normal patients and individuals with an increased risk for the development of colon cancer have been discussed in Chapter 9.

The endoscopic spectrum of colonic cancer can vary from an obstructing friable lesion to an irregular or ulcerative adenomatous polyp. The presence of an ulceration or an adenoma is highly suggestive of malignancy, and a biopsy is mandatory (Figs. 10–23 and 10–24).

REFERENCES

1. Katon RM, Keefe EB, and Melnyk CS: Flexible Sigmoidoscopy. Orlando, FL, Grune & Stratton, 1985.
2. Schrock TR: Examination of the anorectum, rigid sigmoidoscopy, flexible sigmoidoscopy, and diseases of the anorectum. In Gastrointestinal Disease: Pathophysiology, Diagnosis, Management, 4th Ed. Edited by MH Sleisenger and JS Fordtran. Philadelphia, WB Saunders, 1989, pp 1570–1591.

3. Guidelines for the cancer-related checkup. Recommendations and rationale. CA, 30:208, 1980.
4. Luk GD: Colorectal cancer. Gastroenterol Clin North Am, 17:655–945, 1988.
5. Butt JH, Price A, Williams CH: Dysplasia and cancer in ulcerative colitis. *In* Inflammatory Bowel Disease. Edited by RN Allan and R Norman. Edinburgh, Churchill Livingstone, 1983, pp 140–154.
6. Earnest DL, Schneiderman DJ: Other diseases of the colon and rectum. *In* Gastrointestinal Disease. Edited by MH Sleisenger and JS Fordtran. Philadelphia, WB Saunders, 1989, pp 1592–1631.
7. Donaldson RM: Crohn's disease. *In* Gastrointestinal Disease. Edited by MH Sleisenger and JS Fordtran. Philadelphia, WB Saunders, 1989, pp 1327–1358.
8. Meyer CT, Troncale FJ, Galloway S, et al: Arteriovenous malformations of the bowel: An analysis of 22 cases and review of the literature. Medicine, 60:36, 1981.
9. Zuckerman GR, Cornette GL, Clouse RE, et al: Upper gastrointestinal bleeding in patients with chronic renal failure. Ann Intern Med, 102:588, 1985.
10. Waye JD: Hyperplastic colon polyps—are they markers? Ann Intern Med, 109:852, 1988.
11. Achkar E, Carey W: Small polyps found during fiberoptic sigmoidoscopy in asymptomatic patients. Ann Intern Med, 109:880, 1988.
12. Morson, BC: The pathogenesis of colorectal cancer. Introduction. Major Probl Pathol 1978; 10:1–13.
13. Tedesco FJ, Corless JK, Brownstein RE: Rectal sparing in antibiotic-associated colitis: A prospective study. Gastroenterology, 83:1259, 1982.
14. Blaser MJ, Reller B: Campylobacter enteritis. N Engl J Med, 305:1444, 1981.
15. Butlzer JP (ed): Campylobacter Infections in Man and Animals. Boca Raton, FL, CRC Press, 1984.
16. Owen RL: Parasitic diseases. *In* Gastrointestinal Disease. Edited by MH Sleisenger and JS Fordtran: Philadelphia, WB Saunders, 1989, pp 1153–1191.

chapter

11

THE DIAGNOSIS AND MANAGEMENT OF CHRONIC PANCREATITIS

Joseph T. Danzi

The clinical presentation of chronic pancreatitis varies according to the stage of the disease and the amount of destruction of the exocrine and endocrine components of the gland. The early stages of the disease are characterized by recurrent episodes of abdominal pain and inflammatory changes within the pancreas. The early stage of chronic pancreatitis can persist for variable periods and can last up to a decade. In this stage of chronic pancreatitis, no evidence of exocrine or endocrine deficiency is seen.

As the disease progresses, the clinical component becomes characterized by a pain-free period, whereas the histologic changes within the gland show progressive fibrosis and then atrophy of the acinar, ductal, and islet cells of the pancreas. Because of the large functional reserve of the gland, it requires 90 to 95% destruction of the secretory function before the clinical symptoms related to steatorrhea appear.[1] The onset of glucose intolerance usually precedes the development of insulin-dependent diabetes mellitus.

The impressive aspect of chronic pancreatitis is the variability of its clinical presentation. Some patients never experience abdominal pain, yet develop classic signs of pancreatic insufficiency. Importantly, the cause of the patient's chronic pancreatitis does not seem to influence the clinical presentation. It is known that about 50% of patients with alcohol-induced chronic pancreatitis have a painful early phase of their disease, whereas 50% are asymptomatic and present only with clinical evidence of pancreatic endocrine and exocrine insufficiency.[2]

Despite the need for pathologists to classify the varying stages of this disease, little clinical correlation is found with the histologic changes noted within the gland.[3] This is important when considering the diagnosis of chronic pancreatitis by imaging modalities. The poor correlation with histologic features explains the variability of onset of the glucose intolerance and exocrine insufficiency in this disease. The classic description is the diagnosis of diabetes before steatorrhea, but it is found to vary in clinical practice.

Chronic pancreatitis has various causes, but in this country the most common are chronic alcohol ingestion, cystic fibrosis, and "idiopathic" factors.[4] Unfortunately, the most common cause of chronic pancreatitis in both sexes in this country today is alcohol abuse. About 50% of all those suffering with chronic alcoholism have either functional or pathologic changes of chronic pancreatitis.[1]

The exact pathogenesis of alcohol-related chronic pancreatitis is unknown, but it is presumed to be related to changes in the pancreatic ductal and acinar cell secretions, which are more proteinic.[5] This protein precipitates in the ducts, calcifies, and results in duct obstruction, atrophy of the acinar cells, and fibrosis. The time required for the development of a functional chronic pancreatitis is 10 years of chronic alcohol abuse.

The second most common cause of chronic pancreatitis in the United States involves idiopathic factors. It is assumed that most of these cases are related to viral infection. This diagnosis is frequently established in younger patients than those with the cause related to chronic alcohol abuse. Importantly, this group of patients with chronic pancreatitis has a good response of their abdominal pain to pancreatic replacement therapy.[6]

The true incidence and significance of the chronic pancreatitis associated with cystic fibrosis are now being recognized, because these individuals are living longer. It is estimated that 80 to 90% of patients with cystic fibrosis have functional evidence of chronic pancreatitis.[5] The cause of the chronic pancreatitis is related to the altered mucus, which inspissates the ductal secretions and results in secondary changes.

A group of metabolic diseases are associated with chronic pancreatitis, including hemochromatosis, hyperparathyroidism, and hyperlipidemia. Currently, the diagnosis of hemochromatosis can be made more readily and it is a recognized cause of chronic pancreatic insufficiency. The association of chronic pancreatitis with hyperlipidemia and hyperparathyroidism is less certain. Some studies have demonstrated an incidence of association no greater than that expected in the general population, whereas other studies have indicated a causal relationship.[4] When evaluating a patient with a cryptic cause of chronic pancreatitis, it is important to exclude these two possible causes.

DIAGNOSIS

The clinical dilemma with chronic pancreatitis is the usual inability to diagnosis the condition early, before the late manifestations of chronic pancreatic exocrine insufficiency are seen. The early diagnosis of chronic pancreatitis requires the performance of a test painful to the patient, time-consuming to the clinician, and difficult to assess by the pathologist. Despite all its drawbacks, the secretin test is the standard of all diagnostic tests for chronic pancreatitis.[7] Usually, patients with an abnormal secretin test result have a decreased bicarbonate level with a normal volume of their duodenal aspirate. Importantly, the abnormal secretin test result can be noted years before an abnormal endoscopic retrograde cholangiopancreatography (ERCP) is found to diagnose the chronic pancreatitis. Therefore, a functional test is more sensitive and specific for the early diagnosis of chronic pancreatitis.

Major research efforts have involved the development of a tubeless, secretin-like test with the same early diagnostic sensitivity that would be more widely clinically applicable. The Chymex test is clinically available in the United States. The basis of this tubeless pancreatic function test is the ability of the pancreatic enzyme chymotrypsin to cleave bentiromide, a synthetic protein, from para-aminobenzoic acid (PABA). The PABA is then metabolized and excreted in the urine. Urinalysis of the by-products accounts for the diagnostic capabilities of this test. The advantages of this test is that it is well tolerated, inexpensive, and cost-effective. Its major disadvantage is its lack of sensitivity. It is positive only with clinical evidence of pancreatic insufficiency and negative in patients with early chronic pancreatitis. Therefore, it has not replaced the secretin test in its diagnostic sensitivity.

Another indirect tubeless test measures the ability of the pancreatic enzyme elastase to release a fluorescein component from an ingested compound. This test is still experimental but appears to be less sensitive than the bentiromide test; it is positive only in patients with documented pancreatic insufficiency.

The second most sensitive indicator of chronic pancreatitis is not a diagnostic test but a radiologic finding—namely, the presence of diffuse pancreatic calcifications.[1] Their presence suggests that more than 75% of the gland has been damaged, usually by chronic alcohol ingestion.[2] This feature, however, is only found in about 25% of all patients with chronic pancreatitis.[1] Therefore, it is a specific but not a sensitive finding. The presence of local calcification within the pancreas can be attributed to trauma, hypercalcemic states, and islet cell tumors.

The diagnosis of chronic pancreatitis by the demonstration of abnormal ductal morphology using ERCP has a sensitivity of diagnosis lower than that of the secretin test but greater than that of pancreatic calcification. The changes of chronic pancreatitis seen on the pancreatogram are helpful for patients with unexplained chronic abdominal pain secondary to chronic pancreatitis, and for the differential diagnosis of pancreatic cancer. Currently, this combined endoscopic-radiographic test is probably the most widely used clinical diagnostic test for pancreatic disease.

The diagnosis of steatorrhea attributable to chronic pancreatitis can be established by a quantitative fecal fat analysis. The test is not specific for pancreatic disease and is abnormal with any cause of maldigestion of fats. In addition, the sensitivity of this test is low, because it is positive only when more than 90% of the pancreas is destroyed.

It is a relatively unknown clinical fact that about 40% of patients with

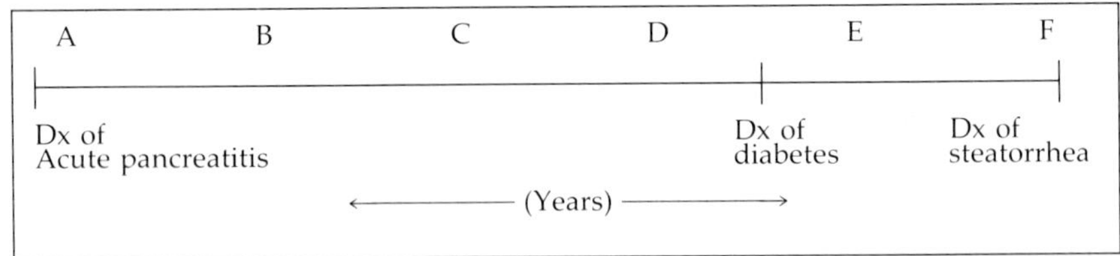

FIG. 11–1. Diagnostic tests and their value in the diagnosis of chronic pancreatitis (A, abnormal secretin test; B, pancreatic calcifications by ultrasound; C, abnormal pancreatogram by ERCP; D, pancreatic calcifications by flat plate of abdomen; E, abnormal bentiromide test; F, abnormal serum trypsin-like activity).

chronic pancreatitis have malabsorption of vitamin B_{12}. The malabsorption of cobalamin results because it is bound to R protein and is not transferred to intrinsic factor until the R protein has been degraded by pancreatic proteases. This transfer does not occur in patients with chronic pancreatitis and decreased protease activity.

Two other diagnostic tests have been developed, the serum trypsin-like immunoreactivity and serum pancreatic polypeptide tests. Serum trypsin-like activity is decreased in patients with chronic pancreatitis and steatorrhea, but normal in patients with chronic pancreatitis and no evidence of steatorrhea.[8] The fasting serum pancreatic polypeptide level is decreased in patients with chronic pancreatitis with steatorrhea, but levels of this hormone after stimulation with cholecystokinin decrease in individuals with early chronic pancreatitis. It is hoped that this latter serologic test has the necessary sensitivity and specificity to replace the secretin test.

Thus, our present diagnostic capabilities for chronic pancreatitis allow for the establishment of a diagnosis of late, severe chronic pancreatitis more easily and readily than early chronic pancreatitis. A summary of the diagnostic tests and their value in the diagnosis of chronic pancreatitis is presented in Figure 11–1.

Other considerations should be addressed. What would be the most efficient and cost-effective approach to a patient with diarrhea, weight loss, and steatorrhea? How do you distinguish a small bowel from a pancreatic origin in regard to the cause of these symptoms? If a bentiromide test is ordered first, and followed by a D-xylose absorption test, the combination allows for the easy differentiation of malabsorption from maldigestion, based on the positivity or negativity of the test results. A positive Chymex test result with a normal D-xylose test indicates a diagnosis of chronic pancreatitis.

Another diagnostic dilemma relates to distinguishing chronic pancreatitis from pancreatic cancer. Most patients have an abdominal ultrasound or CT scan. The performance of an ERCP would be the next diagnostic step. The combination of these two diagnostic modalities should allow for differential diagnosis in over 90% of cases. The addition of a percutaneous aspiration cytologic biopsy increases the distinction further.

A final consideration in the establishment of a diagnosis of chronic

TABLE 11–1. COST OF DIAGNOSTIC MODALITIES FOR CHRONIC PANCREATITIS

Procedure	Cost ($)
Secretin test	>500
Abdominal ultrasound	250
ERCP	820
Flat plate of abdomen	80
Bentiromide test (Chymex)	60

pancreatitis or pancreatic cancer is the cost-effectiveness of the diagnostic test. Table 11–1 lists the average cost of various tests and their reported diagnostic accuracy.

MANAGEMENT

An important area in clinical practice is the management of the three main complications of chronic pancreatitis—insulin-dependent diabetes, cyst formation, and steatorrhea. It is estimated that more than one-third of patients with severe, long-standing chronic pancreatitis have symptomatic diabetes mellitus.[1] The resultant diabetes is not only associated with a relative insufficiency of insulin availability, but also with low glucagon reserves. This combination explains the prolonged and troublesome hypoglycemic episodes and brittleness seen with this type of diabetes. Another observation is the decreased incidence of ketoacidosis and vasculopathy associated with pancreas-related diabetes. Finally, a higher incidence of hyperosmolar-nonketotic coma is found with this type of diabetes than with diabetes not associated with pancreatic disease.

The association of pancreatic pseudocyst with chronic pancreatitis is usually noted early in the disease process. The presence of a pseudocyst is the most common cause of persistent abdominal pain seen in association with an abdominal mass in patients with chronic pancreatitis.[3] The diagnosis of this complication is usually through the use of a radiologic scanning procedure, followed by an ERCP. The pancreatogram is important for documenting the presence or absence of a communication between the main pancreatic duct and the pseudocyst. The presence of such a communication could require pancreatic surgery if medical therapy fails to resolve the pseudocyst.

Steatorrhea develops in about one-third of all patients with chronic pancreatitis.[2] The steatorrhea associated with pancreatic disease is usually greater than that associated with biliary or small intestinal disease. The intensity of the steatorrhea may be so great that only frank oil is passed with the movement. The presence of steatorrhea is generally associated with diarrhea, but about 25% of patients with steatorrhea present with constipation.

The clinician must be aware of the possibility of fat-soluble vitamin deficiencies, as manifested clinically or subclinically. This requires the evaluation of serum calcium and zinc levels, night vision checks, and alertness to the possible existence of osteomalacia.

Steatorrhea is usually easily corrected with pancreatic enzyme replacements and with supplemental bicarbonate to assist in the digestive process. If this regimen does not cure the steatorrhea, the addition of an H_2 antagonist might be necessary to reduce the gastric acid that is inactivating the enzymes.[9,10] Enzymes are required in sufficient dosage to resolve the steatorrhea. The addition of a fat-soluble vitamin replacement is helpful to correct or prevent the manifestation of these insufficiencies. Rarely is the use of antidiarrheal medications necessary to control the symptoms of diarrhea.

The management of the pain aspect of chronic pancreatitis is one of the most important and frustrating aspects in the therapy of patients with chronic pancreatitis.[11] This is especially true when treating an individual with chronic pancreatitis secondary to alcohol abuse who continues to drink. These individuals should be encouraged to use the services of Alcoholics Anonymous or other detoxification and support groups. If this trend continues after considerable time has been spent with the patient discussing the risks involved, a difficult decision must be made about continuing the patient-doctor relationship.

The approach to controlling the abdominal pain of patients with chronic pancreatitis requires the following: (1) documentation of abstinence from alcohol (blood alcohol levels); (2) use of a radiologic scanning modality to exclude complications, such as a pancreatic pseudocyst; (3) performing an ERCP to document the morphology of the pancreatic ductal system and to define the presence or absence of pancreaticoliths; and (4) determination of the patient's possible dependency on analgesic medication.

For those individuals without evidence of pancreatic duct obstruction, pseudocyst, or pancreaticoliths, high-dose pancreatic enzyme replacement is recommended. Usually this dose level is double to triple the average therapeutic dose. The basis of this treatment is the inhibition of the feedback pancreatic secretory mechanism, which should result in decreased stimulation of the gland and decreased abdominal pain.[12] In my limited experience with high-dose therapy, it has been successful but not well tolerated by the patients because of their need to take 30 to 60 tablets daily, at a prohibitive cost.

If high-dose enzyme therapy fails, careful use of analgesic medication is the next treatment step. This should be used judiciously in an attempt to reduce the incidence of dependency but keep the patient functioning actively in society.[1] The effect of the analgesic on the sphincter of Oddi function should be known so that the cure does not exacerbate the symptoms.

A difficult clinical decision involves choosing the best approach for those patients that have failed medical therapy, have stopped their alcohol abuse for some time, and have abnormalities of their pancreatic duct, as demonstrated by ERCP. Formerly, our surgical colleagues would have suggested a decompressive type of surgery, such as a caudal or distal pancreaticojejunostomy. These operations are effective in about 50 to 60% of patients in the control of their abdominal pain.[13,14] The applicability of shock wave lithotripsy therapy for the destruction of pancreaticoliths in the main pancreatic duct has been evaluated. This form of therapy appears to "free" the duct of stones, but the clinical usefulness of this form of therapy in controlling pain symptoms remains to be thoroughly evaluated.

The early recognition of chronic pancreatitis, abstinence from alcohol consumption, and control of pain with advancing disease has resulted in a decreased incidence of morbidity and mortality. The Mayo Clinic experience has demonstrated a 10-year mortality rate of 25%, with only 20% of patients dying of complications directly related to their disease.[13]

REFERENCES

1. Bank S: Chronic pancreatitis: Clinical features and medical management. Am J Gastroenterol, 81:153, 1986.
2. Toskes PP: Diagnosis of chronic pancreatitis and exocrine insufficiency. Hosp Pract, 20:97, 1988.
3. Niedran C, Grendell JH: Diagnosis of chronic pancreatitis. Gastroenterology, 88:1973, 1985.
4. Toskes PP, Greenberger NJ: Acute and chronic pancreatitis. DM, 29:1, 1983.
5. Greenberger NJ: Etiology and pathogenesis of chronic pancreatitis. Hosp Pract, 20:83, 1985.
6. Slaff JL: Management of pain in chronic pancreatitis. Hosp. Pract, 20:53, 1985.
7. Lankisch PG: Exocrine pancreatic function tests. Gut, 23:777, 1982.
8. Jacobson DG, Curington C, Connery K, et al: Trypsin-like immunoreactivity as a test for pancreatic insufficiency. N Engl J Med, 310:1307, 1985.
9. DiMagno EP: Controversies in the treatment of exocrine pancreatic insufficiency. Dig Dis Sci, 27:481, 1982.
10. Graham DV: Pancreatic enzyme replacement. The effect of antacids or cimetidine. Dig Dis Sci, 27:485, 1982.
11. Warshaw AL: Pain in chronic pancreatitis. Gastroenterology, 86:987, 1984.
12. Slaff J, Jacobson D, Tillman CR, et al: Protease-specific suppression of pancreatic exocrine secretion. Gastroenterology, 87:44, 1984.
13. Ammann RW, Akovbiantz A, Largiader F, et al: Cause and outcome of chronic pancreatitis—longitudinal study of a mixed medical-surgical series of 245 patients. Gastroenterology, 86:820, 1984.
14. Scuro LA, Vantini I, Piubello W, et al: Evolution of pain in chronic relapsing pancreatitis: A study of operated and nonoperated patients. Am J Gastroenterol, 78:495, 1983.

chapter

12

THE MANAGEMENT OF THE IRRITABLE BOWEL SYNDROME

Kevin V. Carey, M.D.

The irritable bowel syndrome (IBS) is a disorder defined by its symptoms. The constellation of symptoms is characteristic: abdominal pain and a disorder of defecation in the absence of a structural or chemical cause. The features of the clinical history that best differentiate IBS from organic disease are the following: (1) distention; (2) relief of pain by defecation; (3) looser stools with the onset of pain; (4) more frequent stools with the onset of pain; (5) more than three bowel movements daily; and (6) mucus in the stool.[1,2] Various other symptoms are associated with IBS, although these are less characteristic. They include dyspepsia, gas, bloating, nausea, vomiting, headache, flushing, fatigue, sighing respirations, hyperventilation, dysmenorrhea, headache, and dysuria.

An important part of the definition is that structural or chemical causes of the symptoms have been excluded. That is, alternative diagnoses have been ruled out. Unfortunately, this may create the impression that the diagnosis of IBS is a "wastebasket" diagnosis (one looks for the "real disease" and labels the rest as IBS). Actually, by careful history and physical examination, the experienced clinician ought to be able to make a diagnosis of IBS with a high degree of certainty.

The importance of IBS lies particularly in its great frequency. Between 40 and 70% of patients seen in a gastroenterologist's office suffer with IBS. In a general practice, most patients with gastrointestinal complaints have IBS. The advantage of an efficient and effective approach to the problem is plain.

PATHOGENESIS

IBS is a motility disturbance of the gastrointestinal tract. A number of studies have demonstrated muscular and myoelectric abnormalities:

1. Muscular contractions over long segments of colon and small intestine correlate with pain.[3–5]
2. Increased resting colonic motility is noted in spastic colon patients and decreased motility in those with the painless diarrhea variant.[6]
3. An increased colonic muscular response is found to parasympathetic drugs,[7] an abnormality also found in those with diverticular disease.[8]
4. An increased response is also provoked by cholecystokinin and meals.[9,10]
5. In the colon, the ratio of 3 cycle/min basic electrical rhythm to 6 cycle/min activity is greater in IBS patients than in normal controls.[11]
6. Changes in colonic motility occur in response to stress.
7. An alteration in the perception of colonic distention occurs.[12] IBS patients have an increased sensitivity to balloon distention in the rectosigmoid, which appears to be the result of an associated colonic spasm. Rather than being generally supersensitive to pain, however, they have an increased tolerance of other noxious stimuli.[13]
8. The technique of 24-hour ambulatory monitoring of colonic motility has shown that high-amplitude peristaltic contractions, which begin in the right colon and traverse the whole colon, occur after meals and are associated with bowel movements. These contractions are infrequent during sleep. Patients with constipation and IBS have a marked diminution of these high-amplitude contractions.[14]

Fortunately, measurement of these phenomena is not necessary to establish a diagnosis of IBS, but these observations suggest that IBS is a real physiologic entity, rather than somatization of a psychologic disturbance.

PSYCHOSOCIAL FACTORS

The frequent association of stress with symptoms and the exacerbation of symptoms by stress has led to extensive evaluation of the relationship of IBS to psychologic abnormalities. A study done in North Carolina[15] has examined the difference between IBS patients who sought medical care, IBS sufferers who had IBS symptoms but did not seek medical attention, and normals who did not have IBS symptoms. The patients scored higher on several scales of a standardized psychologic inventory test (the MMPI). They scored higher on scales of hypochondriasis, depression, hysteria, psychasthenia, and lower ego strength, but no typical or characteristic psychological profile was established. In the same study, responses to a "Life Experience Survey" were studied. IBS patients reported lower scores and fewer events for positive experiences and, interestingly, lower scores and fewer events for negative experiences as well. They tended to minimize the import and frequency of both positive and negative experiences. Finally, on an "Illness Behavior Questionnaire," the patients reported greater illness disruption than sufferers and normals, and greater health worries and affective disturbance than normals.

These and the results of similar studies suggest that more psychologic disturbance may occur in patients who come to the office for their IBS symptoms than in patients with other disorders. Psychologic problems, however, do not seem to be the cause of the symptoms. Rather, the psychologic make-up of the individual may affect the perception of symptoms and the likelihood of seeking medical care. Nonetheless, many IBS patients report that emotional upset provokes symptoms and increased sensitivity to dietary indiscretion.

DIAGNOSIS

In the United States and other developed Western countries, the female-to-male ratio in IBS patients who see physicians is approximately 3:1. This appears to be a result of a cultural difference between men and women in their health care-seeking behavior. It is noteworthy that IBS symptoms worsen with menses. In one study,[16] 34% of normal women reported increased flatus, diarrhea, or constipation with menses, whereas nearly twice as many women with IBS reported worsened symptoms with their menstrual period.

Most patients have symptoms before the age of 40 years. It is unusual for a patient to experience the onset of symptoms at an older age. The older the age at onset, the more an alternative diagnosis should be suspected.

The typical history is of a lower abdominal or vaguely localized abdominal pain that is provoked by meals. As already noted, it is related to looser or more frequent bowel movements. It is often relieved by the bowel movements. The bowel movements are generally small in volume. Only mucus or gas may be passed. The evacuation often feels incomplete. Many patients report a pattern of an initial hard, scybalous stool in the morning followed by small, urgent, increasingly loose movements.

The pain should not occur at night. Nocturnal episodes should be rare, and ought not to be the cause of waking.

A history of bleeding is cause for consideration of another diagnosis. Bright red blood on the toilet tissue or other evidence of anal bleeding, however, is not unusual. Fever and weight loss are also not associated with the syndrome, and require a more intense search for a cause.

The physical examination (including a pelvic examination in females) of a patient with IBS should be generally normal. Often, a patient appears tense and shows autonomic symptoms, such as sweaty palms, tachycardia, and blushing. Occasionally, there is tenderness on palpation in the left lower quadrant and suprapubic area.

A sigmoidoscopy examination is essential in the work-up of all patients with symptoms compatible with those of IBS. The patient with colitis has identical symptoms. The patient with proctitis can only be identified by sigmoidoscopy. The patient with proctitis is as likely to have constipation as diarrhea, and may even have alternating diarrhea and constipation. The bleeding appears to be anal in origin and the purulent fecal discharge is indistinguishable grossly from the mucus characteristic of IBS.

Sigmoidoscopy should be done without enema preparation. Erythema and edema are the most subtle changes of proctitis, and these changes can be provoked by an enema. Also, if no enema is given, stool samples may be obtained to test for occult blood, stain for polymorphonuclear cells, and culture and examine for ova and parasites. Reproduction of the pain by air insufflation during the procedure supports a diagnosis of IBS.

A biopsy may be taken at the time of this examination, and is particularly useful when prominent diarrhea occurs. The biopsy may show unsuspected microscopic colitis or collagenous colitis.

Laboratory tests recommended for all patients with compatible symptoms include a complete blood cell count, erythrocyte sedimentation rate, chemistry profile, and urinalysis. These relatively inexpensive and nontraumatic tests provide much information. The hemoglobin and hematocrit should help exclude significant blood loss, as well as screen for iron, folate, or vitamin B_{12} deficiency. The normal white blood cell count helps exclude inflammatory lesions, and the sedimentation rate also checks for inflammation. The chemistry profile helps exclude malabsorptive states if the calcium, phosphorus, and cholesterol levels are normal. The blood glucose level and urinalysis help exclude diabetes. Urinalysis also helps exclude urinary causes of lower abdominal pain.

Much has been made of lactose intolerance as a cause of IBS symptoms. Because lactose intolerance is common, it is easy to overemphasize this association. Patients with IBS are sensitive to bowel distention, so they should avoid all sorts of gas-forming foods. The intake of fruits and vegetables that contain nonabsorbable sugars should be limited. Also, dietetic foods and medications that contain sorbitol and other nonabsorbable sugars should be avoided. Whether a lactose tolerance test should be performed depends on the physician's judgment.

One principle of IBS therapy is that the therapist should be satisfied at the outset that an adequate work-up has been done. Later or repeated testing tends to undermine the credibility of the original diagnosis. Such doubts on the patient's part may increase anxiety and symptoms. Therefore, in considering further testing, one should try to do all necessary tests to be certain of the diagnosis. No further tests than those outlined above are necessary when the symptoms are typical.

If the patient is over 40 at the time of onset of symptoms, a barium enema examination is recommended. If upper intestinal symptoms are prominent, upper gastrointestinal roentgenography is considered with the small intestinal examination. This is especially important if right lower quadrant pain, weight loss or evidence of chronic inflammation suggests Crohn's disease. Upper abdominal pain may also suggest gallstones or pancreatic disease, so measurement of the serum lipase level and ultrasound or CT scan may be warranted.

Prominent pain may be of neuropathic origin, suggesting diabetic neuropathy, syphilis, lead intoxication, or porphyria. Acute intermittent porphyria is particularly suggested by evidence of autonomic dysfunction (e.g., hypertension, orthostatic hypotension, cardiac rhythm disturbance). Psychiatric disturbance is also seen in this disease.

If diarrhea is more voluminous or severe than expected, an extensive work-up for diarrhea may be desired. In addition to the tests listed above, others may be needed. For example, thyroid hormone measurements, thyroid scan for medullary carcinoma of the thyroid, gastrin levels, and cortisol levels help exclude endocrine causes of diarrhea. The urinary 5-HIAA level measurement helps diagnose carcinoid tumor, which can also be evaluated by ultrasound or CT scan of the liver. Laxative abuse is determined by careful questioning of the family and patient, as well as by alkalinization of the stool and other stool analyses. Stool collections for volume and fat determinations may also be helpful.

After considering such a long list of possibilities, it should be noted that this extensive work-up is seldom warranted.

TREATMENT

IBS is, at present, not "curable." It is a chronic disorder that, hopefully, may be controlled.

PATIENT EDUCATION

The mainstay of therapy is patient education. Patients tend to judge their physicians by results, just as one judges a plumber or car repairman. If a leaky faucet still leaks after the plumber's visit, the plumber is incompetent. No physician can stand up to the test, however, if the job is to make the IBS symptoms disappear. Patients need to know that a cure is not to be expected, and that they will continue to suffer symptoms. It is hoped that their frequency and severity are reduced. They also need to learn that improvement requires their active involvement in therapy. The patient who expects to take a pill for 1 or 2 weeks and be cured will certainly be disappointed. One goal of therapy should be to prevent the continuing search for a "good" physician to cure the symptoms.

Given that the patient is not to have the physician's competence proven by the immediate result, it is easy to appreciate how much the patient relies on the physician's demeanor in conducting the diagnostic testing and on the ability to communicate. A hurried and disorganized approach does not elicit the confidence necessary for successful treatment.

The patient needs to know that the physician believes that the symptoms are real. Patients who are told that their symptoms are just "nerves" may try to believe it for a while, but the next attack convinces them otherwise. A diarrheal stool is good evidence that the symptoms are not imagined. It is helpful to make an analogy with cramps in other muscles. The explanation that a charleyhorse of the gut is present clarifies the idea that a muscle cramp of the intestine can produce pain and disruption of function. Also, it makes the point that the pain is not imagined, but does not indicate serious underlying pathology.

The patient who is to be reassured must know that the physician has fully heard his or her complaints. It is important not to reassure the patient prematurely. Only when the testing is complete should the patient be told the diagnosis and its prognosis. Of course, the prognosis is excellent. IBS is not associated with a shortened life expectancy. That is the good news, with the bad news being that it cannot be cured.

Often, literature about IBS is helpful. Booklets, available through pharmaceutical firms, or one of many books available on the subject can confirm the points that the physician has made. Although these materials are not suitable for every patient, they can significantly improve communication and win patient support.

Modification of lifestyle may also be suggested at this time. Regular eating habits and adequate sleep may help control symptoms. If symptoms are significantly related to stress, various stress reduction techniques can be recommended. Relaxation techniques, hypnosis, and meditation are useful, if available. A program of regular exercise or walking can also be beneficial.

Avoidance of stimulating foods or beverages (e.g., coffee) should be suggested. Also, if certain foods are particularly troublesome, especially fatty foods and the gas-forming foods mentioned above, these should be restricted. Often, these foods can be taken at times of reduced symptoms or stress, but must be avoided when IBS is more active.

IBS has a wide spectrum of severity. More than 15% of the normal population has reported symptoms of IBS and does not seek medical attention.[15,17] At the other end of the spectrum lies the extremely demanding, hypochondriac patient who has focused on the gastrointestinal symptoms and demands relief. Frequently, more than education, reassurance, support, dietary adjustments, and lifestyle changes are required.

SPECIFIC THERAPY

A number of agents have been proposed as therapy for IBS. This suggests that none has been particularly effective in treating the condition. In fact, Klein has published a review and analysis of controlled trials of therapy for IBS.[18] Trials of antispasmodics, anticholinergic-barbiturate combinations, antidepressants, bulking agents, carminatives, dopamine antagonists, opioids, tranquilizers, and a miscellaneous category were reviewed. The author states that, "In my opinion not a single study has been published that provides compelling evidence that any therapeutic agent is efficacious in the global treatment of IBS. This is not to say that no effective therapies exist; only that none have been documented."[18] Problems with the studies included difficulties with the definition of IBS, measuring efficacy, trial design, generalizing studies done on well-defined subgroups to the general population, and statistical considerations. It was not believed that the problems were insurmountable.[18] Hopefully, effective therapy can be found and validated.

It is worthwhile to attempt to find effective symptomatic therapy.

Because the symptoms are the disease and do not indicate progressive underlying pathology, control of symptoms represents effective therapy. At the same time, tremendous expense or significant side effects represent too high a price to pay for drugs of unproven benefit.

Fiber Supplements. Increasing dietary fiber and taking fiber supplements have long been the foundation of treatment for IBS. Five of six studies reviewed by Klein and a more recent study[19] have failed to demonstrate an effect on the global syndrome. In all studies, the placebo treatment yielded remarkably good results. About 70% of placebo-treated patients reported relief of symptoms. This prominent placebo benefit is seen in most IBS treatment programs, but makes it more difficult to demonstrate the efficacy of therapy. It also emphasizes the value of paying attention to patients and their symptoms to help alleviate those symptoms. The attention and heightened interest of a formal study appear to yield remarkable benefits.

Despite a lack of scientific confirmation of its global benefit for IBS, fiber usually provides relief to the constipated patient and, paradoxically, often even reduces diarrhea. Initially, fiber may increase the symptoms of bloating and distention. It might be helpful to start at a low dosage and increase as tolerated, or to start with a high dose and reduce to a tolerable dose. Symptoms often resolve when the fiber is continued for 2 or 3 weeks.

Patients with hard, scybalous stools can be helped if the fiber is taken with meals. This allows better mixing of the water-absorptive bulk with the food. Patients who are overweight may want to take the fiber before meals to reduce their appetite. Underweight individuals may want to take the supplement after meals. In addition, psyllium taken before meals can help reduce LDL cholesterol levels.[20]

Anticholinergics. Anticholinergics are frequently used to prevent or control the spasm thought to be at the root of IBS pain. Dicyclomine or propantheline bromide are frequently given 30 to 45 minutes before meals when symptoms occur postprandially. The long delay before effective blood levels are attained can be avoided by the use of hyoscyamine which, when taken sublingually, produces effective blood levels in minutes. Thus, unpredictable attacks may be treated. Propantheline bromide is preferred over dicyclomine in patients with diarrhea. The greater antisecretory effects of the propantheline may help reduce the diarrhea.

Anticholinergics are contraindicated in patients with glaucoma and obstructive uropathy. They may worsen constipation, and side effects are frequent. These include dry mouth, blurred vision, nausea, dizziness, lightheadedness, drowsiness, nervousness, and weakness.

Tranquilizers. Many trials have shown that IBS patients feel "better" on tranquilizers, but this does not address whether their symptoms have actually been reduced. The issue of whether tranquilizers are indicated depends on whether abnormal anxiety deserves treatment in its own right, independent of intestinal symptoms. These drugs clearly have addictive potential, and long-term use is to be avoided, if possible. Without convincing proof of efficacy for the relief of IBS, tranquilizers should not be used for IBS alone.

Combination drugs containing tranquilizers are even more difficult to use. Now the patient is instructed not to take the drug for anxiety, but to take it for IBS symptoms. Often, the doses prescribed for these agents are subtherapeutic. Patients may begin using large numbers of tablets in an attempt to obtain the desired effect. This obviously increases addictive potential.

Opioids. Loperamide and diphenoxylate with atropine are effective for controlling diarrhea. They seem particularly helpful in patients with painless diarrhea. Patients who have been unable to perform at work, travel, or enjoy dining out or other activities may be able to lead a more normal life, with the drug providing "social insurance."

As with the other agents, opioids have not been proven effective at relieving the other symptoms of IBS.

Antidepressants. Again, no scientific proof of efficacy has been found, but these drugs can be useful adjuncts. I have found the tricyclics to be particularly useful in the control of pain. As with other chronic pain disorders (e.g., chronic headache, fibrositis), tricyclic antidepressants may be effective at doses well below those that are therapeutic for depression. It is unclear whether this is a placebo effect, an anticholinergic effect, an antihistamine effect, or some combination.

Clearly, if clinical depression is present, appropriate use of these agents is warranted, and this may help control gastrointestinal symptoms.

Psychotherapy. The decision to refer a patient for psychiatric consultation is sometimes difficult. If a clear depression or anxiety disorder is noted, the decision to seek psychiatric assistance is straightforward and can be discussed directly with the patient. When a somatization disorder is suspected, or a psychiatric diagnosis is not clear, however, this is a problem. Somatization disorder patients are resistant to the suggestion that they don't have organic disease, and they are also unlikely to benefit from psychotherapy.

In difficult cases, psychiatric evaluation can be requested without a prejudgment as to whether further psychotherapy can be recommended. Explaining to the patient that emotional factors have a significant impact on the gastrointestinal tract may gain patient understanding and compliance.

Most patients do not need psychiatric help. In fact, the suggestion that their distress is caused by a psychiatric disorder may lead them to suspect that the physician has not given their complaints proper attention. Lifestyle modification is important in the therapy of IBS, but a psychiatrist is not usually needed to foster it.

ADDITIONAL CONSIDERATIONS

The management of patients with IBS presents a real challenge to the physician, one that many physicians do not relish. It is interesting to reflect on what your feelings are when you learn that the next patient waiting in the office probably has IBS. Many physicians have a negative reaction, perhaps because IBS is so different from our cultural expectation of the physician-patient interaction. The model is acute illness: the pneumonia cured by a course of antibiotic, the cholecystitis cured by an operation. The patient expects a clear diagnosis, confirmed by an irrefutable laboratory test, to be cured by a prescription if possible, or an operation if necessary. The physician would like to live up to that model. The patient then expresses gratitude, both verbally and monetarily.

IBS deviates from the model in many ways. It is not an acute illness. No test can confirm it. No pill or surgery can cure it. Patients are not "made" better by the physician, but rather must participate to make themselves better. Depending on the patients' psychologic make-up they may be resistant to this.

Clearly, this represents a challenge. The art of medicine is far more important than the science. The interaction of the physician and the patient is the treatment. Patient education is essential. The patient must understand that the disorder is common and chronic, and is not permanently disabling nor progressive. The patient does not have cancer or a disease related to it. A number of factors, including diet, stress, lifestyle, and hormonal effects, can produce troublesome symptoms because of gas and spasm. Modifying these factors can help control the symptoms. When the symptoms are particularly disabling, medications can be used to ameliorate them. Scientific studies have shown a remarkable placebo effect in IBS patients, which tends to confirm the value of the physician-patient interaction in those settings.

Successful treatment requires time, energy, and empathy. It may be worth recalling that the physician enjoyed a higher status years ago, when the art of medicine was practiced more expertly, and the science was more primitive.

REFERENCES

1. Manning AP, Thompson WG, Heaton KW, Morris AF: Towards positive diagnosis of the irritable bowel. Br Med J, 2:653, 1978.
2. Talley NJ, Phillips SF, Melton J 3rd, et al.: A patient questionnaire to identify bowel disease. Ann Intern Med 111:671, 1989.
3. Connell AM, Jones FA, Rowlands EN: Motility of the pelvic colon. IV. Abdominal pain associated with colonic hypermotility after meals. Gut, 6:105, 1965.
4. Horowitz DJ, Farrar JT: Intraluminal small intestinal pressure in normal patients and in patients with functional gastrointestinal disorders. Gastroenterology, 42:455, 1962.
5. Kellow JE, Phillips SF: Altered small bowel motility in irritable bowel syndrome is correlated with symptoms. Gastroenterology, 92:1885, 1987.
6. Chaudhary MB, Truelove SC: Human colonic motility: A comparative study of normal subjects, patients with ulcerative colitis, patients with the irritable colon syndrome. I. Resting patterns of motility. Gastroenterology, 40:1, 1961.
7. Chaudhary MB, Truelove SC: Human colonic motility: A comparative study of normal subjects, patients with ulcerative colitis, patients with the irritable colon syndrome. II. The effect of prostigmine. Gastroenterology 40:18, 1961.
8. Painter NS, Truelove SC: The intraluminal pressure patterns in diverticulosis. Part III: The effect of prostigmine. Gut 5:365, 1964.
9. Connell AM, Jones FA, Rowlanes EN: Motility of the pelvic colon. Part IV. Abdominal pain associated with colonic hypermotility after meals. Gut 6:105, 1965.
10. Harvey RF, Read AE: Effect of cholecystokinin on colonic motility and symptoms in patients with the irritable bowel syndrome. Lancet 1:1, 1973.

11. Snape WJ Jr, Carlson GM, Cohen S: Colonic myoelectric activity in the irritable bowel syndrome. Gastroenterology 70:326, 1976.
12. Whitehead WE, Engel BJ, Schuster MM: Irritable bowel syndrome: Physiological and psychological differences between diarrhea-predominant and constipation-predominant patients. Dig Dis Sci 25:404, 1980.
13. Cook IJ, van Eeden A, Collins SM: Patients with irritable bowel syndrome have greater pain tolerance than normal subjects. Gastroenterology 93:727, 1987.
14. Crowell MD, Whitehead WE, Cheskin LJ, Schuster MM: Twenty-four hour ambulatory monitoring of peristaltic activity from the colon in normals and constipation-predominant IBS patients. Gastroenterology 96:A103, 1989.
15. Drossman DA, Sandler RS, McKee DC, Lovitz AJ: Bowel patterns among subjects not seeking health care. Gastroenterology 83:529, 1982.
16. Whitehead WE, Cheskin LF, Heller BR, et al.: Evidence for exacerbation of irritable bowel syndrome during menses. Gastroenterology 98:1485, 1990.
17. Thompson WG, Heaton KW: Functional bowel disorders in apparently healthy people. Gastroenterology 79:283, 1980.
18. Klein KB: Controlled treatment trials in the irritable bowel syndrome: A critique. Gastroenterology 95:232, 1988.
19. Cook IJ, Irvine EJ, Campbell D, et al.: Effect of dietary fiber on symptoms and rectosigmoid motility in patients with irritable bowel syndrome: A controlled, crossover study. Gastroenterology 98:66, 1990.
20. Anderson JW, Zettwoch N, Feldman T, et al: Cholesterol-lowering effects of psyllium hydrophilic mucilloid for hypercholesterolemic men. Arch Intern Med 148:292, 1988.

chapter

13

NONSURGICAL TREATMENT OF GALLSTONES

Joseph A. Scopelliti

Gallstones represent a common diagnosis in all Western countries. It is estimated that, at present, 20 million Americans have been diagnosed with gallstones and, of these, 500,000 cholecystectomies are performed annually for the relief of symptomatic stones.[1] In addition, many patients with stones would rather not undergo surgery because of personal preference, concomitant medical problems, or other reasons. As a result, nonsurgical methods of dealing with gallstones have become popular.

CLINICAL MANIFESTATIONS

Gallstones are characterized by the predominant symptom of biliary colic, which is typically located in the right upper quadrant. It is of sudden onset and can be severe. The pain often radiates to the chest or right infrascapular region. Typical biliary colic is a restless discomfort. Patients report that they can find no comfortable position, and often desire to walk the floors. The pain usually lasts for some time, from 30 minutes to 2 days. A characteristic symptom is that of nocturnal episodes of pain that often awaken patients from sleep, even though they have been fasting for hours before retiring to bed. The pain can be associated with nausea and vomiting, and is sometimes associated with episodic diarrhea.

Symptoms of common duct obstruction should be evaluated. These are symptoms that suggest jaundice, such as alcoholic stools or dark urine. In addition, pruritus can be associated. The presence of fever with pain is particularly ominous because it might indicate such problems as cholangitis or emphysematous cholecystitis.

HISTORY AND PHYSICAL EXAMINATION

Background data, including family history and past medical problems predisposing to the formation of gallstones, are necessary parts of the history. The typical patient with gallstones has a strong family history. Medical problems that may be associated with the diagnosis of gallstones include hereditary spherocytosis, cirrhosis, Crohn's disease or other ileal diseases, ileal resection, and intestinal bypass surgery.

The main focus in the physical examination should be on the evaluation of right upper quadrant tenderness. The patient with gallstones is generally found to have a normal physical examination between episodes of pain. With an acute episode of pain, however, patients usually are found to have deep tenderness in the right upper abdomen. Murphy's sign is a sudden halt in inspiration when deep pressure is held in the right subcostal region, and this is typical of acute cholecystitis. Evidence of guarding or rebound tenderness indicates severe, acute cholecystitis, and suggests an associated pancreatitis. Such a patient should be hospitalized immediately. Peripheral findings such as icterus or fever are rarely found in the typical patient with symptomatic cholelithiasis.

PATHOGENESIS

Pathogenesis of gallstones reveals two types. Cholesterol stones are those comprised of more than 50% cholesterol by weight. Pigment stones contain generally less than 30% cholesterol by weight.

CHOLESTEROL GALLSTONES

Cholesterol stones account for 75% of all gallstones in Western countries. These can be broken down further into true cholesterol stones, those with more than a 90% cholesterol content, and mixed cholesterol stones, those with a 50 to 90% cholesterol content.

Risk factors for cholesterol gallstones include gender, with women being afflicted significantly more often than men. Cholesterol gallstones are rare before the ages of 20 years, and risk increases with age. The use of exogenous female hormones, such as birth control pills, is another risk factor. Obesity and prolonged periods of weight loss, as well as sudden massive weight changes, are also known risk factors. Finally, native American Indians have a predisposition to the development of cholesterol gallstones.

Cholesterol gallstones are formed through two pathways. The normal secretion of cholesterol in the bile is 1 to 2 g/day. Hypersecretion of biliary cholesterol results in a supersaturated bile and causes cholesterol crystallization in the bile, which eventually leads to the formation of cholesterol gallstones. This is the most common method by which cholesterol gallstones form, and several mechanisms are involved. Increased hepatic lipoprotein uptake as a result of constitutional factors or estrogens is one mechanism. Decreased cholesterol synthesis as a result of obesity or hyperlipidemia also results in the hypersecretion of biliary cholesterol. Decreased degradation of cholesterol occurs with age. Finally, progesterones can cause decreased hepatic storage of cholesterol, and results in increased secretion rates.

The second pathway, hyposecretion of bile salts, results in excess cholesterol concentration in the bile. This can be caused by increased gastrointestinal losses of bile salts, such as in ileal diseases or resection, or in intestinal bypass surgery. Note that 98% of bile salts are reabsorbed by way of the enterohepatic circulation. Ineffective synthesis, such as in those patients with liver diseases, results in decreased bile salt pools.

Finally, gallbladder motility and emptying have been studied and may play a role in the initiation of sludge formation, although this is not clear at present.

PIGMENT GALLSTONES

Noncholesterol gallstones are of two types, black and brown stones. Black stones occur in a sterile bile and are a result of the supersaturation of bile with calcium bilirubinate and calcium carbonate-phosphate. They typically occur because of hemolytic disease, with the increased production and excretion of pigments. Patients with cirrhosis are also at risk for the development of black stones, although the reason for this is unclear. Increasing age yields a statistically greater probability of developing black stones.

Brown stones are soft and greasy, indicating a high content of calcium soaps, and contain a greater amount of cholesterol. They occur in infected intrahepatic and extrahepatic bile ducts and in the gallbladder. They are usually infected with anaerobic organisms as a result of stasis or obstruction of the bile ducts. Bacteria are typically found in the center of these stones, and they serve as the nidus for formation of stones in a patient who would otherwise be a low-risk patient.

NONSURGICAL OPTIONS FOR THERAPY

The nonsurgical treatment of gallstones generally involves two approaches, dissolution or lithotripsy.

DISSOLUTION THERAPY

Bile salts are basically detergents for biliary cholesterol. Their function is to solubilize cholesterol in a liquid state. Adding to the bile acid pool is part of the effort to diminish crystallization of cholesterol in the bile.

Oral Treatment

Chenodeoxycholic acid was the first bile acid agent available for general use in the United States. Its mechanism of action is to extend the bile acid pool and to inhibit cholesterol synthesis and secretion. It thereby reduces cholesterol saturation of the bile.

The complete dissolution rate has been found to be approximately 50% in selected patients in whom its efficacy was studied.[2] Several factors need to be present for this agent to be effective. The gallstone composition needs to be predominantly cholesterol, with a minimal degree of calcium. Stones that are found to float at the time of oral cholecystography are the most likely to be dissolved. In addition, the gallstone needs to be less than 1.5 cm in diameter. The gallbladder should be a functioning gallbladder—again, as determined by oral cholecystography. Finally, chenodeoxycholic acid works best when the patient is of ideal body weight or less, female, and with a serum cholesterol level lower than 227 mg/d.[2]

Indications for this agent are mild to moderate symptoms in a patient who is a poor surgical candidate or an increased surgical risk. Patient preference should also be considered when treatment decisions are made. As noted, an approximate 50% rate can be expected for complete dissolution in these selected patients.

Side effects include diarrhea, which appears to be dose-related. Elevation of the serum LDL cholesterol level has been noted. More importantly, abnormal liver function tests, especially ALT levels, are found in as many as 30% of patients receiving this medication. These abnormalities are transient, and reverse with discontinuation of the medication. Regular monitoring with liver function testing and lipid profiles is generally necessary.

Therapy should be continued for a period of 1 year, at which time re-evaluation for a change in the presence and size of gallstones is necessary. It may, however, be useful to continue therapy for as long as 3 years. Gallstones do recur once this medication is stopped. One study has found a 50% rate of recurrence within 7 years in patients followed by ultrasonography.[3]

Ursodeoxycholic acid is a 7β-epimer chenodeoxycholic acid that has been released for use more recently in the United States. Its mechanism of action appears to be primarily through the inhibition of cholesterol secretion, so it reduces the cholesterol saturation of bile.

Its efficacy appears to be similar to that of chenodeoxycholic acid when used in a dose of 10 mg/kg/day. Again, however, patient selection is extremely important, and the factors noted above should be considered.

More important is the side effect profile of this medication, which is more promising than that of chenodeoxycholic acid. This agent does not cause diarrhea nor elevations in the serum cholesterol level. At present, it also appears to be free of any hepatotoxicity, although periodic measurements of liver function tests are still recommended.[8] Long-term follow-up of this agent is not yet clearly documented, although results similar to those for chenodeoxycholic acid should be expected.

Two promising developments have been reported. The first is the combination of chenodeoxycholic acid and ursodeoxycholic acid in the same patient. Because of their different mechanisms of action, dissolution may be accelerated when they are used in this manner.[3] The second factor is the identification of reduced recurrence rates in patients taking nonsteroidal anti-inflammatory drugs.[4] These two developments, if found to be conclusive, would substantially improve the long-term usefulness of these agents.

Patient selection for oral dissolution therapy is the most difficult part of the decision. As noted, specific characteristics should be examined, including stone composition, size of the gallstones, function of the gallbladder, and patient characteristics. Patient selection and patient preference, however, are distinctly different.

It seems prudent at this point to weigh the benefits and risks of traditional cholecystectomy against those of nonsurgical measures. In view of the natural history of gallstones, it appears that only symptomatic patients should be treated medically or surgically. The single indication for treatment of asymptomatic gallstones—that is, recurrent symptoms in a diabetic patient—has now been retracted. It has been clearly shown that no increased risk for complications of gallstones occurs in diabetic patients.[5]

Patients with complicated gallstones, including those who have acute cholecystitis, pancreatitis, or cholangitis, require surgical therapy. The delay between the onset of therapy and successful dissolution is simply too long for these patients. In addition, it is unclear whether gallstones in the common bile duct are affected by oral agents, and it is suspected that they may not respond.

Patients who have symptomatic gallstones without any complications are certainly candidates for oral agents, but they must be apprised of the necessity of long-term therapy and regular follow-up.

Finally, patients who have an absolute or relevant contraindication to surgery are good candidates for oral agents, because their benefit-to-risk ratio would be favorable.

Contact Dissolution Therapy

It has now been recognized that the instillation of substances directly into the gallbladder can dissolve cholesterol crystals and stones. The most widely recognized of these substances is methyl tert-butyl ether.

This substance is an aliphatic ether that is a liquid at body temperature. When stored in the gallbladder, it has a high capability for dissolving cholesterol. At present, it is an investigational substance only, but early reports have indicated it to be a promising therapy.[6]

Treatment criteria for patients receiving this substance are similar for those receiving oral agents. A patent cystic duct is necessary for effective clearing of the gallbladder. Small stones, size, composed primarily of cholesterol, are optimum.

Therapy is carried out after a catheter is placed into the gallbladder using ultrasound or CT guidance. Sedation necessary for this procedure is minimum. The gallbladder is then infused with the dissolving agent in a continuing cycle of infusion and aspiration; this minimizes overflow out of the gallbladder so that the ether compounds cannot be absorbed. Once stained dissolution is complete, the catheter is removed and the patient observed for any adverse side effects. Generally, the procedure is well tolerated, but some pain may occur because of catheter placement, as well as occasional nausea. If gallbladder overflow does occur, sedation can result. In addition, intravascular hemolysis and duodenitis have been identified as potential side effects.

Initial reports have shown that complete dissolution of gallstones can be expected in greater than 90% of selected patients.[6] Long-term follow-up studies for recurrence are incomplete at this time.

EXTRACORPOREAL SHOCK WAVE LITHOTRIPSY

The technique of crushing gallstones with extracorporeal shock waves is the same as that for kidney stone fragmentation. The shock waves are generated by various methods, such as electromagnetic, piezoelectric, or spark gap generators. No matter what generator is used, it produces a shock wave that focuses on the gallstone and results in its fragmentation.

Patient selection is again a critical part of the decision process. Gallstones with a total diameter greater than 3 cm cannot be crushed by this method. Radiolucent gallstones are preferable, and densely calcified gallstones should not be attempted. The presence of multiple small stones may also be a deterrent to successful therapy.

Results of investigational trials so far have focused on selected groups of patients. Stone fragmentation rates have been high, more than 90% in this patient population.[7] The addition of ursodeoxycholic acid, before and after the lithotripsy, has enhanced the success rate even further. A large, multicenter study has indicated that 21% of patients using ursodeoxycholic acid and receiving entracorporeal shock wave lithotripsy were free of stones after 6 months. Among the group not receiving bile acid therapy, 0% were free of stones at 6 months. Few adverse side effects were associated with this therapy. Biliary pain was the most frequent, but was not severe. Acute cholecystitis and pancreatitis were reported in 1 and 1.5%, respectively.[7]

At present, the cost of this therapy is considerable, and its exact place in the scheme of decisions is unclear.

Currently, the patient with symptomatic gallstones has a wide array of treatment choices available. Those patients who are at high risk for surgery should be considered for the nonsurgical approach. Options include both FDA-approved and investigational treatments. With these choices, treatment can be individualized to the patient's needs.

REFERENCES

1. Holzbach RT: Pathogenesis and medical treatment of gallstones. *In* Gastrointestinal Disease. 4th Ed. Edited by MH Sleisenger and JS Fordtran. Philadelphia, WB Saunders, 1989, pp. 1668–1691.

2. Schoenfield LJ, Lachin JM: The Steering Committee of the National Cooperative Gallstone Study Group: Chenodiol (chenodeoxycholic acid) for dissolution of gallstones: the National Cooperative Gallstone Study: a controlled study of efficacy and safety. Ann Intern Med 95:257, 1981.
3. Villanova N, Bazzoli F, Taroni F, et al.: Gallstone recurrence after successful oral bile acid treatment. Gastroenterology 97:726, 1989.
4. Hood K, Ruggin DC, Gleeson D, et al.: Prevention of gallstone recurrence by non-steroid anti-inflammatory drugs. Lancet 2:1223, 1988.
5. Ransohoff DF, Miller GL, Forsythe SB, Herman RE: Outcome of acute cholecystitis in patients with diabetes mellitus. Ann Intern Med 106:829, 1987.
6. Thistle JL, May GR, Bender CE, et al.: Dissolution of cholesterol gallbladder stones by methyl tert-butyl ether administered by percutaneous transhepatic catheter. N Engl J Med 320:633, 1989.
7. Schoenfield LJ, Berci G, Carnovale RL, et al.: The effect of ursodiol on the efficacy and safety of extracorporeal shock-wave lithotripsy of gallstones. N Engl J Med 323:1239, 1990.
8. Roda E, Bazzoli F, Morselli Labate AM, et al.: Ursodeoxycholic acid vs. chenodeoxycholic acid as cholesterol gallstone-dissolving agents: a comparative randomized study. Hepatology 2:804, 1982.

c h a p t e r

14

THE DIAGNOSIS AND TREATMENT OF VIRAL HEPATITIS

Mark Flemmer

Viral hepatitis is a common disease with an estimated yearly incidence of 1 to 2 in 1000.[1] Thus, after gastroenteritis, it is probably the most common infectious disease seen by office gastroenterologists. Although an enormous variety of agents can be responsible for viral hepatitis, most are caused by the five forms of hepatitis virus mentioned in this chapter. Of all the other types of viral hepatitis, probably cytomegalovirus and the Epstein-Barr virus occur with sufficient frequency to give diagnostic confusion. The Centers for Disease Control (CDC) have estimated that 29% of hepatitis cases are caused by hepatitis A, 44% by hepatitis B, and 27% by non-A, non-B hepatitis.[2] It is hoped that the clumsiness of the term "non-A, non-B hepatitis" will be replaced by hepatitis C (for the post-transfusional form) and hepatitis E (for the enteric form).

The signs and symptoms of the different types of viral hepatitis are generally not distinctive enough to separate them clinically. Where these differences exist they are mentioned in the text (e.g., the abrupt onset of hepatitis A, the serum sickness prodrome of hepatitis B). Figure 14–1 shows the representative signs and symptoms of acute viral hepatitis.

Similarly, the biochemical profile of all forms of viral hepatitis is similar (e.g., elevation of the alanine aminotranferase [ALT] level). Certain clues may suggest a particular virus. For example, dual ALT peaks are more often associated with hepatitis D (delta), whereas wide fluctuations of ALT are more frequently found with hepatitis C. Also, prolonged elevation of the alkaline phosphatase level is seen most commonly with hepatitis A. Figure 14–2 shows representative biochemical patterns of liver injury.

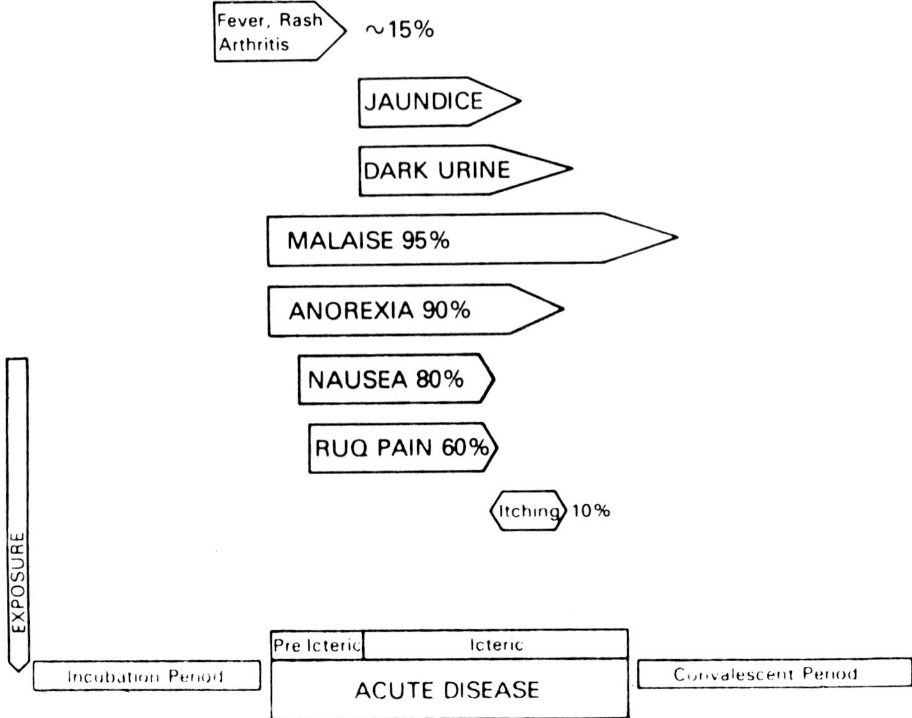

FIG. 14–1. Signs and symptoms of acute viral hepatitis. (From Hoofnagle JH: Acute viral hepatitis. *In* Principles and Practice of Infectious Disease. Edited by G Mandell, RG Douglas, and JE Bennett. 3rd Ed. New York, Churchill Livingstone, 1990, pp 1001–1017.

HEPATITIS A

Hepatitis A virus (HAV) causes about 20% of cases of clinical viral hepatitis worldwide.[3] The virus is a single-stranded RNA picornavirus. Unlike hepatitis B, it has a direct cytopathic effect, and is almost never associated with chronic hepatitis.

EPIDEMIOLOGY

Hepatitis A is primarily spread by the fecal-oral route, so most cases are caused by ingestion of contaminated food and water. The virus has no known carrier state, and infection is therefore maintained by person-to-person spread.[4] Viral excretion and infectivity occur 2 weeks before clinical jaundice to less than 1 week after it, so isolating icteric patients is of little value in preventing the spread of an epidemic.

The prevalence of antibodies to hepatitis A (reflecting previous hepatitis A infection) varies among countries, reflecting standards of sanitation and

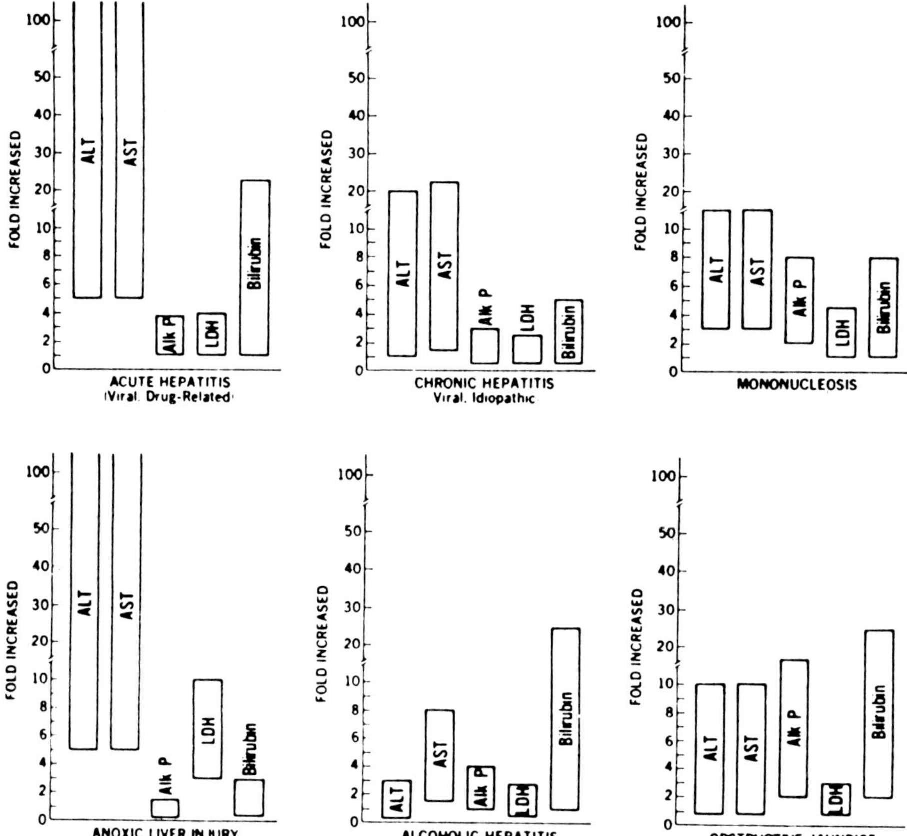

FIG. 14–2. The range of elevation of key serum enzyme levels in acute viral hepatitis and other common liver diseases (ALT, alanine aminotransferase; AST, asparate aminotransferase; Alk P, alkaline phosphate; LDH, lactic dehydrogenase). (From Hoofnagle JH: Acute viral hepatitis. *In* Principles and Practice of Infectious Disease. Edited by G Mandell, RG Douglas, and JE Bennett. 3rd Ed. New York, Churchill Livingstone, 1990, pp 1001–1017.

socioeconomic class, and increases with increasing age. For example, antibodies to hepatitis A (anti-HAV) are found in 23.5% of Canadian Forces personnel[5] and in 96.9% of urban Yugoslavian adults.[3]

Other risk factors for hepatitis A include being in a day care center or in an institute for custodial care (e.g., prison, nursing home, home for the developmentally disabled), sibship of greater than 5,[6] and IV drug abuse.[7] It is thought that the unifying epidemiologic mechanism for the above is poor personal care and hygiene. Because hepatitis A has such a short viremic phase parenteral transmission is rare, although it has been reported.[8]

Recent epidemics of hepatitis A have been associated with the eating of shellfish.[9] Clams and mussels are thought to become infected by ingesting offshore water that has been contaminated by sewage. Steaming the mollusks may not inactivate the virus because the temperature achieved in the shells may not be sufficiently high.

MANIFESTATIONS

In general, severity is related to age. In children, most cases are anicteric and are passed off as flu or gastroenteritis. In contrast, most infected adults become symptomatically ill with jaundice.

The incubation period averages 4 weeks and the relationship among viral excretion, symptoms, and antibody response is depicted in Figure 14–3. The onset of symptoms is characteristically more abrupt in hepatitis A than in other types of viral hepatitis but, like other forms of hepatitis, a flu-like prodrome is frequently followed by mild gastrointestinal symptoms. Right upper abdominal pain reflecting distention of the liver capsule, accompanied by dark urine and light stools, is often seen. Alcohol and nicotine intolerance are variable. A serum sickness-like picture is seen less frequently than in hepatitides B and C.

Laboratory results reflect a hepatitis with raised transaminase levels and a modestly elevated alkaline phosphatase level (usually less than three

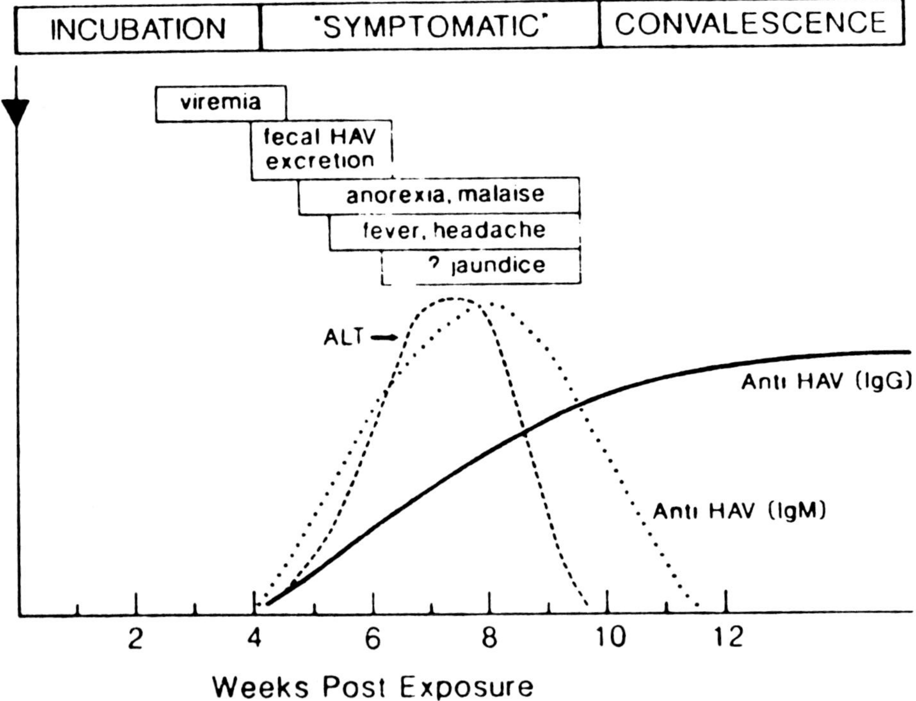

FIG. 14–3. Phases of hepatitis A infection. (From Balisteri WF: Viral Hepatitis. Pediatr Clin North Am, 35:376, 1988.)

times normal). Maximum transaminase levels usually occur 2 to 3 days before the jaundice. As with most viral diseases usually a mild leukopenia and lymphopenia are present. Prolonged cholestasis is surprisingly more common with hepatitis A than with the other hepatitides.[9]

Liver biopsy is not specific for acute hepatitis A. Panlobular infiltration with mononuclear cells, hepatic cell necrosis, hyperplasia of Kupffer cells, and erosion of the limiting plate can all be seen. As mentioned above, cholestasis can be particularly marked.

DIAGNOSIS

Although virus can be recovered from the feces, this is transient and rarely accomplished. A high index of suspicion is present when a patient has elevated transaminase levels, with or without icterus. The diagnosis is confirmed by finding an elevated IgM titer to HAV, which usually lasts up to 12 weeks after exposure (Table 14–3). An elevated IgG titer to HAV means previous infection and immunity. Of interest is the fact that saliva

TABLE 14–1. VIRAL HEPATITIS MARKERS AND THEIR SIGNIFICANCE

Marker	Significance
Hepatitis A	
IgM anti-HAV	Acute hepatitis A
IgG anti-HAV	Immune to hepatitis A
Hepatitis B	
HBsAg	Acute or chronic hepatitis B carriage
IgM anti-HBc	Acute hepatitis B (high titer); chronic hepatitis B (low titer)
IgG anti-HBc	Past exposure to hepatitis B (with negative HBsAg); chronic hepatitis B (with positive HBsAg)
Anti-HBs	Immune to hepatitis B
HBeAg	Acute hepatitis B; persistence means continued infectious state
HBV-DNA	Continued infectious state
Delta (can only occur if HBsAg-positive)	
IgM anti-delta	Low titer with anti-HBc IgM– positive (acute, coinfection)
IgM anti-delta	High titer (anti-HBc IgM negative), chronic or acute superinfection
IgG anti-delta	Past delta infection
HDV-RNA	Ongoing viral replication (research laboratories only)
Hepatitis C	
Anti-HCV	Previous, ongoing infection

Adapted from Sherlock S: *Diseases of the Liver and Biliary System, 7th ed.* Cambridge, MA, Blackwell Scientific Publications, 1986.

can be tested for anti-HAV (IgG) and anti-HAV (IgM), with a similar degree of sensitivity to serum testing.[10]

PROGNOSIS

The prognosis is generally excellent. The case fatality rate of clinical hepatitis A is 1 in 1000, which is caused by the occasional fulminant hepatitis and hepatic failure. For all practical purposes, chronic hepatitis does not occur. The average young adult with icteric hepatitis can anticipate 6 weeks of illness, and this rarely exceeds 3 months.

TREATMENT

In general, no treatment is required except attention to nutrition and hydration. For the rare fulminant hepatitis interferons have been used, but the data are insufficient to allow commentary.[11]

For prolonged cholestasis, some authorities use a trial of steroids (steroid whitewash).[3] Although this can hasten normalization of the bilirubin level, and improve patient morale, no evidence has been found to show that it hastens resolution of the hepatitis.

PREVENTION

Lifestyle

Good socioeconomic status and high levels of personal hygiene confer a low risk of developing hepatitis A. An unpolluted supply of drinking water is also vital in prevention. As can be inferred, these goals are difficult to accomplish in third world countries. Those addicted to eating shellfish should realize that they are a potent vector of disease, and that even the current "purification" techniques do not guarantee safety from hepatitis A transmission.[12]

Vaccine

Although currently not available commercially, promising reports have described a killed vaccine made from HAV propagated in diploid human fibroblast cells.[13] In the cohort of volunteers vaccinated a 100% response rate was found. It is anticipated that a similar vaccine may soon be available for general use.

Pre-Exposure. For travellers visiting developing countries, the CDC has recommended a single dose of immunoglobulin (IG), 0.02 ml/kg given IM. This confers immunity for 3 to 5 months.[14] Repeat injections need to be given if travel is more prolonged. If repeated injections are envisaged it would be cost-effective to test for total anti-HAV to determine whether the individual is susceptible. Hopefully, the availability of a vaccine might make these recommendations obsolete.

Postexposure. Because hepatitis A cannot be diagnosed clinically, serologic confirmation of the index patient is required. Serologic screening of contacts for anti-HAV is not recommended because it is not cost-effective and would delay administration. For all close personal contacts of those with hepatitis A, IG should be administered as above. Giving IG more than 2 weeks after exposure does not have any benefit. An excellent review about determining to whom to give IG has been published.[14]

HEPATITIS B

Hepatitis B virus (HBV) is a disease of global importance in that at least 300 million people are infected worldwide.[15] This places an intolerable burden on public health services, particularly in developing countries, whose health services are already overburdened. HBV causes up to 80% of cases of primary liver cancer and, as such, is second only to tobacco as a cause of cancer mortality.[15] Routes of transmission include percutaneous inoculation or direct transfusion of HBV-containing blood or serum, and transmucosal spread from infected semen. Although saliva can transmit HBV, this is probably uncommon.

VIRAL STRUCTURE

A detailed discussion of the HBV genome might not be relevant to office gastroenterology, but a limited understanding is necessary to unravel the complexities of its serologic diagnosis. HBV is one of a group of animal viruses known as the hepadnaviridae, which are small DNA viruses. With the exception of some higher primates, it is only known to infect humans. It is not thought to exert any direct cytopathic effect, with liver damage being mediated by immune effects.

The causative virus consists of an envelope and a nucleocapsid. The principal component of the capsule is hepatitis B surface antigen (HBsAg) which, although immunogenic, is not infectious, and forms the basis for HBV vaccines. The nucleocapsid contains a DNA polymerase and a circular, double-stranded DNA molecule.[16] The latter consists of two important antigenic determinants, the HBV core antigen (HBcAg) and the HBV e antigen (HBeAg).

EPIDEMIOLOGY

Although it has long been known that HBV is spread by parenteral contact with blood and blood products (serum hepatitis), it became evident in the 1970s that this is not the major route of spread in developed countries.[17] Most HBV in the United States is sexually acquired, both heterosexually and homosexually. Homosexual men in general have a higher incidence of infection than their heterosexual counterparts, with the exception of female prostitutes.[18] It is thought that the number of sexual partners is the unifying concept, more than the mode of transmission (i.e., anal versus vaginal intercourse), which is of lesser importance. One study has suggested that the incidence of HBV infection in homosexual men may be declining, reflecting the greater awareness of AIDS and condom usage.[19]

Intravenous drug users (IVDU) show the highest infection rates in developed countries, with from 65 to 90% showing markers for HBV infection.[18] As is the case with AIDS, the sharing of needles and other drug paraphernalia probably accounts for the spread of HBV. In addition, many IVDU resort to prostitution to finance their drug habits, which compounds the epidemiologic problem.

In developing countries, the spread of HBV in areas of high endemicity occurs primarily by vertical spread from an infected mother to her child perinatally. Because the probability of chronic carriage of HBV increases dramatically with childhood and neonatal infection, this route of transmission has the most important global consequences for the chronic sequelae of HBV.[15] In areas of low endemicity spread is usually by sexual contact, occurs in adult life, and has a lower risk of chronicity.

MANIFESTATIONS

The course of the disease may be subclinical and icteric or acute and rarely fulminant. Similarly, in approximately 10% of patients, the disease may become chronic, with its risk of cirrhosis and hepatocellular carcinoma. The possible sequelae are outlined in Figure 14–4.

The incubation period varies from 30 to 180 days, with a mean of 2 to 3 months. Although HBV tends to be more severe than hepatitis A or C, the overall clinical picture is similar. Features differentiating HBV from hepatitis A are a less abrupt onset and the infrequent occurrence of a cholestatic hepatitis. HBV infection can also be complicated by a serum sickness-like picture in the prodrome, which occurs in 10 to 20% of patients. It consists of rash, fever, urticaria, arthralgias, and sometimes arthritis. It is thought that HBsAg-antibody complexes are trapped and bind complement in involved areas.[20]

The icteric phase of HBV rarely lasts more than 4 weeks,[16] and recovery tends to be complete in 90% of patients. Approximately 10% develop chronic hepatitis B, and 1% have fulminant hepatic failure (FHF). FHF is defined as the onset of hepatic encephalopathy within 8 weeks of clinical illness.[21] It is generally believed that the more severe the attack of hepatitis, the lower the chance of developing chronic HBV. Thus, survivors of FHF only rarely develop chronic HBV, whereas anicteric HBV becomes chronic more frequently. This paradigm may explain why FHF resulting from HBV infection is often associated with absent HBsAg, and can only be diagnosed by a high IgM titer HBcA.[22] These findings are in accord with the belief that the immune system mediates most of the damage in HBV.

The usual clinical course of HBV and its serologic diagnosis are summarized in Figure 14–5.

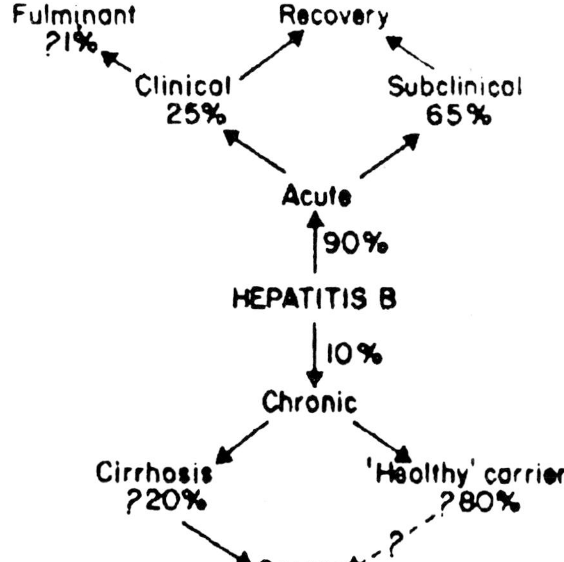

FIG. 14–4. Natural history of hepatitis B infection in adults. (From Sherlock S: Hepatitis B: The disease. Vaccine, 8(Suppl):7, 1990.)

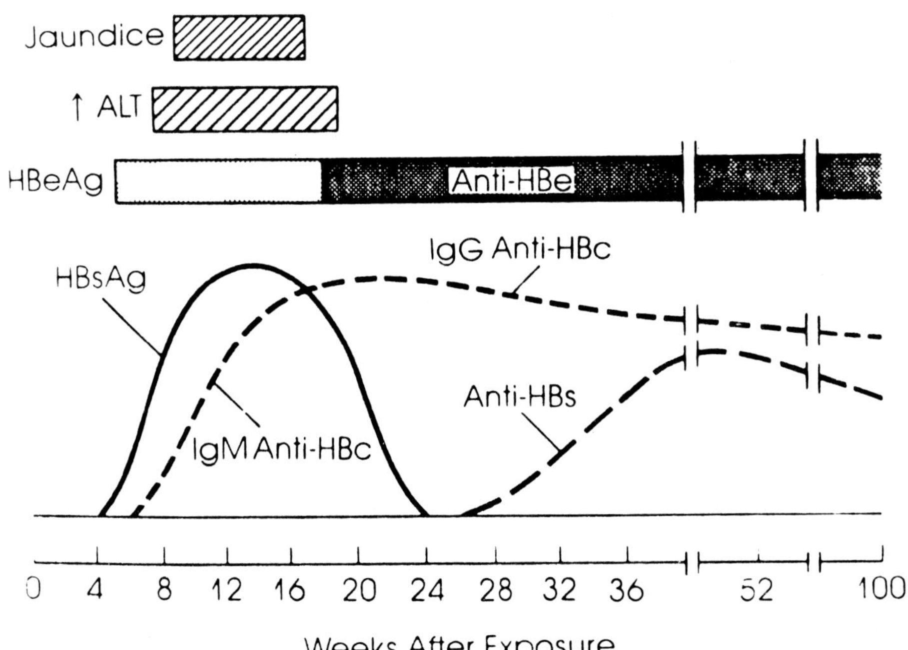

FIG. 14–5. Schematic of typical clinical and laboratory features of acute viral hepatitis type B. (From Wilson JD, Braunwald E, Isselbacher KJ, et al.: Harrison's Principles of Internal Medicine, 12th Ed. New York, McGraw Hill, 1991.)

COMPLICATIONS

Complications include chronic hepatitis, primary hepatocellular carcinoma, and extrahepatic immune disease.

Chronic Hepatitis

As mentioned above, approximately 10% of patients who develop HBV become chronic carriers of HBsAg. Of these, about 70% develop chronic persistent hepatitis (CPH), and the remainder (or 3% of the total) have chronic active hepatitis (CAH).

Chronic persistent hepatitis, when associated with HBV, is usually a benign disease, and patients are generally in good health. Mild hepatomegaly is common but usually no progression to cirrhosis is seen.[23] Laboratory abnormalities are episodic elevations of the transaminase levels without jaundice. A variant of CPH known as chronic lobular hepatitis can be differentiated histologically, and has the same excellent prognosis. Occasionally, its development has been temporally related to the seroconversion from hepatitis B e antigen to hepatitis B e antibody.[3]

CAH is frequently a silent disease, with minimal correlation between symptoms and liver damage. In about 50% of patients the clinical presentation is jaundice, portal hypertension, and ascites—all late manifestations of liver disease.[16] CAH is more likely to progress in males and in patients who present at more than 40 years of age. Sometimes, apparently stable CAH may have a relapse, which can be fatal. This can occur spontaneously but is more often associated with the withdrawal of corticosteroids or immunosuppressives.[24] It appears that viral replication occurs during periods of immunosuppression, with subsequent immune rebound on discontinuation that causes liver injury. A disordered immune response is also believed to underlie the development of CAH. It has been postulated that lack of HLA type 1 and HBc antigen expression, together with poor cytotoxic T-cell function, may prevent the clearance of HBV-infected hepatocytes.[25]

If cirrhosis develops with CAH, it is recommended that ultrasound and α_1-fetoprotein examinations be done at 6-month intervals to diagnose hepatoma while it is still potentially resectable.[16]

Primary Hepatocellular Carcinoma

It has been irrefutably shown that chronic HBV infection is linked to primary hepatocellular carcinoma (PHC). In Taiwan and South Africa, 60 to 80% of patients with PHC are HBsAg-positive, as compared to approximately 10% of the general population.[26] Molecular hybridization experiments have shown that HBV-DNA integration occurs early in chronic HBV infection and, coupled with a hepatocyte DNA sequence, resembles both an oncogene and a retinoic acid receptor gene.[27] This agrees well with the generally held theories of oncogene derepression and the subsequent development of cancer.

The clinical manifestations of PHC are protean, but it should be suspected in any patient with chronic HBV who undergoes sudden deterioration. The most common features include abdominal pain, upper abdominal mass, ascites, edema of the lower extremities, hematemesis, melena, and fever. Jaundice is a relatively uncommon complaint.[28] Various paraneoplastic syndromes, such as hypoglycemia, hypercalcemia, erythrocytosis, hypercholesterolemia, and hyperthyroidism, can confound the diagnosis, making PHC another example of the "internist's tumor."

Extrahepatic Immune Disease

Extrahepatic immune diseases are usually associated with circulating immune complexes containing HBsAg. The accompanying liver disease is usually mild.[3] The best-defined syndromes are the following:

1. Polyarteritis nodosa—"classic" type (approximately 10%)
2. Glomerulitis—almost all types of lesions can be seen, but this is rare
3. Miscellaneous conditions (e.g., as essential cryoglobulinemia, myocarditis, Guillain-Barré syndrome, polymyalgia rheumatica[3])

PATHOLOGY

For acute HBV, hepatitis histology is nonspecific and may resemble that of any other viral hepatitis. Frequently, a panlobular infiltrate is present with mononuclear cells and hepatic cell necrosis, with evidence of hepatocyte regeneration.

Chronic persistent hepatitis is distinguished by expansion of the portal zone by mononuclear cells without disruption of the limiting plate. This is the layer of cells between the portal zones and the liver cell columns. Piecemeal necrosis is not seen.

Chronic lobular hepatitis resembles acute viral hepatitis, but lasts more than 3 months. Most of the infiltrate of mononuclear cells is found in the intralobular areas, with varying degrees of necrosis.[3] Bridging necrosis and cirrhosis are not seen.

Chronic active hepatitis shows considerable expansion of the portal tract by mononuclear cells, with disruption of the limiting plate and bridging necrosis. Bridging necrosis is the loss of the reticulin framework between lobules or central veins, and results from large areas of hepatocyte death. In addition, areas of piecemeal necrosis with varying amounts of fibrosis are present. If severe enough, regenerating nodules of hepatocytes are seen.

DIAGNOSIS

As always, a high index of suspicion is necessary with the clinical picture of an acute or a chronic hepatitis in the appropriate epidemiologic setting. Transaminase levels are usually elevated at some point in the course of HBV, and represent the hallmark of its diagnosis.

The diagnosis is predominantly serologic and is summarized in Figure 14–5. Highly sensitive tests for HBsAg, anti-HBs, anti-HBc, anti-HBc IgM, HBeAg, and anti-HBe are commercially available. HBcAg is not found in serum and is consequently not measured. Tests specific for HBV-DNA polymerase or for the complete HBV virion (Dane particle) are only available in research laboratories.

In general, screening for active HBV requires the measurement of HBsAg together with HBc IgM. The latter marker should always be used, because sometimes a window period occurs when HBsAg and anti-HBs are negative, and only measuring the titers of HBc IgM allows diagnosis. HBeAg implies relative infectivity, and has its most useful clinical application in deciding whether a steroid "primer" is needed (see below).

TREATMENT

Acute HBV

Because this is usually a benign and self-limiting disease, no treatment is required. No specific treatment is available for fulminant HBV hepatitis. Corticosteroids have not been shown to have a significant impact on survival, and most authorities believe that their known adverse effects outweigh their marginal benefits.[29] Interferons have not been shown to be helpful. This is understandable, because active viral replication may have ceased at the time of presentation.[29]

Chronic HBV

Of all the agents studied (steroids, levamisole, adenosine arabinoside, acyclovir, interleukin-2), only interferon (IFN) has shown promise. IFNs have potent immunomodulatory and antiviral effects. An intriguing report has suggested that lymphocytes of patients with chronic HBV have deficient amounts of IFN in blood mononuclear cells,[30] which may explain their efficacy.

The following generalizations can be made about IFN therapy for chronic HBV:

1. The greatest chance of success is before the HBV genome has become integrated with the host DNA. It is not known when this occurs, but it is probably within the first few years of HBV carriage. It follows, therefore, that perinatally acquired infection does not respond to IFN.
2. The greatest chance of success can be anticipated in patients who have markers for active viral replication (i.e., HBeAg, HBV-DNA, HBV-DNA polymerase). In addition, these markers are associated with ongoing liver damage, and their absence may help predict the "healthy" carrier state.[31]
3. A steroid "primer" may enhance the effect of IFN, perhaps because withdrawal of prednisone produces a rebound stimulation of the immune response. Steroids tend to be used in patients with normal

transaminase levels (alanine transaminase <100 IU/dl), as this is thought to identify patients with a disordered pattern of immune response.[32] Steroids should not be used alone, as noted above.
4. Although usually well tolerated, IFN therapy is potentially hazardous. At present it should not be used in decompensated cirrhosis outside of clinical trials. In addition, the FDA has not yet approved IFN for general use.

Thus, it can be seen that IFN is not yet part of the treatment regimen available for use by the office gastroenterologist. A large, controlled study using IFN for chronic HBV has shown that α_{2B}-IFN (5 million units/day, for 16 weeks) is effective in inducing a sustained loss of viral replication and in achieving remission in one-third of patients.[33] In addition, 10% of patients lost HBsAg from their serum. Although the use of IFN therapy is a major advance, IFN is ineffective in two-thirds of patients eligible for therapy. Hopefully, further refinements of IFN therapy may improve these somewhat dismal findings.

PREVENTION

Modification of Lifestyle

Lifestyle changes are probably helpful in reducing the incidence of sexual transmission of HBV because of the current AIDS "phobia," but this does not appear to be the case with IVDU. Programs to provide drug users with free, sterile needles have not been universally implemented, and thus do not significantly aid in prevention.

Vaccine

Vaccination to prevent HBV is fully described in Chapter 17.

HEPATITIS C

The serologic test for hepatitis C virus (HCV) has only recently become available, so what formerly was a "wastebasket" diagnosis of non-A, non-B (NANB) hepatitis can now be confirmed. Hepatitis C is recognized to be a RNA virus with properties similar to those of flaviviruses. Hepatitis C is not, however, synonymous with a viral hepatitis-like picture associated with negative markers for hepatitis A and B infection. The enteric form of NANB hepatitis is now classified as hepatitis E (see below).

EPIDEMIOLOGY

Hepatitis C has two distinct epidemiologic patterns, post-transfusional and sporadic.[34]

Post-Transfusional Hepatitis

This occurs after the intravenous administration of blood or blood products. Numerically packed cell transfusion produces the most cases, with the incidence averaging approximately 5% of those receiving such blood transfusions. With pooled blood products, such as factor VIII concentrate, hepatitis C has developed in almost all recipients in some series.[35] Intravenous drug users and medical workers are also at increased risk, presumably because of percutaneous inoculation with the virus.

Sporadic

At least 50% of cases of HCV occur in patients in whom no blood transfusion or remembered percutaneous exposure has occurred. Because at least 1% of healthy blood donors in the United States probably harbor HCV,[36] it follows that nonparenteral routes of transmission are active. One study[37] has demonstrated the importance of promiscuous heterosexuality as a risk factor for transmission of the virus, although a limitation of this study was that HCV serology was not used. Curiously, this same article found no correlation between male homosexuality and HCV. Although it is possible, no evidence has yet been found to show that HCV is spread horizontally in families.

MANIFESTATIONS

Much of what is known about hepatitis C has been gathered from data relating to the post-transfusional form and, unless otherwise, these data are used here. The incubation period (defined by elevation of the ALT level) averages 7 weeks, but can vary from 20 to 90 days. Like most viral hepatitides, a prodrome of constitutional signs preceding the jaundice by 1 to 2 weeks can occur. This includes fever, myalgias, arthralgias, nausea, vomiting, and anorexia. On average, HCV has a more protracted and indolent course than hepatitis B,[38] and is frequently associated with wide fluctuations in the ALT level. Generally, the hepatitis is mild but can occasionally present as fulminant hepatic failure (1%). It was claimed that most cases of hepatitis-associated aplastic anemia are related to NANB,[39] but this association seems not to hold for HCV.[40]

Unlike other forms of hepatitis, at least 50% of hepatitis C patients continue on to a chronic hepatitis.[34] Of this subgroup, approximately 25% develop cirrhosis, with its attendant risk of hepatocellular carcinoma. Therefore, of 100 patients receiving a blood transfusion, 5 go on to develop hepatitis C, and 1 of these 5 goes on to develop cirrhosis. In contrast, the risk of developing AIDS after a transfusion has been estimated as 1 in 100,000.[41]

The role of HCV in various other liver diseases is the subject of ongoing debate and scrutiny. A study from Spain has found that 44% of patients with autoimmune hepatitis and 45% of patients with alcoholic hepatitis are positive for antibodies to HCV.[42] These observations are probably the result of international differences in diagnostic criteria for liver diseases, because other studies have failed to show these associations.[43] A similar study, again from Spain, has found evidence of HCV in 70% of patients with hepatocellular carcinoma.[44] It seems that the exact role of HCV in various liver diseases awaits clarification as the antibody test becomes more widely available.

PATHOLOGY

Liver histology is not specific for hepatitis C. Biopsy specimens can show acute hepatitis, chronic persistent hepatitis, chronic active hepatitis with or without cirrhosis, and hepatocellular carcinoma.

DIAGNOSIS

The diagnosis should be pursued in any viral hepatitis-like picture, particularly in the appropriate risk group or in any patient with cryptogenic liver disease. HCV diagnosis has been revolutionized by the discovery of an antibody to hepatitis C.[45] This antibody is positive in up to 90% of patients with post-transfusion hepatitis (hepatitis C) and in up to 50% of patients with sporadic (presumed) hepatitis C. Unfortunately, anti-HCV conversion usually occurs up to 6 months after transfusion, and can take up to 1 year. The current antibody kits are: a first generation enzyme-linked immunosorbent assay (ELISA), which measures antibodies to a recombinant nonstructural HCV protein called C100, which is not part of the circulating virus, and a confirmatory second generation test (both provided by Ortho Diagnostic Systems). The latter is a four-antigen recombinant immunoblot assay (RIBA) that measures antibodies to both structural and nonstructural antigens.

Perhaps the greatest pitfall of the anti-C100 ELISA is that it measures previous exposure to HCV, and not infectivity. Only a small proportion (17%) of anti-C100 positive blood donations are infectious for HCV as determined by two studies.[47,48] The office-based gastroenterologist, thus, cannot decide whether the patient is infectious, has convalescent antibody titers, or has ongoing viral replication when faced with positive anti-C100. Correlation with transaminase levels might help clarify this, but, at least for infectivity, has been shown to yield equivocal results.[47] The RIBA test is more specific, and one study showed that only 22% of HCV C-100 ELISA-positive samples, which also tested positive with the RIBA, were subsequently found to be clinically infectious.[46] This same study found none of the HCV C-100 positive, RIBA-negative blood samples to be infectious.

The most reliable method of diagnosing HCV infection is by identifying its genomic RNA in serum. This has been done successfully in research laboratories using the polymerase chain reaction,[47] but is too time-consuming and costly to have universal application. Hopefully, the anti-HCV RIBA test will help the clinician unravel the uncertainties of anti-C100 positivity, although more studies are needed.

PREVENTION

Over about the last 10 years the incidence of post-transfusion hepatitis C has been steadily decreasing. This has followed the voluntary self-exclusion of high-risk groups for AIDS (American Blood Transfusion Service, 1983) from blood donation, as well as the adoption of "surrogate" markers for hepatitis C. These markers are elevated ALT and HBCAb positivity. It should be realized that only HBCAb positivity denotes previous hepatitis B infection with its risk factors, which to some extent are shared by HCV. Also, the two most common causes of a raised ALT level are obesity and alcohol consumption, not hepatitis. These practices have decreased the incidence of hepatitis C from 10 to 15% to 5% over the last decade.

It is anticipated that the introduction of routine anti-HCV screening can further decrease the incidence of post-transfusion hepatitis C, although the 4- to 6-month screening gap before seroconversion is still cause for concern.

THERAPY

It is hoped that the dictum of prevention being better than cure may soon be realized, at least in regard to the post-transfusional form of HCV. This seems unrealistic, though, in IV drug abusers.

Currently, it is believed that steroids, with their propensity of enhancing viral replication, have little place in the treatment of hepatitis C. They may aggravate it. The most promising therapy for hepatitis C seems to be the use of the interferons, particularly recombinant α-IFN. Trials sponsored by the NIH using α-IFN have yielded the following conclusions:[49]

1. Interferons decrease ALT levels in from 50 to 75% of patients (the higher the dose, the greater the response).
2. Serial liver biopsies have shown that a decrease in the ALT level is reflected by a decrease in liver inflammation. As expected, liver fibrosis is unaffected by therapy.
3. Most patients experience a biochemical relapse on cessation of therapy. The optimal duration or dose of interferon therapy is not known.
4. Interferons, apart from mild, flu-like symptoms, are generally well tolerated.

Interferons are currently licensed by the FDA for the treatment of chronic HCV hepatitis.

It is difficult to write definitively about hepatitis C because the whole subject is in such a state of flux. Although it is believed that post-transfusional hepatitis is synonymous with hepatitis C, this has not been proven. Some authorities still maintain that at least two forms of post-transfusional hepatitis exist.[50] Uncertainty also prevails in regard to the sporadic form of hepatitis C. It is only with more research and better serologic testing that, in the future, we may view non-A, non-B hepatitis as only of historic interest.

HEPATITIS D

Since its discovery in 1977, the hepatitis D (delta-virus HDV) has assumed worldwide importance as a cause of acute and chronic hepatitis.[51] It is a defective RNA virus that requires the hepatitis B surface antigen (HBsAg) to replicate and survive. HDV thus contains an outer core of HBsAg surrounding an internal delta antigen (HDVAg), which is associated with a circular molecule of RNA.[52] The structure and replication of HDV make it absolutely unique as an animal virus. Clinical HDV can only exist in a setting of hepatitis B virus (HBV) infection.

EPIDEMIOLOGY

This is as complex as the virus itself. Although HDV is linked with HBV infection, it nonetheless has three distinct patterns of spread.[53]

First, HDV is endemic in certain areas of the world, particularly the Mediterranean basin and the Middle East.[54] A 20 to 40% prevalence of hepatitis D in HBsAg-positive carriers has been reported from Kuwait and Saudi Arabia.[53] It is thought that the mode of transmission is predominantly horizontal, through families and close contacts of the index case.[55] Thus, the probability of infection clearly increases when persons are crowded together in unhygienic circumstances and exposed to infectious body fluids. Paradoxically, not all areas with a high incidence of hepatitis B have a high incidence of hepatitis D. In the Far East, where about 10% of the population has HBsAg, the incidence of hepatitis D is low.[56] This intriguing observation has not been explained.

Second, hepatitis D occurs in epidemics in underdeveloped areas in isolated areas of the world.[57] This hepatitis is characterized by its severity and frequently fulminant course. Illness involves children the most severely, and has a 10 to 20% mortality.[53]

Finally, in developed countries, hepatitis D is a rare disease that occurs in populations at high risk for hepatitis B (e.g., intravenous drug users, hemophiliacs, dialysis patients). Homosexual men are probably only at a slightly increased risk for developing hepatitis D.[58,59]

MANIFESTATIONS

These occur in two forms, namely co-infection and superinfection.

Co-Infection

This is the simultaneous infection of acute HBV and acute HDV. It tends to be a self-limiting hepatitis with clearance of both agents, because HDV cannot "outlive" HBV. Evolution to chronicity probably occurs in fewer than 5% of patients.[60] A characteristic observation with this form of hepatitis is the occurrence of a dual peak of transaminases. It has been hypothesized that the initial peak is a result of HDV replication rapidly overwhelming the synthetic capabilities of HBV and direct HDV hepatotoxicity.[60] The subsequent peak is then related to the simultaneous immunologic clearance of both HDV and HBV. If the two necrotic events occur closely in time, the chances of a fulminant hepatitis are greater. This may explain why one-third of cases of fatal hepatitis is associated with co-infection.[3]

Superinfection

This occurs when an HBsAg carrier (often asymptomatic) becomes exposed to HDV. The incubation period is unknown in humans but, in carrier chimpanzees, is 3 to 6 weeks.[61] Acute HDV superinfection, like co-infection, tends to be an unusually severe and accounts for a large proportion (30 to 60%) of cases of fulminant, HBsAg-positive hepatitis.[62] Of even greater concern is that up to 80% of patients with superinfection develop chronic hepatitis.[63] This contrasts with the approximately 10% risk of chronicity from HBV. Chronic hepatitis is again severe and, in a large series, about 70% of patients developed cirrhosis, and most of these died.[64] The progression to cirrhosis usually takes about 10 years, but an abrupt interval of 2 years has been described.[63] HDV is not believed to result in an incremental risk for hepatocellular carcinoma above that of HBV infection alone.

Of interest is the association of chronic HDV hepatitis with splenomegaly,[64] unrelated to the degree of portal hypertension. Another unexplained immune phenomenon is the finding of antibodies to microsomal membranes of liver and kidney.[65] These antibodies are associated with the presence of chronic active hepatitis.

PATHOLOGY

Like most viral hepatitides, the pathology of HDV is nonspecific. The most frequent histologic feature is that of chronic active hepatitis with varying degrees of cirrhosis, reflecting the chronic nature of the disease. Some authorities have claimed that acute HDV infection is characterized by a cytopathic lesion of foamy degeneration of hepatocytes (microsteatosis), similar to the pathology of Reye's syndrome.[56]

DIAGNOSIS

Diagnostic confirmation is best sought in the relevant clinical setting. HDV infection should be suspected in a patient who has an acute hepatitis with a biphasic illness and undue severity, or a chronic hepatitis with a progressive course in the setting of HBsAg positivity.

The definitive diagnosis of HDV infection is based on the detection of HDVAg and/or HDV-RNA in the liver or serum of infected patients. These results indicate active viral replication. Unfortunately, these tests are not generally commercially available, and diagnosis in the office rests on serologic responses to the virus (see Table 14–1). Usually, acute HDV is associated with weak and variable antibody responses, whereas chronic HDV is associated with high antibody levels. Because the antibody titers in HDV co-infection can take up to 8 weeks to develop, it is recommended that multiple blood samples be collected.[66] Also, HDV co-infection is associated with HBV serology, indicating an acute infection (i.e., IgM anti-HBc).

HDV can induce striking repression of HBV replication,[67] so occasionally in HDV co-infection patients are negative for HBsAg but remain IgM anti-HBc–positive.[68] This fact emphasizes the need for doing HDV testing in HBsAg-negative hepatitis in the appropriate epidemiologic setting. Also, a small percentage of patients with chronic HDV hepatitis might be HBsAg-negative at some time in its course, which is another reason for obtaining HDV serology in a patient with cryptogenic liver disease.

TREATMENT

A) Acute HDV like most forms of fulminant hepatitis, no effective therapy is available, and steroids and interferons have no benefit. Results of liver transplantation have been good,[69] and this therapy should be considered.

B) Chronic HDV is more susceptible to drug therapy but, as yet, this has not been definitively established. The only medication showing any benefit is recombinant α-interferon, with currently available studies suggesting a decrease in liver necroinflammatory injury in 25% of patients.[70] The responders tended to relapse with discontinuation of therapy, however, so this therapy may have to be indefinite. The optimal dosage schedule and duration have yet to be determined.

PREVENTION

Because HDV transmission is inescapably liked with HBV, it follows that vaccination of all those at risk for the latter can prevent HDV infection. This is the only feasible method, because no HDV vaccine is available. Regrettably, HBV vaccination may not have a significant impact on HDV infection, because the population most at risk is the asymptomatic HBsAg carrier. The only advice that can be offered is that they abstain from high-risk behavior.

HEPATITIS E

For many years it has been known that a form of hepatitis exists that is distinct from hepatitis A but has similar epidemiology.[71] This was previously known as epidemic non-A, non-B hepatitis but, shortly after the isolation of the hepatitis C virus, the epidemic non-A, non-B hepatitis agent was cloned and provisionally called the hepatitis E virus.[72] Hopefully, this is the last agent in the alphabet of viral hepatitis. Hepatitis E virus (HEV), an RNA virus, is thought to be related to the calciviruses (e.g., Norwalk virus), which usually cause diarrhea.

EPIDEMIOLOGY

HEV is spread by the fecal-oral route, and is thus a disease of poor sanitation. Epidemics have not occurred in developed societies, but large epidemics have occurred in the Soviet Union, India, Burma, and Nepal. The first reported epidemic of HEV was in India in 1956, and involved approximately 30,000 people.[73] This outbreak was retrospectively confirmed to be caused by a non-A, non-B hepatitis agent.[74]

Although HEV usually occurs in epidemics, infection among household contacts can occur, although the secondary attack rate is low.[75] The disease usually affects either sex and the highest attack rate is in those between 15 and 40 years of age. HEV is generally a benign disease and is not associated with chronic hepatitis. An important exception is pregnant women in whom it is associated with a 20% mortality, particularly if contracted in the third trimester.[76]

It is believed that immunity from HEV is short-lived, because the neutralizing antibody response is poor and transient.[77]

MANIFESTATIONS

The incubation period varies from 2 to 9 weeks (mean, 6 weeks). Like hepatitis A, the disease is usually benign but may be associated with a slightly higher mortality, 1 to 2%.[78] Viral particles thought to be HEV were recovered from the feces of a volunteer 9 days before clinical illness to 8 days after.[79] In epidemics,[77] initial symptoms are typical of acute viral hepatitis, consisting of anorexia, malaise, abdominal discomfort, occasional vomiting, and fever. Jaundice is usually mild, and the mean duration of disease is 24 days. Elevations of transaminase levels are variable. It is currently not known whether subclinical forms of HEV exist, but these are suspected.

Liver histology shows two main patterns of damage, a cholestatic picture and a "standard" viral hepatitis pattern. In both types, frequent areas focal necrosis suggest a toxic liver injury.[80]

DIAGNOSIS

It is unlikely that an epidemic can ever occur in the United States, so the only exposure to HEV that the office-based physician might expect are sporadic cases in travellers returning from developing countries, including

Mexico. Although HEVAg has been isolated in primate models, and a fluorescent antibody blocking assay for anti-HEVAg has been developed, it is not known whether this will become commercially available.[80] Any physician wishing to confirm a case of HEV serologically should contact the CDC.

THERAPY

Only supportive therapy is available at present. More specific treatment (e.g., steroids, interferon) might be used in pregnant women but, because HEV remains a disease of underdeveloped countries, it is unlikely that therapeutic trials are to be undertaken.

PREVENTION

A vaccine might be developed in the future, but none is likely to be available soon. Because most fatalities occur in pregnant women, it is recommended that they be strongly discouraged from travelling to endemic areas. Ensuring a clean source of drinking water is probably the single most important step in the prevention of disease transmission.

Immunoglobulin has been reported to prevent severe clinical disease, but these reports need to be verified in larger, controlled studies.[81] Immunoglobulin prepared in industrialized societies is unlikely to be protective, because such populations do not have antibody.[78]

REFERENCES

1. Koff RS, Chalmers TC, Culhane PO, et al.: Underreporting of viral hepatitis. Gastroenterology 64:1194, 1973.
2. Centers for Disease Control: Hepatitis surveillance report 51:13, 1987.
3. Sherlock S: Diseases of the Liver and Biliary System. 7th Ed. London, Blackwell Scientific Publications, 1986, pp 257–285.
4. Balisteri WF: Viral hepatitis. Pediatr Clin North Am, 35:376, 1988.
5. Embil JA, Manley K, White LA: Hepatitis A: A serological study in the Canadian Armed Forces. Milit Med, 154:461, 1989.
6. Green MS, Zaaido Y: Sibship size as a risk factor for hepatitis A infection. Am J Epidemiol, 129:800, 1989.
7. Hepatitis among drug users. MMWR 37:297, 1988.
8. Hollinger FB, Naravan CK, Oefinpe PE. Post transfusion hepatitis A. JAMA, 250:2313, 1983.
9. Gordon SC, Reddy KR, Panday S: Prolonged intrahepatic cholestasis secondary to acute Hepatitis A. Ann Intern Med, 101:635, 1984.
10. Parry JV, Perry KR, Panday S, et al.: Diagnosis of hepatitis A and B by testing saliva. J Med Virol, 28:255, 1989.
11. Levin S, Leibowitz E, Tortan J, et al.: Interferon treatment in acute progressive and fulminant hepatitis. Isr J Med Sci, 25:364, 1989.

12. Mele A, Rastelli MG, Gill ON: Recurrent epidemic hepatitis A associated with consumption of raw shellfish, probably controlled by public health measures. Am J Epidemiol, 130:540, 1989.
13. Flehmig B, Heinricy U, Pfisterer M: Immunogenicity of a killed hepatitis A vaccine in seronegative volunteers. Lancet, 1:1039, 1989.
14. Protection against viral hepatitis. MMWR, 39:2, 1990.
15. Maynard JE: Hepatitis B: Global importance and need for control. Vaccine, 8(Suppl):18, 1990.
16. Sherlock S: Hepatitis B: The disease. Vaccine, 8(Suppl):7, 1990.
17. Hersh T, Melnick LI, Goval RK, et al.: Nonparenteral transmission of viral hepatitis type B (Australia antigen-associated serum hepatitis). N Engl J Med, 285:1363, 1971.
18. Piot P, Goilay C, Kegels E: Hepatitis B transmission by sexual contact and needle sharing. Vaccine 8(Suppl): S37, 1990.
19. Couthino RA, VanGrievsen GJP, Leentvar Kuipers A, et al.: Decline of HIV attack-rate in homosexual men corresponds best with male incidence of hepatitis B (abstract 4581). Presented at the Fourth International Conference on AIDS, Stockholm, June 1988.
20. Wards JR: The pathogenesis of arthritis associated with acute hepatitis B surface antigen-positive hepatitis. Complement activation and characterization of circulating immune complexes. J Clin Invest 55:930, 1975.
21. Trey C, Davidson LS: The management of fulminant hepatic failure. *In* Progress in Liver Disease. Edited by H Popper and F Schaffner. New York, Grune & Stratton, 1970, pp 282–298.
22. Gimson AES, Tedder RS, White YS, et al.: Serological markers in fulminant hepatitis B. Gut 24:615, 1983.
23. Redeker AG: Viral hepatitis: Clinical aspects. Am J Med Sci 270:9, 1975.
24. Bird GLA, Smith H, Portmann B, et al.: Acute liver decompensation on withdrawal of cytotoxic chemotherapy and immunosuppressive therapy in hepatitis B carriers. Q J Med 270:895, 1989.
25. Thomas HC, Jacyna M, Waters J, et al.: Virus-host interactions in chronic hepatitis B virus infections. Semin Liv Dis 8:342, 1988.
26. Song E, Dusheiko GM, Bowyer S, et al.: Hepatitis B viral replication in Southern African Blacks with HB_5Ag-positive hepatocellular carcinoma. Hepatology, 3:817, 1983.
27. Tiollais P, Buenda MA, Brechot C, et al.: Structure, genetic organization and transcription of hepadna viruses. *In* Viral Hepatitis and Liver Disease. Edited by A Zuckerman. New York, Alan R. Liss, 1988, pp 295–300.
28. Dusheiko GM: Hepatocellular carcinoma associated with chronic viral hepatitis. Br Med Bull 46:492, 1990.
29. Fagan EA, Williams R: Fulminant viral hepatitis. Br Med Bull 46:462, 1990.
30. Peters M, Davis GL, Dooley JS, et al.: The interferon system in acute and chronic viral hepatitis. *In* Progress in Liver Diseases. Edited by H Popper and F Shaffner. New York, Grune & Stratton, 1986, pp 453.
31. Hoofnagle JH, Shafritz DA, Popper H, et al.: Chronic type B hepatitis and "healthy" HB_5Ag carrier state. Hepatology, 7:758, 1987.
32. Silva MO, Schiff ER: Progress in treating chronic viral hepatitis. Contemp Intern Med, 000:25, 1990.
33. Perillo RP, Schiff ER, Davis GL, et al.: A randomized controlled trial of interferon alpha-2b alone and after prednisone withdrawal for the treatment of chronic hepatitis B. N Engl J Med 323:295, 1990.
34. Mattson L: Chronic non-A, non-B hepatitis with special reference to the transfusion-associated form. Scand J Infect Dis(Suppl), 59:1, 1989.
35. Fletcher ML, Trowell JM, Craske J: Non-A, non-B hepatitis after transfusion of factor VIII in infrequently treated patients. Br Med J, 287:1754, 1983.
36. Dienstag JL: Non-A, non-B hepatitis. 1. Recognition, epidemiology and clinical features. Gastroenterology, 85:439, 1983.

37. Alter MJ, Coleman PJ, Alexander WJ, et al.: Importance of heterosexual activity in the transmission of hepatitis B and non-A, non-B hepatitis. JAMA, 262:1201, 1989.
38. Hoofnagle JH: Acute viral hepatitis. *In* Principles and Practice of Infectious Disease. Edited by G. Mandell, RG Douglas, and JE Bennett. 3rd Ed. New York, Churchill Livingstone, 1990, pp 1001–1017.
39. Zeldis JB, Dienstag JL, Robert PG: Aplastic anemia and non-A, non-B hepatitis. Am J Med, 74:64, 1983.
40. Pol P, Driss F, Devergie A, et al.: Is hepatitis C involved in hepatitis-associated aplastic anemia? Ann Intern Med 113:435, 1990.
41. Bove JR: Transfusion-associated hepatitis and AIDS. What is the risk? N Engl J Med 317:242, 1987.
42. Esteban JI, Esteban R, Viladomiu L, et al.: Hepatitis C virus antibodies among risk groups in Spain. Lancet, 2:294, 1989.
43. Jacyna MR, O'Neill J, Brown R, et al.: Hepatitis C virus antibodies in subjects with and without liver disease in the United Kingdom. Q J Med, 282:1009, 1990.
44. Bruix J, Barrera JM, Calvet X, et al.: Prevalence to antibodies to hepatitis C virus in Spanish patients with hepatocellular carcinoma and hepatic cirrhosis. Lancet, 2:1004, 1989.
45. Kuo G, Choo QL, Alter HJ, et al.: An assay for circulating antibodies to a major etiologic virus of non-A, non-B hepatitis. Science, 244:362, 1989.
46. Van der Poel CL, Cuypers HTM, Reesink HW, et al.: Confirmation of hepatitis C virus infection by a new four-antigen recombinant immunoblot assay. Lancet, Vol. 237, Feb. 9, 1991.
47. Garson JA, Preston FE, Makris M, et al.: Detection of hepatitis C viral sequences in blood donations "nested" polymerase chain reaction and prediction of infectivity. Lancet, 335:1419, 1990.
48. Van der Poel CL, Reesink HW, Schaasberg W, et al.: Infectivity of blood seropositive for hepatitis C virus antibodies. Lancet, 335:558, 1990.
49. DiBisceglie AM, Martin P, Kassiandes C, et al.: Recombinant interferon alpha therapy for chronic hepatitis C: a randomized, double-blind, placebo-controlled trial. N Engl J Med, 321:1506, 1989.
50. Editorial: The A to F of viral hepatitis. Lancet 2:000, 1990.
51. Rizetto M, Canese MG, Arico S, et al.: Immunofluorescence detection of a new antigen-antibody system associated to the hepatitis B virus in the liver and in the serum of HBsAg carriers. Gut, 18:997, 1977.
52. Rizzetto M: The delta agent. Hepatology, 1:127, 1981.
53. Hoofnagle J: Type D (delta) hepatitis. JAMA, 261:1321, 1989.
54. Rizzetto M, Purcell RH, Gerin JL: Epidemiology of HBV-associated delta antigen: Incidence of anti-delta in HBsAg carriers and evidence for a transmissible agent. Lancet, 1:1215, 1980.
55. Bonino F, Caporaso N, Dentico P, et al.: Familial clustering and spreading of hepatitis delta virus infection. J Hepatol, 1:221, 1985.
56. Bonino F, Negro F, Brunetto MR, et al.: Hepatitis delta virus infection. Prog Liver Dis 9:485, 1990.
57. Hadler SC, DeMonzon M, Ponzetto A, et al.: Delta virus infection and severe hepatitis: An epidemic in the Yucpa indians of Venezuela. Ann Intern Med, 100:339, 1984.
58. Bodsworth NJ, Donovan B, Gold J, et al.: Hepatitis delta infection in homosexual men in Sydney. Genitourin Med, 65:235, 1989.
59. Judson FN, Ostrow DG, Altman NL: Delta hepatitis in homosexual men in the United States. Hepatology, 6:872, 1989.
60. Bonino F, Smedile A, Verme G: Hepatitis delta virus infection. Adv. Intern Med, 32:345, 1986.
61. Rizzetto M, Canese MG, Gerin J: Transmission of hepatitis B virus-associated delta antigen to chimpanzees. J Infect Dis 14:590, 1980.

62. Smedile A, Farci P, Verme G, et al.: Influence of delta infection on severity of hepatitis B. Lancet, 2:945, 1982.
63. Rizzetto M, Gerin JL, Purcell RH (eds): Hepatitis Delta Virus and Its Infection. New York, Alan R Liss, 1987.
64. Rizzetto M, Verme G, Recchia S, et al.: Chronic HBsAg hepatitis with intrahepatic expression of delta antigen. An active and progressive disease unresponsive to immunosuppressive treatment. Ann Intern Med 98:437, 1983.
65. Crivelli O, Lavarini C, Chiaberge E, et al.: Microsomal antibodies in chronic infection with the HB_5Ag-associated delta agent. Clin Exp Immunol, 54:232, 1983.
66. DiBisceglie A, Negro F: Diagnosis of hepatitis delta virus infection. Hepatology, 10:1014, 1989.
67. Rizzetto M, Ponzetto A, Bonino F, et al.: Hepatitis delta virus infection: Clinical and epidemiological aspects. *In* Viral Hepatitis and Liver Disease. Edited by AJ Zuckerman: New York, Alan R. Liss, 1988, pp. 389–394.
68. Rizzetto M, Bonino F, Verme G: Hepatitis delta virus infection of the liver: Progress in virology, pathobiology, and diagnosis. Semin Liver Dis, 8:350, 1988.
69. Rizzetto M, Chiaberge E, Negro F, et al.: Liver transplantation in hepatitis delta virus disease. Lancet, 2:469, 1987.
70. Rosina F, Rizzetto M: Treatment of chronic type D (delta) hepatitis with alpha-interferon. Semin Liver Dis 9:264, 1989.
71. Balayan MS, Andzhaparidze AG, Savinskaya SS, et al.: Viral hepatitis. Similar in clinical picture to hepatitis A but differing from it etiologically. Zh Mikrobiol Epidemiol Immunobiol, 8:79, 1982.
72. Reyes GR, Purdy MA, Kim JP, et al.: Isolation of a cDNA from the virus responsible for enterically transmitted non-A, non-B hepatitis. Science, 247:1335, 1990.
73. Viswanathan R: Infectious hepatitis in Delhi (1955–56): A critical study; epidemiology. Indian J Med Res 45(Suppl):1, 1957.
74. Wong DC, Purcell RH, Sreenivasan MA, et al.: Epidemic and endemic hepatitis in India: Evidence for non-A, non-B virus etiology. Lancet 2:876, 1980.
75. Zuckerman AJ: Hepatitis E virus. The main cause of enterically transmitted non-A, non-B hepatitis. (Editorial). Br Med J 300:1475, 1989.
76. Bradley DW, Krawczynski K, Cook EH, et al.: Enterically transmitted non-A, non-B hepatitis: Etiology of disease and laboratory studies in non-human primates. *In* Viral Hepatitis and Liver Disease. Edited by AJ Zuckerman. New York, Alan R. Liss, 1988, pp. 138–147.
77. Panda SK, Datta R, Kaur J, et al.: Enterically transmitted non-A, non-B hepatitis: Recovery of virus-like particles from an epidemic in south Delhi and transmission studies in Rhesus monkeys. Hepatology, 10:466, 1989.
78. Purcell RH: Enterically transmitted non-A, non-B hepatitis. Prog Liver Dis, 9:497, 1990.
79. Balayan MS, Andzhaparidze AG, Savinskaya SS, et al.: Evidence for a virus in non-A, non-B hepatitis transmitted via the fecal oral route. Intervirology, 20:23, 1983.
80. Krawczynski K, Bradley DW: Enterically transmitted non-A, non-B hepatitis: Identification of virus-associated antigen in experimentally infected cyanomolgus macaques. J Infect Dis 159:1042, 1989.
81. Tandon BN, Joshi YK, Jain SK, et al.: An epidemic of non-A, non-B hepatitis in North India. Indian J Med Res, 75:739, 1982.

chapter

15

THE MANAGEMENT OF CHRONIC ACTIVE HEPATITIS

Sheila Sherlock

Chronic hepatitis is usually defined as a chronic inflammatory disease of the liver that lasts for at least 6 months.[1] The time frame is usually stated to prevent diagnosis close to an acute attack of viral hepatitis when the hepatic histology is that of an unresolved hepatitis and difficult to interpret. In the absence of a history of an acute attack, it is not as necessary to wait and diagnosis may be earlier, although a follow-up of 6 months is wise before chronicity is deemed certain.

CLINICAL MANIFESTATIONS

The patient comes to the clinician through general circumstances, symptoms, physical signs, or abnormal serum biochemical test results. The most important general symptom is fatigue. Physical signs include jaundice, rarely vascular spiders, a large or small liver, and splenomegaly. Suggestive abnormal biochemical test results are a modestly raised serum bilirubin level, increased transaminase and gammaglobulin values, and a moderately raised serum alkaline phosphatase level. The next step is to test for serum hepatitis B surface antigen (HBsAg) and anti-HCV. Management depends on whether these are positive or negative (Fig. 15–1).

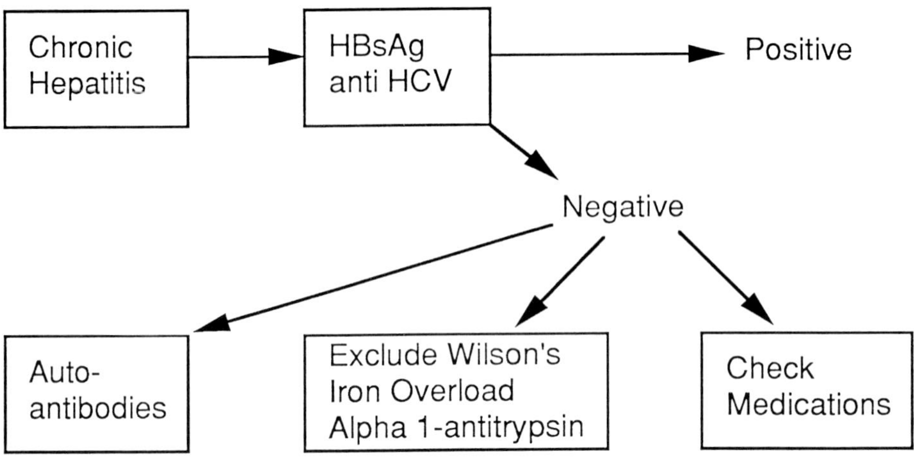

FIG. 15–1. Stages in the diagnosis of chronic hepatitis.

SUGGESTIVE CLINICAL PROFILE

CHRONIC HEPATITIS B

This is suggested by the ethnic origin of the patient, male homosexuality, drug abuse, or a likely contact with the blood of patients carrying hepatitis B (Table 15–1). The patient may present because of fatigue. Serum transaminase levels may be found at a routine medical check or by biochemical screening for some unrelated condition. Hepatitis B can be diagnosed at the time of blood donation. In a known hepatitis B carrier, a relapse, with jaundice and high transaminase values, may indicate superinfection with hepatitis D (delta) virus.

HEPATITIS C

The history of receiving a blood transfusion or blood products, however distant, suggests non-A, non-B hepatitis (hepatitis C).[2,3] The patient may bring a chart recording fluctuating serum transaminase levels over many months or years. The disease is insidiously progressive toward cirrhosis.

AUTOIMMUNE CHRONIC ACTIVE HEPATITIS

This should be expected in women, usually aged 15 to 25 years, when amenorrhea is usual, or in women of menopausal age.[4] The patient is mildly jaundiced and well nourished with vascular spiders. Splenomegaly is usual. Serum aspartate transaminase and gammaglobulin levels are high. Associated features may include fever, arthralgias, lymphadenopathy, and Coombs'-positive hemolytic anemia.

TABLE 15–1. CLASSIFICATION OF CHRONIC HEPATITIS				
	Predominant			
Cause	**Age**	**Sex**	**Associations**	**Diagnostic Tests**
Hepatitis B	All	Male	Immigrants from the Orient, Africa, and Mediterranean area; health care workers; male homosexuals; drug abusers; immuno-suppressed individuals	HBsAg, Ig Manti, HBc, HBeAg, IgM anti-HBe, HBV-DNA, anti-HDV
Hepatitis C	All	Equal	Blood transfusion, use of blood products, drug abuse	Anti-HCV
Autoimmune	14–25 years and post-meno pausal	Female	Multisystem disorders (e.g., diabetes, arthralgia, hemolytic anemia, nephritis)	ANA-positive* (diffuse); SMA-positive; serum gamma-globulin level high; "florid" liver histology
Wilson's disease	10–30 years	Equal	Family history, hemolysis neurologic signs	Kayser-Fleischer rings; serum copper, cerulo-plasmin levels; urinary copper and liver copper levels
Drug	Middle-aged and elderly	Female	Usually occurs within 3 months; includes INAH*, methyl-dopa, furantoin, dantrolene, anti-thyroid drugs, NSAIDs.	History, liver histology

*ANA, ______________________; SMA, ______________________;
INAH, ______________________.

DRUG-RELATED CHRONIC ACTIVE HEPATITIS

This most frequently affects older persons, often women. The patient has usually been taking the drug for more than 1 month. Drugs incriminated include isoniazid, methyldopa, dantrolene, ketoconazole, and nonsteroidal anti-inflammatory drugs (NSAIDs), but any drug should be suspected.

WILSON'S DISEASE

This usually presents before the age of 25 years, sometimes with hemolysis and ascites. A family history can be obtained, and siblings may have suffered or died from liver disease. Parental consanguinity may be present. Neurologic features such as slurred speech or tremor may be present or absent in young people with hepatic Wilson's disease. Serum ceruloplasmin and copper levels are reduced, and the 24-hour urinary copper level is increased. If a liver biopsy is performed, the copper content must be quantitated, and is increased.

LIVER BIOPSY

This is essential to confirm the diagnosis, to assess activity, to determine the presence or absence of cirrhosis, and to indicate a possible cause. Usually a distinction is made between chronic persistent hepatitis, in which inflammation is confined to the portal zone (zone 3) and the limiting plate between liver cell columns and portal zones is intact and chronic active hepatitis, in which the portal zones are expanded by a cellular, largely mononuclear infiltrate and the limiting plate is eroded by piecemeal necrosis. Cirrhosis, defined as widespread nodular formation and fibrosis with a destruction of a zonal architecture, may coexist with chronic hepatitis. Whatever the type of chronic hepatitis, the same basic, underlying liver histology is seen. Superimposed are histologic features related to the cause.

MANAGEMENT

CHRONIC HEPATITIS B

Most patients with chronic hepatitis B lead normal lives; strong reassurance can prevent introspection by the patient. Excessive fatigue should be avoided, but bed rest is not helpful. Physical fitness is encouraged by graduated exercises.

A distinction must be made between the replicative and integrated stages of the disease. During the phase of acute viral replication, the patient's serum is positive for HBeAg and HBV-DNA. At some stage, the hepatitis B viral genome becomes an integral part of the host's genome, so

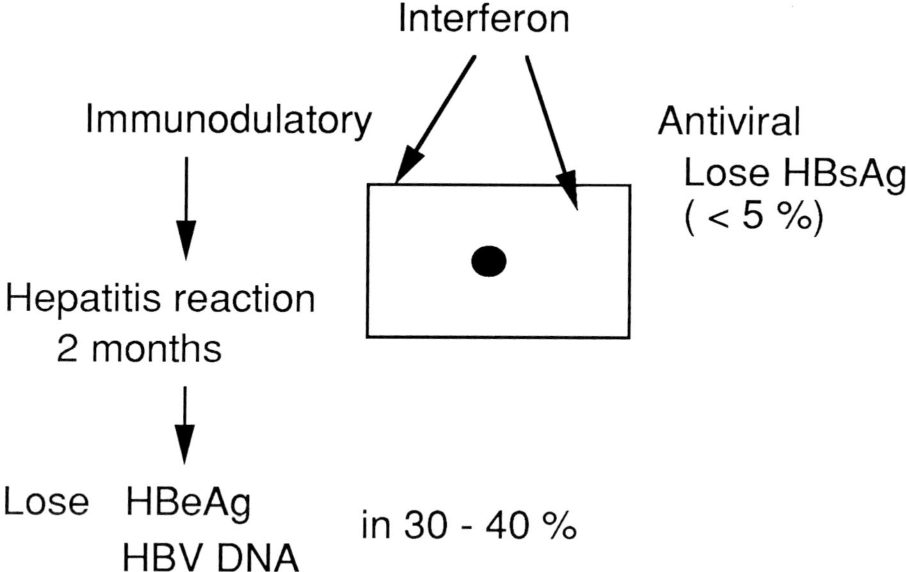

FIG. 15–2. Interferon, used to treat chronic hepatitis B, acts as an immunomodulatory agent, resulting in loss of circulating HBeAg and HBV-DNA in 30 to 40% of patients and, to a lesser extent, acts as an antiviral agent, resulting in loss of HBsAg in less than 5% of patients.

that viral genes are transcribed, along with those of the host. The hepatocytes secrete HBsAg but serum HBeAg is absent, anti-HBe develops, and HBV-DNA can no longer be detected. Treatment is aimed at controlling infectivity, eradicating the virus, and preventing the development of cirrhosis and hence, possibly, of hepatocellular carcinoma. It is unusual with any treatment to rid the patient of the hepatitis B virus.

In the replicative stage (HBeAg and HBV-DNA–positive), reduction or cessation of the inflammatory necrosis of hepatocytes may be achieved by successful antiviral therapy. In these patients, the use of α-interferon, whether lymphoblastoid or recombinant, must be considered.[5] The full course is 10 million IU three times weekly, for 12 weeks. Side effects include malaise, fever, and small decreases in white cell and platelet counts. A positive response is shown by the loss of HBeAg and HBV-DNA and a transient rise in transaminase levels at about 8 weeks, as infected cells are lysed. Ultimately, liver biopsy specimens reveal less inflammation and hepatocellular necrosis. Serum HBeAb appears after about 6 months. HBsAg is cleared in only 5 to 10% of patients, usually when the patient is treated soon after acquiring the disease.

Antiviral treatment must be considered for the HBe antigen-positive patient who is likely to disseminate hepatitis B. Adults seen early after infection, HIV-negative, with low serum HBV-DNA values, high transaminase levels, and active liver biopsy appearances are likely to respond. In well-chosen patients, a 30 to 40% response rate can be expected (Fig. 15–2). A good candidate is a person with a clear exposure who develops an acute attack of hepatitis B and remains HBsAg- and HBeAg-positive after 6 months. Orientals do not respond. Corticosteroids enhance viral replication and, after withdrawal, an immunologic rebound results in a fall of viral markers, including HBV-DNA. Immunocompetence is restored, and cells expressing target viral antigens are destroyed. Following the use of corticosteroids, a full course of interferon is given. This routine, however, can be dangerous; enhancing the immune response by corticosteroids followed by withdrawal can lead to hepatocellular failure. This therapy should therefore not be used for ill patients with severe liver disease, as evidenced by such features as jaundice or ascites.

A controlled trial comparing interferon alone with prednisolone followed by interferon has shown no benefit for the combination therapy.[6] A subgroup with serum transaminase levels lower than 100 IU/dl, however, showed improved results when prednisolone treatment was used. The dose is 30 mg daily, reduced to 0 mg over 2 weeks to allow a rest of 2 weeks, and then giving the interferon in the usual 3-month course.

Apart from general measures, no well-defined treatment is available for the HBeAg- and HBV-DNA–negative patient in the integrated stage of the disease. If the patient is symptom-free, or has only mild symptoms, conservative measures are all that should be offered.

No established treatment is available for the hepatitis D (delta) virus-positive patient. α-Interferons have been tried, but without equivocal results. Relapse follows cessation. The results of large, prospective controlled trials are awaited.

Patients who are HBsAg-positive, with chronic hepatitis or cirrhosis, especially if male and more than 45 years old, should be screened regularly so that hepatocellular carcinoma may be diagnosed early, when surgical resection is still possible. The serum α-fetoprotein level should be measured and an ultrasound examination performed at 6-month intervals.

HEPATITIS C

The use of interferons is being assessed. They should not be given except in the context of controlled clinical trials. The use of lymphoblastoid or recombinant interferon seems to yield equivalent results (Fig. 15–3). The usual course is 3 million IU by SC injection, three times weekly, for 6 months or even 1 year.

In a large, controlled trial, 46% normalized or near-normalized serum transaminase levels and histology showed regression of cellular infiltration.[7] The beneficial effect on transaminase levels is usually seen within 4 weeks of starting therapy, so that a decision whether to continue for the full 6 months can be made early. Relapse within 6 months of completion of therapy has been noted in 51% of treated patients (Fig. 15–4),which yields an overall good response rate of 25%.[8] This has to be measured against the usual mild nature of the illness, and the cost and side effects of the interferon. Clearly, different strategies have to be considered. These might include long-term interferon treatment in small doses for life, and intermittent treatment when serum transaminase levels rise and viremia probably increases.

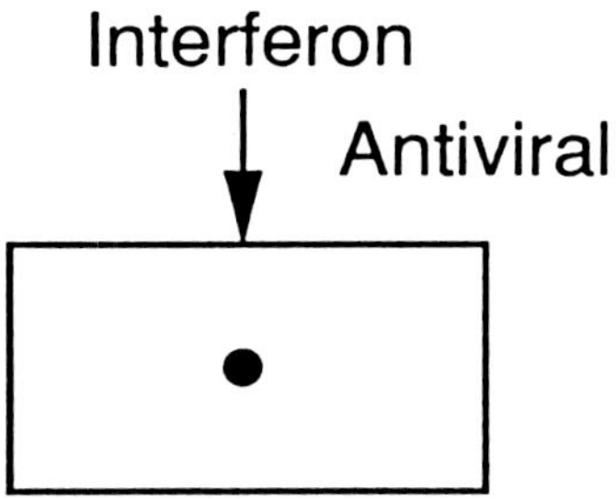

Transaminase

Persistently normal 50%
Partially normal 25%
Relapse 50-80%

FIG. 15–3. Interferon, used to treat chronic hepatitis C, acts as an antiviral agent, resulting in persistently normal or partially normal serum transaminase levels in 25% of patients and a relapse in 50 to 80%.

AUTOIMMUNE CHRONIC ACTIVE HEPATITIS

Drugs that alter immunologic processes are particularly effective, especially prednisolone. Benefit is seen especially in the first 2 years. Well-being is increased, appetite improves, and fever and arthralgias are controlled. Biochemical changes are less constant, although serum bilirubin transaminase and gammaglobulin levels usually decrease and serum albumin concentrations rise. The effect on hepatic histology is variable and unconvincing. Certainly, progression from chronic hepatitis to cirrhosis does not seem to be prevented. The usual dosage is 30 mg prednisolone daily for 1 week, reducing to a maintenance dosage of 10 to 15 mg daily. The initial course lasts 6 months. If a remission has ensued and been judged clinically, biochemically and, if possible, by a further liver biopsy, the drug should be tapered off slowly over a period of about 2 months. In general, however, prednisolone therapy extends over 2 to 3 years and often longer, sometimes for life. Premature withdrawal leads to relapse. Although control is usually re-established, occasional fatalities occur. It is difficult to decide when to withdraw therapy. Long-term, low-dose prednisolone maintenance is probably preferable. Alternate-day prednisolone therapy is not recommended, because the incidence of serious complications is higher and histologic remission is less frequent.

The cosmetic complications of corticosteroid treatment are particularly unwanted by female patients. More severe complications include diabetes, bone thinning, and serious infections. None is usually a problem if the dose of prednisolone is no more than 15 mg daily.

If 20 mg of prednisolone has not produced a remission, azathioprine, (Imuran) 50 to 100 mg daily, may be added. It is not given routinely. Other indications include gross cushingoid features, associated diseases such as

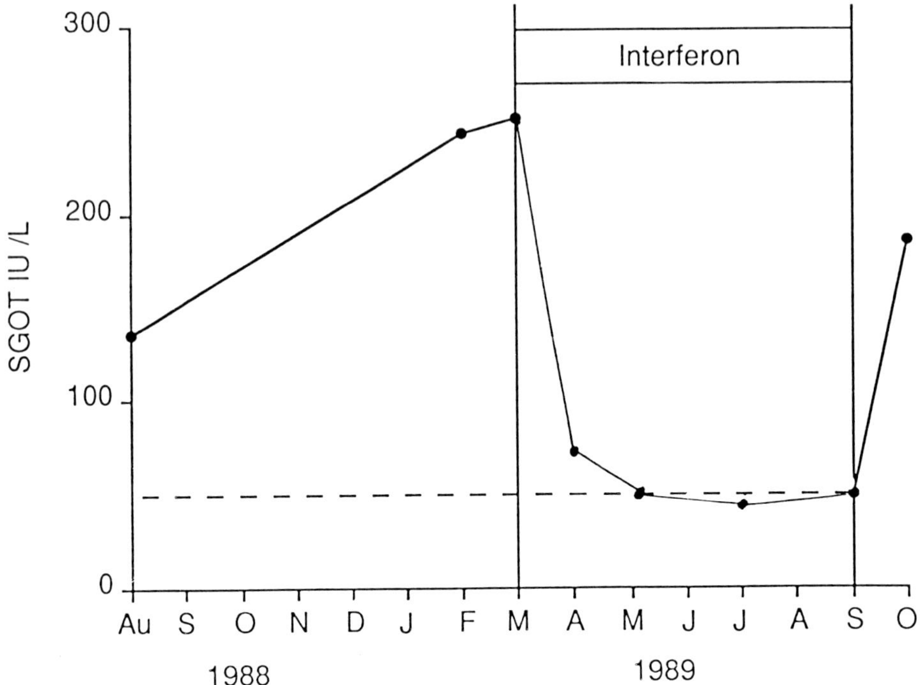

FIG. 15–4. Interferon, 2 million IU SC, three times a week for 6 months, used to treat chronic hepatitis C, resulted in a fall to normal of the serum transaminase levels within 2 months, but with relapse on stopping treatment.

diabetes, and other side effects developing at doses required to induce a remission. Azathioprine should never be given alone. Corticosteroid therapy prolongs life, but most patients eventually reach the end stage of cirrhosis.

The patients are young, often physically attractive, women. With treatment, menses return, and they may become pregnant. This is not contraindicated. Liver function may deteriorate but, after delivery, soon returns to its previous level. The fetal loss rate is about 33%, and babies might be born prematurely but are normal. The coexistence of liver disease with pregnancy should not per se indicate termination. Corticosteroids may be continued during pregnancy. Management in a special Obstetric Unit and hepatologic back-up are essential.

DRUG-RELATED CHRONIC ACTIVE HEPATITIS

A drug cause should be considered in any patient presenting with chronic hepatitis. Clinical and biochemical improvement follow withdrawal. Therefore, all drugs that the patient is receiving, if not actually life-saving, should be stopped, until the nature of the chronic hepatitis has been established. Recovery follows stopping the drug, but fatal, subacute hepatic necrosis may ensue if therapy is continued after the hepatic reaction has commenced.

WILSON'S DISEASE

Initially, penicillamine in doses of 1 to 2 g daily are mandatory. Maintenance is about 1 g daily, and should not be discontinued. Fatal liver disease can follow noncompliance, even after 20 years of successful penicillamine treatment. Oral zinc is given to block the intestinal uptake of copper. The dose is 50 mg elemental zinc (as the acetate salt) tid, between meals. It can be given in the initial stages, but should not replace penicillamine as long-term therapy.

REFERENCES

1. Sherlock S: Chronic hepatitis. *In* Diseases of the Liver and Biliary System. 8th Ed. Oxford, Blackwell Scientific Publications, 1989, pp 339–371.
2. Alter HJ, Purcell RH, Shih JW, et al: Detection of antibody to hepatitis C virus in prospectively followed transfusion recipients with acute non-A, non-B hepatitis. N Engl J Med, 321:1494, 1989.
3. Alter MJ, Sampliner RE: Hepatitis C and miles to go before we sleep. N Engl J Med, 321:1538, 1989.
4. Maddrey WC: Subdivisions of idiopathic autoimmune chronic active hepatitis. Hepatology, 7:1372, 1987.
5. Hoofnagle JH, Peters M, Mullen KD, et al: Randomized, controlled trial of recombinant human alpha-interferon in patients with chronic hepatitis B. Gastroenterology, 95:1318, 1988.
6. Perrillo RP, Regenstein FG, Peters MG, et al: Prednisolone withdrawal followed by recombinant alpha-interferon in the treatment of chronic type B hepatitis. A randomized controlled trial. Ann Intern Med, 109:95, 1988.
7. Davis GL, Balart LA, Schiff ER, et al: Treatment of chronic hepatitis C with recombinant interferon alpha. A multicenter randomized, controlled trial. N Engl J Med, 321:1501, 1989.
8. Di Bisceglie AM, Martin P, Kassianides C, et al: Recombinant interferon alpha therapy for chronic hepatitis C. A randomized, double-blind, placebo-controlled trial. N Engl J Med, 321:1506, 1989.

chapter

16

THE DIAGNOSIS AND THERAPY OF CIRRHOSIS AND ITS COMPLICATIONS

Philip G. Holtzapple, M.D.

Complications of chronic liver disease or cirrhosis are most often manifested as metabolic or hemodynamic consequences. The central role of the liver in its hormonal, synthetic, extraction, and metabolic functions is reflected in the alteration of one, a few, or all these functions in cirrhosis. No set, orderly progression of complications can be easily anticipated, as chronic liver disease and cirrhosis advance and hepatocyte function is gradually reduced. It is difficult to be dogmatic about the sequence of events when differing causes of cirrhosis also contribute to metabolic decompensation, making more unpredictable the complications that are most troublesome to the patient's quality of life. Although many of these complications have an acute onset and are often initially diagnosed and managed on an inpatient basis, in contemporary practice all these complications, with the exception of the hemodynamically unstable gastrointestinal hemorrhage and the patient in unresponsive coma, are treatable in the ambulatory setting.

ASCITES

Ascites, as a manifestation of chronic liver disease and portal hypertension, is a common problem, regardless of the cause of the liver damage. As chronic liver disease progresses, ascites is generally the first and most persistent clinical problem. To understand the rational approach to the management of ascites, one must have a general understanding of the mechanism of ascitic fluid formation.

MECHANISM OF FORMATION

It is impossible to understand the formation of ascites by examining hepatic or portal pressure disturbances alone. The considerable impairment of sodium and water homeostasis suggests a significant, perhaps a primary, role of the kidney in the initial phases. A peripheral arterial vasodilation hypothesis has been advanced to unify two pre-existing theories—"underfill" and "overflow." The role of hemodynamic characteristics and of humoral and renal function emphasized by this theory reflect the significance of the kidney, even in the earliest stages of ascites formation.

The underfill theory proposes that, as portal hypertension progresses, an imbalance of the Starling forces in the hepatic sinusoids and splanchnic capillaries causes excessive lymph formation in the liver and intestinal interstitium. When the capacity of the thoracic duct in returning lymph to the systemic circulation is exceeded, this causes exudation of fluid into the peritoneal cavity. As ascites accumulates, a diminished effective vascular volume develops, in turn stimulating various mechanisms (e.g., increased plasma renin, aldosterone, norepinephrine, and vasopressin), resulting in severe restriction of renal sodium excretion.

Over the years, several observations have raised doubts as to the validity of the underfill theory.[1] First, measurements of plasma volume in patients have consistently demonstrated an expansion rather than a diminution of plasma volume.[2–4] Second, many patients with decompensated cirrhosis fail to respond with a natriuresis when plasma volume is expanded.[5] Third, in measuring endocrine and hemodynamic parameters, ascites is consistently observed in patients with elevated portal pressure, renal sodium retention, and activation of the renin-angiotensin-aldosterone system. No differences in mean arterial blood pressure, peripheral vascular resistance, and other hemodynamic parameters have been noted.[6]

The overflow theory suggests that the primary event is an inappropriate retention of sodium, followed by expansion of the plasma volume. With increased portal and diminished oncotic pressures, ascites forms by overflowing into the peritoneal cavity.[4] Support for this theory comes more from animal than human observations. In following the progression of cirrhosis and ascites formation in dogs, avid sodium retention occurred a few days before the first appearance of ascites.[7] Frequently, in patients with decompensated cirrhosis, activation of the renin-angiotensin-aldosterone and sympathetic nervous systems and nonosmotic release of vasopressin are observed. If overflow accounts for ascites, activation of these factors would be expected to be suppressed by hemodynamic regulatory processes. The differences in these two theories are depicted in Figure 16–1.

The peripheral arterial vasodilation theory,[8] combining many components of the underfill and overflow theories, has suggested the initial event of peripheral arterial vasodilation. Patients with severe cirrhosis are known to have peripheral vasodilation with increased cardiac output and lowered peripheral vascular resistance. Arteriovenous fistulas occur frequently in the skin, lungs, and muscle of cirrhotics, but increased

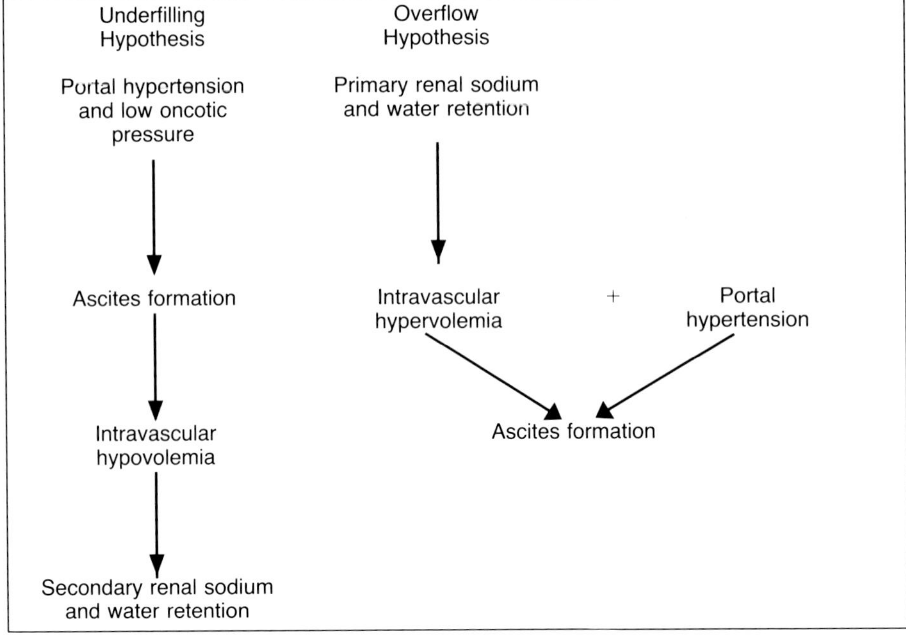

FIG. 16–1. Classic hypothesis for ascites formation.

splanchnic blood flow is the major contributor to arteriolar dilation. All other subsequent events—decreased effective blood volume, increased plasma renin, aldosterone, norepinephrine, and vasopressin concentrations and renal vasoconstriction with sodium retention—lead to plasma volume expansion (Fig. 16–2). This stage of cirrhosis is denoted as compensated. With more severe peripheral vasodilation, the compensatory hormonal responses are inadequate to normalize renal hemodynamics and sodium retention is maintained. In the presence of hypoalbuminemia, ascites formation is progressive.[8]

RATIONAL APPROACH TO TREATMENT

Patients with compensated cirrhosis may be avid sodium retainers.[9] As long as the dietary sodium exceeds the capability for sodium excretion, ascitic formation and weight gain continue; with sodium restriction, weight gain and ascitic formation cease.

The fluid overload condition of the cirrhotic patient with ascites differs considerably from that of the cardiac patient with congestive heart failure. With the former, rigid dietary sodium restriction (250 mg, or 10 mEq/day) is necessary, whereas the cardiac patient can easily sustain diuresis on 1000 to 1500 mg of sodium daily. It is extremely difficult, however, to maintain a sodium restriction of 10 to 20 mEq (250 to 500 mg) in the ambulatory or home environment. Liberalization to a 45- to 65-mEq (1000- to 1500-mg)

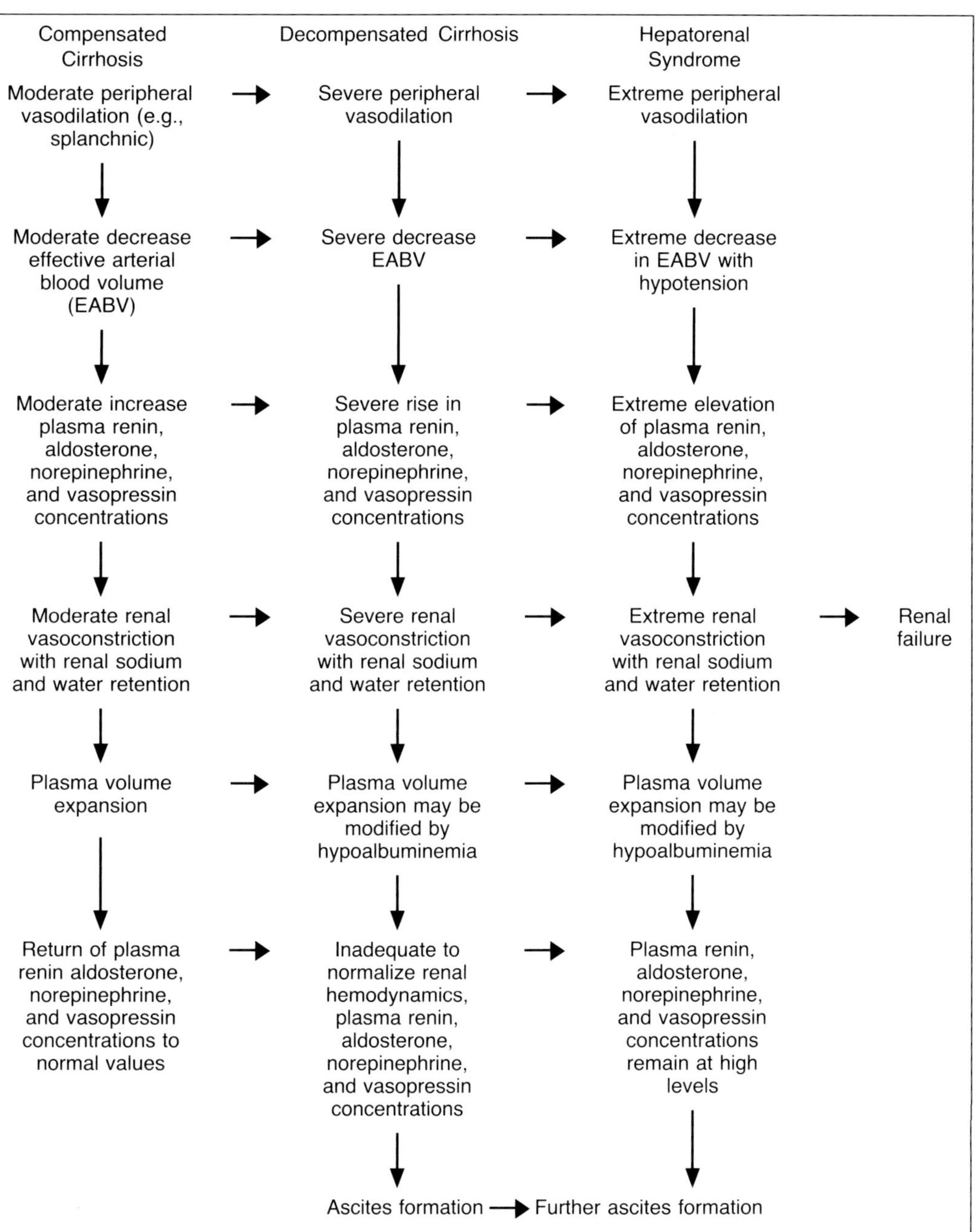

FIG. 16–2. Hypothesis for peripheral arterial vasodilation. (Adapted from Schrier RW, Arroyo V, Bernardi M, et al: Peripheral arterial vasodilation hypothesis: A proposal for the initiation of renal sodium and water retention in cirrhosis. Hepatology, 8:1151, 1988.)

sodium diet is often the compromise reached in office management of the cirrhotic with ascites. (For an example of a 1000-mg sodium diet, see Appendix.)

It is tempting to strive for rapid fluid and weight loss, knowing that up to 25 L of ascitic fluid or edema can be sequestered in the cirrhotic. Limitation of ascitic fluid absorption from the peritoneal cavity, however, prevents rapid weight loss; with spontaneous diuresis (bed rest and sodium restriction), the absorption of ascitic fluid averages 300 to 500 ml/day. If diuretics are used, reabsorption of 900 ml/day of ascitic fluid can be expected.[10] Thus, a steady weight loss of 1 to 2 kg daily is the maximal therapeutic outcome that might be expected. Weight loss more rapid than 2 kg/day can occur when edema is present and being mobilized; in the absence of edema, any excessive diuresis comes as a consequence of plasma volume contraction. In approximately 30% of patients with cirrhosis, spontaneous diuresis can be achieved with bed rest and dietary sodium restriction.[11] Such a conservative approach to the management of ascites could be used exclusively in up to 15% of patients.[12]

DIURETICS

Because continued bed rest at home is often impossible, given the need to maintain other functional activities, diuretic therapy is necessary in most patients. Whereas both proximal and distal renal tubular sodium reabsorption is increased, the more important process occurs in the distal site. A distally acting, potassium-sparing agent is the drug of choice. The potassium-sparing effect is desirable, because many cirrhotics are malnourished, with depleted potassium stores.[13] Also, with increased plasma aldosterone levels, potassium losses prior to diuretic therapy are likely to have occurred.

When a diuretic is used, spironolactone is the recommended agent. Spironolactone has two effects: (1) inhibition of aldosterone synthesis[14] and (2) blockade of the aldosterone effect on the distal renal tubule. Approximately 50% of patients respond to 100 to 200 mg daily. The action results in a mild natriuresis, which takes effect after 3 to 4 days. Patients with urine sodium-to-potassium ratios greater than 1 usually respond to this traditional dosage schedule.[15] When the urine sodium-to-potassium ratio is lower than 1, larger dosages are needed. Spironolactone can be given in the range of 300-600 mg daily; on occasion, up to 1000 mg daily may be used in refractory ascites to initiate a diuresis. The safety of these higher dosage levels has been established.[16]

The use of spironolactone rather than more powerful loop or distal tubular diuretics has clinical advantages. Although hyperaldosteronism is only one of many alterations that produce sodium retention, blocking the aldosterone effect or inhibiting its synthesis theoretically represents a physiologic approach to the management of ascites. The natriuresis induced by spironolactone is mild. Thus, this agent avoids rapid water and potassium loss at a critical time, when additional potassium loss from the already potassium-depleted state could induce cardiac arrhythmias. In avoiding rapid sodium and water loss from the use of loop diuretics, the tendency to deplete plasma volume and induce prerenal azotemia is lowered.

Occasional side effects, however, can occur. Spironolactone may cause uncomfortable gynecomastia, especially with protracted, high-dosage administration. Hyperkalemia may also develop in time, especially in those patients using potassium-containing salt substitutes. Rarely, hyperchloremic acidosis develops.

Some cirrhotics have impaired water excretion, secondary to increased plasma vasopressin activity and decreased delivery of filtrate to the distal tubular diluting sites (decreased glomerular filtration rate, GFR, and increased reabsorption of filtrate in the proximal tubule).[17,18] This impairment in diluting ability is clinically manifested by a decrease in the serum sodium concentration when diuresis is accomplished while allowing unlimited intake of water. A serum sodium level below 135 mEq/L indicates a dilutional hyponatremia and may exist even before diuretic therapy is initiated. If water restriction is not instituted at the start of diuretic therapy, a further decrease in the serum sodium concentration can be expected. Water intake should be restricted to 1000 to 1200 ml daily; if hyponatremia persists, diuretic therapy should be temporarily halted. The symptoms of hyponatremia—apathy, decreased mental concentration, anorexia, headache, and occasionally seizures—are similar to and may be confused with those of impending hepatic encephalopathy.

If weight loss and diuresis are not accomplished after reaching the maximal dosage level with spironolactone, furosemide, 40 to 80 mg/day, may be added. Incremental increases in furosemide administration, up to 240 mg/day, may be necessary. The potassium-wasting effects of this diuretic may counteract the potassium-sparing effect of the spironolactone. A cautionary reminder: whenever aggressive diuretic therapy is attempted, the BUN (blood urea nitrogen) and electrolyte levels should be monitored frequently to avoid prerenal azotemia, hyponatremia, and electrolyte imbalance.

If progressive weight loss (0.75 to 1.0 kg/day) has not been achieved after several weeks, especially with a cooperative patient who restricts sodium and water intake, a more direct approach to the removal of ascites should be considered. Formerly, large-volume abdominal paracentesis was not encouraged. Concern was expressed for various complications,[19] including a rapid depletion of plasma volume,[20] an accentuated reaccumulation of ascites,[10] and asymptomatic hyponatremia.[21]

The use of large-volume paracentesis has been re-examined. The removal of 4 to 6 L/day is rapidly effective in eliminating ascites, but hyponatremia or renal functional impairment occurs in 20% of patients. The intravenous infusion of 6 to 8 g albumin/L ascitic fluid removed during and after the paracentesis eliminated hyponatremia and impairment of renal function.[22] The complication rate of patients undergoing repeated large-volume paracentesis with intravenous albumin infusion is considerably lower (17%) as compared to patients receiving conventional diuretic treatment during hospitalization (61%).[23] Hospitalization stays were shorter—11 days—as compared to 31 days in the diuretic group.[23]

Although these studies were conducted on hospitalized patients, ambulatory, large-volume paracentesis may become acceptable in the future. Diuretic therapy and sodium and water restriction must then be instituted to prevent the reaccumulation of ascites.

SPONTANEOUS BACTERIAL PERITONITIS

A common complication of cirrhosis and ascites is spontaneous bacterial peritonitis (SBP). The "spontaneous" terminology for this infection indicates that an easily identifiable source for the bacterial contamination cannot be found. In cirrhotics, the incidence of spontaneous bacterial peritonitis outnumbers nonspontaneous peritonitis (i.e., ruptured viscus) by 9:1.[24] Ascites appears to be a critical component for the syndrome, because SBP is infrequently seen in the absence of fluid. This syndrome is not confined to the portal hypertension and ascites of alcoholic cirrhosis, but has been found in patients with cirrhosis of other causes.[24–26]

SOURCE OF BACTERIA

Because spontaneous bacterial peritonitis is not associated with an established infection elsewhere in the body, or with an easily recognizable intra-abdominal source, it may be supposed that the infection in the peritoneal fluid has arisen from a hematogenous source or from the transmural migration of organisms. Evidence for a hematogenous source has been supported by a prospective study of infections in 41 cirrhotics, in whom ascitic fluid and blood cultures were obtained simultaneously. Bacteria were isolated from systemic blood at three times the rate as from the ascitic fluid.[27] In normals, spontaneous bacteremia occurs frequently after relatively mild trauma. Portal bacteremia probably also occurs frequently, especially when mucosal integrity is disturbed following intestinal investigative procedures or gastrointestinal hemorrhage. It is conceivable that the congestive enteropathy of portal hypertension may alter mucosal integrity and allow the entrance of enteric bacteria into the portal vein. The normal liver, with a well-functioning reticuloendothelial (RE) system, clears a portal bacteremia. In the cirrhotic, phagocytic activity of the RE system is reduced;[28] those cirrhotics with the most severe reduction in RE function are most likely to acquire a systemic bacteremia. Also, in the cirrhotic liver, intrahepatic and extrahepatic portosystemic shunts may contribute to the frequency by which systemic bacteremia occurs. Intrahepatic (septal) shunts large enough (25 μm) to allow bacteria to pass through the liver have been described in two patients with SBP.[29] Blood-borne organisms could enter ascites by either of two ways: (1) by transfer from the sinusoids of the liver into hepatic lymph; or (2) across the capillary bed of the intestines, gaining access to the interstitial fluid of the intestinal wall. Evidence favoring the concept of organisms crossing the intestinal wall directly includes the demonstration of translocation from the lumen to the peritoneal cavity of radioactively labelled Escherichia coli.[30]

TABLE 16–1. BACTERIAL ISOLATES FROM ASCITIC FLUID

Bacteria	Number of Isolates	%
Escherichia coli	131	43
Klebsiella pneumoniae	26	8
Streptococcus pneumoniae	24	8
α-Hemolytic streptococcus	17	5
Group D streptococcus	17	5
Streptococcus, unclassified	13	4
β-Hemolytic streptoccus	12	4
Enterobacteriacae	8	3
Pseudomonas spp.	6	2
Staphylococcus aureus	5	2
Miscellaneous	48	16
Total	307	100

Data from Hoefs JC, Runyon BA: Spontaneous bacterial peritonitis. DM, 31:1, 1985.

Although a broad spectrum of organisms exists in the gastrointestinal tract, a single species is isolated in 90% of patients. Three-quarters of infections are caused by enteric organisms. Multiple organisms have occasionally been recovered (10% of cases), more noticably in patients receiving vasopressin infusions;[31] anaerobes are cultured in a small minority (6%) of cases.[32] Anaerobic growth may be inhibited by the relatively high P_{O_2} of ascitic fluid or by antibacterial properties directed toward gram-negative bacteria in general.[33] Bacterial isolates from ascitic fluid in 260 episodes of spontaneous bacterial peritonitis in 246 patients are listed in Table 16–1.

IMMUNOLOGIC DISTURBANCES IN CIRRHOTICS

The cirrhotic, particularly the alcoholic, has several defects in immunocompetence. The protein content of the ascitic fluid of cirrhosis tends to be low. Patients with an ascitic protein concentration lower than 1 g/dl are more likely to develop SBP than those whose protein concentration exceeds 1 g/dl.[34] Ascitic fluid "deficient" in opsonic activity is predisposed to becoming infected.[35] Complement activity and immunoglobulin and fibronectin levels are decreased in the ascitic fluid of cirrhotics compared to those in ascitic fluid of noncirrhotic cause.[36,37] Although infection does not increase opsonic activity, diuresis does result in a twofold increase in protein concentration and a tenfold increase in opsonic activity; C3, C4, and total hemolytic complement activity also increase.[38]

Multiple defects in cellular immune function in cirrhotics have been described. Inhibitors to leukocyte chemotaxis have been found by several investigators.[39–41] Multiple, serum-dependent defects in leukocytic ingestion and subsequent oxygen-dependent bactericidal metabolic events, although found most frequently in alcoholic-related cirrhosis, are also seen occasionally with cryptogenic cirrhosis.[42] In general, cirrhotics have an increased tendency for bacterial infections elsewhere, other than in the peritoneum. The incidence of bacterial endocarditis is two to three times higher in the cirrhotic than in the noncirrhotic.[43] Spontaneous bacterial empyema, meningitis, arthritis, and pericarditis have all been reported. The multiplicity of immune dysfunctional activities may also be responsible for these infectious complications.

CLINICAL FEATURES

Fever, abdominal pain, and tenderness should always alert the physician to the possibility of SBP. Deteriorating renal function, worsening liver failure, or the progression of encephalopathy may indicate the infection. Nausea, vomiting, and diarrhea are common complaints. Up to one-third of patients, however, may have no symptoms at all.

When any of these signs or symptoms develop in a previously stable patient with ascites, a diagnostic paracentesis is indicated. The risk of complications is low. Although the main concern is bleeding from coagulopathy, the risk of bleeding from paracentesis is lower than 1%. In the experience of one large center, prophylactic transfusion of fresh-frozen plasma or platelets has never been considered.[44] Needle perforation of the bowel occurs even less commonly (0.6%) than bleeding.[45]

Cell counts and bacterial culture are the two most important tests for confirming the diagnosis. An elevated polymorphonuclear (PMN) cell count (PMN > 250/mm^3) and a positive culture are sufficient for establishing the diagnosis. Occasionally, a high cell count and a negative culture ("neutrocytic" ascites) are seen; treatment is warranted, because the cell count rapidly decreases following the administration of antibiotics.[46] Despite numerous reports attesting to the usefulness of measuring the ascitic fluid pH or lactate level, and of determining the arterial blood-ascites lactate level or pH gradient, the sensitivity of a cell count greater than 250/mm^3 (87%) is better than other proposed tests.[47] The culture yield can be improved by inoculating blood culture bottles[48] or by centrifuging the ascitic fluid and culturing the pellet.[47]

TREATMENT

Unless treated, most patients with SBP die. The inpatient mortality rate of cirrhotic patients with the initial episode of SBP has been estimated as between 30 and 50%.[49,50] Antibiotic therapy must consider several goals—broad-spectrum coverage, with achievable ascitic fluid drug levels, and the avoidance of renal toxicity and superinfections. Presently, intravenous administration of antibiotics is the recommended therapy. Third-generation cephalosporin appears to be safer, with improved efficacy (19 of 22 patients cured), as compared to a group of patients receiving ampicillin and an aminoglycoside (11 of 18 cured).[51] Cefotaxime,

2 g IV every 4 to 8 hours, depending on renal function, is the drug of choice. Even after cure, the probability of a recurrent infection has been estimated as 69%.[49] In one study, the use of a fluoroquinolone reduced the incidence of reinfection from 33 to 12% during the 6 months following the initial infection.[52] One study has suggested that SBP can be treated in an ambulatory setting using a combination of a quinolone antibiotic with trimethoprim-sulfomethoxazole, amoxicillin, or metronidozole.[53] Further studies are necessary before uniformly adopting this therapeutic program.

Aminoglycosides should be avoided, when possible, because cirrhotics with ascites are particularly susceptible to nephrotoxicity.[54] Although a diagnostic paracentesis can be done on an outpatient basis, antibiotic therapy is usually administered intravenously in an inpatient setting. Many of these patients are severely ill, with decompensating liver and/or renal function, so additional therapeutic and care programs can be instituted at the same time. Indicators of a poor outcome (91% mortality) for patients with SBP include the following: hyperbilirubinemia greater than 8 g/dl, creatinine greater than 2.1 mg/dl.[45] Even if patients survive the hospitalization, the mortality in the following 12 months has been estimated as 60 to 80%. This outcome is more reflective of the severe hepatocellular dysfunction (44% of deaths secondary to liver failure), even though a significant number of deaths have occurred with recurrence of SBP (33%).[48]

HEPATIC ENCEPHALOPATHY

Hepatic encephalopathy (HE) is a reversible, altered state of consciousness with neurologic symptoms and signs. It is seen with both acute and chronic hepatic failure.

Increasing signs of neural inhibition characterize the progressive clinical spectrum of coma. A rapid, progressive loss of neural function occurs with acute fulminant hepatic failure when the hepatic metabolic function is being destroyed. Hepatic encephalopathy occurs in cirrhotics and is known as portal-systemic encephalopathy when significant shunting of portal blood bypasses the hepatic sinusoids, thus reducing the hepatic extraction of nitrogenous substances. Shunts occur naturally with the progression of cirrhosis, or may be synthetic. The varying patterns of neural abnormalities are thought to result from the impaired hepatic metabolism of nitrogenous products delivered to the liver from digestive and absorptive activity in the intestine and colon.

MANIFESTATIONS

Depending on the type and progression of liver failure, the syndrome can be considered as acute, subacute, chronic, or even episodic. Most commonly recognized, the episodic nature of the syndrome occurs in decompensated cirrhotics as gastrointestinal bleeding suddenly delivers a high digestible protein load to the intestines. The patient rapidly pro-

TABLE 16–2. GRADING SYSTEM FOR HEPATIC ENCEPHALOPATHY

Grade of Encephalopathy	Level of Consciousness	Intellectual Function	Neurologic Abnormalities
0	Normal	Normal	None
1	Trivial lack of awareness; personality change; day-night reversal	Short attention span; easy forgetfulness	Slight tremor; uncoordination; asterixis
2	Lethargic; inappropriate behavior	Loss of orientation	Asterixis; abnormal reflexes
3	Asleep but rousable; confused when awake	Loss of ability to calculate; loss of meaningful communication	Asterixis; abnormal reflexes
4	Unrousable	Absent	Babinski response; decerebrate; pupillary responses preserved

gresses through the phases of hepatic coma (Table 16–2). Often, the onset or episodic intensification of HE is related to a precipitating cause. On these occasions, correction of the precipitating cause is the only form of therapy necessary.

In the chronic form, the manifestations are more of a psychiatric nature, including mild impairment of intellectual ability, deterioration of job function, personality change, and short attention span. Neurologic examination at this time may be normal, or may demonstrate mild incoordination. Determining the neuropsychiatric deficits accurately allows for comparisons to be made in optimizing therapy.

TREATMENT

The first responsibility of the physician is to reverse those conditions that induced the HE. Iatrogenic causes can be found, such as the prescribing of hypnotics or sedatives. Using a sedative when the patient is irritable or disruptive only results in advancement of the neurologic disturbance. Allowing a patient to become constipated contributes to an increase in amine absorption from the colon and induction of the syndrome. An asymptomatic urinary tract infection with urea-splitting organisms allows the absorption or return of ammonia into the systemic circulation, thus increasing the demand on hepatic urea synthesis. With the vigorous use of

TABLE 16–3. COMMON PRECIPITATING FACTORS IN HEPATIC COMA
Drugs, especially tranquilizers and sedatives
Gastrointestinal bleeding
Azotemia
Hypokalemia
Constipation
Diuretics, metabolic alkalosis
Anesthesia
Hypoxia
Infections, especially urinary tract

diuretics, contraction of extracellular volume, induction of hypokalemia, and alkalosis increase ammonia production by the kidney and drive un-ionized extracellular ammonia into the cells, especially neurons. Other commonly encountered precipitating factors are listed in Table 16–3.

After reversible causes have been identified and corrected, attempts to reduce the arterial ammonia level are instituted. Withdrawal of all dietary protein and removal of blood and protein from the digestive system constitute first-line efforts. If blood is present in the stomach from a recent variceal or gastric bleed, the insertion of a nasogastric tube and removal and lavage of the gastric contents prevent further protein digestion. Instilling a cathartic, such as the nonabsorbable carbohydrate lactulose, quickly induces diarrhea. Metabolism of this sugar by colonic bacteria generates hydrogen ions, which reduces the pH of the colonic fluid and causes additional ammonia to be trapped within the lumen of the colon, thus preventing absorption. Other possible mechanisms for the effectiveness of lactulose in treating hepatic coma is a decreased production or uptake of ammonia by colonic bacteria. Lactulose can be continued during the chronic phase, using a sufficient amount (30 to 60 ml PO) each day to keep stools frequent and loose.

Prior to the discovery of lactulose, poorly absorbed antibiotics, such as neomycin, were used to decrease ammonia and amine production in the colon. Neomycin actually inhibits those bacteria (enterobacteria, enterococci, and staphylococci) that are poor degraders of lactulose, rather than anaerobic bacteria, which effectively metabolize lactulose. It has been found that the combination of lactulose and neomycin can be additive in the treatment of HE.[55]

On recovery from the severe phases of hepatic coma, the absolute dietary protein restriction can be lifted. Usually, a protein intake between 40 and 80 g daily can be tolerated. The source of protein is important in determining the amount that can be consumed safely; larger amounts of vegetable protein can be consumed than meat protein before changes in mental status occur.[56] By working closely with a dietician, and by having the patient keep an occasional 3-day food diary, the physician can fine-tune the eating behavior of the patient. Often, the physician balances a program by adjusting the level of protein intake and the amount of lactulose necessary to maintain stability. Because increased levels of "false neurotransmitters" might be involved in the development of hepatic coma, and an imbalance of plasma branched-chain amino acids or aromatic amino acids contribute to the production of false neurotransmitters, formulations designed to increase plasma branched-chain amino acid concentrations were developed. A review of published studies has failed, however, to show any benefit from branched-chain amino acid supplementation in patients with acute, subacute, or chronic forms of hepatic encephalopathy.[57]

APPENDIX 1000-MG SODIUM DIET PLAN

Food		Sodium Content (approx.; in mg)
Breakfast		
1 cup milk		120
¾ cup shredded wheat cereal		2
Banana		1
4 oz orange juice		1
8 oz coffee		7
1 slice toast		123
1 tsp unsalted margarine		5
Lunch		
2 slices bread		246
3 oz unsalted meat (e.g., roast beef)		48–75
½ oz unsalted mayonnaise		5
Fresh apple		1
½ cup milk		60
1 cup mixed green salad		5
Unsalted oil and vinegar dressing		tr
Tea		0
Dinner		
3 oz. unsalted meat, fish (e.g., haddock) or poultry		51–75
Baked potato		16
½ cup unsalted green beans		11
1 slice bread		123
3 tsp unsalted margarine		15
½ cup sherbet or gelatin		25–54
½ cup milk		60
Tea		0
Snacks		
Fruit cocktail		7
Cola drink, 12 oz		14
	Total sodium:	946–1,026 mg

REFERENCES

1. Rocco VK, Ware A: Cirrhotic ascites: Pathophysiology, diagnosis and management. Ann Intern Med, 105:513, 1986.
2. Perera GA: The plasma volume in Laennec's cirrhosis of the liver. Ann Intern Med, 24:643, 1946.
3. Eisenberg S: Blood volume in patients with Laennec's cirrhosis of the liver as determined by radioactive chromium-tagged red cells. Am J Med, 20:189, 1956.
4. Lieberman FL, Ito S, Reynolds TB: Effective plasma volume in cirrhosis with ascites: Evidence that a decreased volume does not account for renal sodium retention, a spontaneous reduction in glomerular filtration rate (GFR) and a fall in GFR during drug-induced diuresis. J Clin Invest, 48:975, 1969.
5. Tristani FE, Cohn JN: Systemic and renal hemodynamics in oliguric hepatic failure: Effect of volume expansion. J Clin Invest, 46:1894, 1987.
6. Bosch J, Arroyo V, Betrin A: Hepatic hemodynamics and the renin-angiotensin-aldosterone system in cirrhosis. Gastroenterology, 78:72, 1980.
7. Levy M: Sodium retention and ascites formation in dogs with experimental cirrhosis. Am J Physiol, 238(F):353, 1977.
8. Schrier RW, Arroyo V, Bernardi M, et al: Peripheral arterial vasodilation hypothesis: A proposal for the initiation of renal sodium and water retention in cirrhosis. Hepatology, 8:1151, 1988.
9. Naccarato R, Messa P, D'Angelo A, et al: Renal handling of sodium and water in early chronic liver disease. Evidence for a reduced natriuretic activity of the cirrhotic urinary extracts in rats. Gastroenterology, 81:205, 1981.
10. Shear L, Ching S, Gabuzda GJ: Compartmentalization of ascites and edema in patients with hepatic cirrhosis. N Engl J Med, 282:1391, 1970.
11. Bosch J, Arroyo V, Rodes J, et al: Compensación espontanea de la ascites en la cirrhosis hepatica. Rev Clin Esp, 133:441, 1974.
12. Linas SI, Anderson RJ, Miller PD, Sabirer RW: The rational use of diuretics in cirrhosis. *In* The Kidney in Liver Disease. 2nd Ed. Edited by MD Epstein. New York, Elsevier, pp 555–567, 1983.
13. Podolsky S, Zimmerman HJ, Burrows BA, et al: Potassium depletion in cirrhosis: Impaired growth-hormone and insulin response. N Engl J Med, 288:644, 1973.
14. Conn JW, Hinerman DJ: Spironolactone-induced inhibition of aldosterone biosynthesis in primary aldosteronism. Morphological and functional studies. Metabolism, 26:1293, 1977.
15. Eggert RC: Spironolactone diuresis in patients with cirrhosis and ascites. Br Med J, 4:401, 1970.
16. Campra JL, Reynolds TB: Effectiveness of high-dose spironolactone therapy in patients with chronic liver disease and relatively refractory ascites. Am J Dig Dis, 23:1025, 1978.
17. Epstein M (ed): The Kidney in Liver Disease. 2nd Ed. New York, Elsevier, pp 35–53.
18. Chiandusi L, Bartoli E, Arras S: Reabsorption of sodium in the proximal renal tubule in cirrhosis of the liver. Gut, 19:497, 1978.
19. Liebowitz HR: Hazards of abdominal paracentesis in the cirrhotic patient (Part III). NY State J Med, 62:2223, 1962.
20. Knauer CM, Lowe HM: Hemodynamics in the cirrhotic patient during paracentesis. N Engl J Med, 276:491, 1967.
21. Nelson WP, Rosenbaum JD, Strauss MB: Hyponatremia in hepatic cirrhosis following paracentesis. J Clin Invest, 30:738, 1951.
22. Titó L, Ginès P, Arroyo V, et al: Total paracentesis associated with intravenous albumin management of patients with cirrhosis and ascites. Gastroenterology, 98:146, 1990.
23. Ginès P, Arroyo V, Quintero E, et al: Comparison between paracentesis and diuretics in the treatment of cirrhotics with tense ascites. Gastroenterology, 93:234, 1987.
24. Conn HO: Cirrhosis in Diseases of the Liver. 5th Ed. Edited by L Schiff and ER Schiff. Philadelphia, JB Lippincott, 1982. p 951.

25. Epstein M, Calia FM, Gabuzda GJ: Pneumococcal peritonitis in patients with postnecrotic cirrhosis. N Engl J Med, 278:69, 1968.
26. Pinzello G, Simonetti R, Craxi A, et al: Spontaneous bacterial peritonitis: A prospective investigation in predominantly nonalcoholic cirrhotic patients. Hepatology, 3:545, 1983.
27. Rimola A, Bovy F, Teres J: Oral nonabsorbable antibiotics prevent infection in cirrhotics with gastrointestinal hemorrhage. Hepatology, 5:463, 1985.
28. Rimola A, Soto R, Borg F, et al: Reticuloendothelial system phagocytic activity in cirrhosis and its relation to bacterial infections and prognosis. Hepatology, 4:53, 1984.
29. Hoefs JC, Reynolds TB, Sakimura I, et al: A new method for the measurement of intrahepatic shunts. J Lab Clin Med, 103:446, 1984.
30. Schweinberg FB, Seligman AM, Fine J: Transmural migration of intestinal bacteria: A study based on the case of radioactive Escherichia coli. N Engl J Med, 242:747, 1950.
31. Bar-Meir S, Conn HO: Spontaneous bacterial peritonitis induced by intra-arterial vasopressin therapy. Gastroenterology, 70:418, 1976.
32. Targan SR, Chow AW, Guze LB: Role of anaerobic bacteria in spontaneous peritonitis of cirrhosis. Report of two cases and review of the literature. Am J Med, 27:364, 1977.
33. Fromkes JJ, Thomas FB, Mekhjian HS, Evans M: Antimicrobial activity of human ascitic fluid. Gastroenterology, 73:668, 1977.
34. Runyon BA: Low-protein-concentration ascitic fluid is presdisposed to spontaneous bacterial peritonitis. Gastroenterology, 91:1343, 1986.
35. Runyon BA: Patients with deficient ascitic fluid opsonic activity are predisposed to spontaneous bacterial peritonitis. Hepatology, 8:632, 1988.
36. Runyon BA, Morrissey R, Hoefs JC, et al: Opsonic activity of human ascitic fluid: A potentially important protective mechanism against spontaneous bacterial peritonitis. Hepatology, 5:634, 1985.
37. Simberkoff MS, Moldover NH, Weiss G: Bactericidal and opsonic activity of cirrhotic ascites and nonascitic peritoneal fluid. J Lab Clin Med, 91:831, 1978.
38. Runyon BA, Van Epps DE: Diuresis of cirrhotic ascites increases its opsonic activity and may help prevent spontaneous bacterial peritonitis. Hepatology, 6:396, 1986.
39. Van Epps DE, Strickland RJ, Williams RC: Inhibitors of leukocyte chemotaxis in alcoholic liver disease. Am J Med, 59:200, 1975.
40. Maderazo EG, Ward PH, Quintiliani R: Defective regulation of chemotaxis in cirrhosis. J Lab Clin Med, 85:621, 1975.
41. DeMeo AN, Andersen BR: Defective chemotaxis associated with a serum inhibitor in cirrhotic patients. N Engl J Med, 266:735, 1972.
42. Feliu E, Gougerot M, Hakim J, et al: Blood polymorphonuclear dysfunction in patients with alcoholic cirrhosis. Eur J Clin Invest, 7:571, 1977.
43. Snyder N, Atterbury CE, Correia JP, Conn HO: Increased occurrence of cirrhosis and bacterial endocarditis, a clinical and postmortem study. Gastroenterology, 73:1107, 1977.
44. Runyon BA: Paracentesis of ascitic fluid: A safe procedure. Arch Intern Med, 146:2259, 1986.
45. Hoefs JC, Runyon BA: Spontaneous bacterial peritonitis. DM, 31:1, 1985.
46. Runyon BA, Hoefs JC: Culture-negative neutrocytic ascites: A variant of spontaneous bacterial peritonitis? Hepatology, 4:1209, 1984.
47. Wright TS, Boyer TD: Diagnosis and management of cirrhotic ascites. *In* Hepatology: A Textbook of Liver Disease. 2nd Ed. Edited by D Zakim and TD Boyer. Philadelphia, WB Saunders, 1990, p 616–634.
48. Runyon BA, Umland ET, Merlin T: Inoculation of blood culture bottles with ascitic fluid: Improved detection of spontaneous bacterial peritonitis. Arch Intern Med, 147:73, 1987.
49. Titó L, Rimola A, Ginès P, et al: Recurrence of spontaneous bacterial peritonitis in cirrhosis frequency and predictive factors. Hepatology, 8:27, 1988.
50. Runyon BA: Spontaneous bacterial peritonitis: An explosion of information. Hepatology, 8:171, 1988.

51. Felisart J, Rimola A, Arroyo V, et al: Cefotaxime is more effective than is ampicillin-tobramycin in cirrhotics with severe infections. Hepatology, 5:457, 1985.
52. Gines P, Rimola A, Planas, R, et al: Norfloxacin prevents spontaneous bacterial peritonitis recurrence in cirrhosis: Results of a double-blind, placebo-controlled trial. Hepatology, 12:716, 1990.
53. Silvain C, Breux JP, Grollier G, et al: Les septicemies et les infections du liquide d'ascite du cirrhotique peuvant-elles etre traitées exclusivement par voie orale? Gastroenterol Clin Biol, 13:335, 1989.
54. Cabrera J, Arroyo V, Ballesta AM, et al: Aminoglycoside nephrotoxicity in cirrhosis: Value of urinary B_2-microglobulin to discriminate functional renal failure from acute tubular damage. Gastroenterology, 82:97, 1982.
55. Pirotte G, Guffens JM, Devos J: Comparative study of basal arterial ammonemia and of orally induced hyperammonemia in chronic portal systemic encephalopathy, treated with neomycin, lactulose, and an association of neomycin and lactulose. Digestion, 10:435, 1974.
56. Greenberger NJ, Carley J, Schenker S, et al: Effect of vegetable and animal protein diets in chronic hepatic encephalopathy. Am J Dig Dis, 22:845, 1977.
57. Eriksson LS, Conn HO: Branched-chain amino acids in the management of hepatic encephalopathy: An analysis of variants. Hepatology, 10:228, 1989.

chapter

17

HEPATITIS IMMUNOPROPHYLAXIS

Steven Yu Villanueva
Kevin V. Carey

HEPATITIS A

The hepatitis A virus (HAV) is a small, spherical, nonenveloped, 27-nm, RNA-containing virus belonging to the picornavirus family.

TRANSMISSION AND RISK FACTORS

Viral A hepatitis (formerly called infectious hepatitis, short-incubation hepatitis) is highly contagious. It is spread by the fecal-oral route. Exposure to infected stool is necessary for transmission to occur. Transmission is facilitated by poor personal hygiene, poor sanitation, intimate (household or sexual) contact, and overcrowding.[1–4] Exposure may be direct (person-to-person exposure) or indirect through the ingestion of contaminated food or water (common source exposure).

It is not associated with a carrier state and, therefore, relies on person-to-person spread to continue. HAV infection does not result in chronic liver disease, including cirrhosis or hepatocellular carcinoma. Although hepatitis A does not lead to chronicity, it is a cause of significant morbidity and loss of productivity, accounting for 25% of cases of clinical hepatitis in developed countries.[2] The disease is self-limited. Fatalities in the acute icteric form are exceedingly rare (0.6%).[1] Occasionally, a prolonged cholestasis may complicate the picture but this, too, resolves within 2 to 4 months.

Fecal viral shedding is maximal 1 to 2 weeks prior to the onset of jaundice. Once jaundice occurs, viral excretion declines rapidly. Patients sick enough to be hospitalized for viral A hepatitis are usually not infectious, because viral excretion is absent or minimal once symptoms occur. Patients are usually hospitalized because of protracted vomiting, coagulation abnormalities, or development of fulminant hepatic failure.

Approximately 10 to 20% of Americans have antibody against HAV (anti-HAV) by the age of 20 and 50% by the age of 50,[3] yet most do not recall an episode of jaundice.

Although diminishing in importance in developed countries, specific risks in the United States associated with HAV infection include contact with another person with hepatitis (26%), male homosexuality (15%), foreign travel (14%), contact with children attending a day care center (11%), and illicit drug use (10%). In many cases (40%), no specific risk factors have been identified.[3] Post-transfusion HA infection is rare because of the limited duration of HA viremia. The prevalence of type A hepatitis is not increased among health care workers, but outbreaks in hospital nurseries have been reported.

Day care centers contribute to a significant proportion of HAV outbreaks. Infants are ideal hosts for enteric pathogens and may serve as silent vectors of HAV infection.[4] Lack of toilet training, oral behavior, and poor hygiene[3,4] lead to enhanced transmission of HAV. Infected children often transmit the virus to older siblings and parents. Characteristically, infected children of primary and nursery school age have a mild infection, whereas affected adults (parents, older siblings, day care workers) are symptomatic.

Immune Globulin

Immune globulin (IG) (formerly called immune serum globulin or gamma globulin; Gamastan, Gammar) is a sterile protein solution of antibodies obtained from pooled human plasma that is negative for hepatitis B surface antigen (HBsAg). The process of cold ethanol fractionation, in use since World War II, produces a richer gamma globulin fraction[6] and also denatures viral particles, including those of the human immunodeficiency virus (HIV). The administration of IG has not been reported to lead to the development of acquired immunodeficiency syndrome (AIDS).

IG has been known for over 40 years to provide protection against hepatitis A. It is most effective when given early. It has an efficacy of 87% in preventing symptomatic hepatitis if administered within 2 weeks of exposure.[7]

Passive Active Immunization

The ability of IG to prevent the development of clinically significant hepatitis is probably a result of the phenomenon of passive active immunization. The intramuscular administration of IG transfers antibodies, which modifies the acute disease to a more benign form. At the same time, the resultant subclinical infection actively stimulates antibody production, thus conferring lifelong protection against HAV.[4]

Pre-Exposure Prophylaxis. For travelers, a single dose of IG, 0.02 ml/kg, is recommended if travel to developing countries is for less than 2 months. For prolonged travel, 0.06 ml/kg should be given every 5 months. Pre-exposure prophylaxis is also advised for travelers who eat in settings with poor sanitary conditions.[1] For individuals who require repeated IG prophylaxis, screening for total anti-HAV before IG administration is cost-effective and helps eliminate unnecessary immunization in those who have natural immunity against HAV.

Animal handlers who work with higher apes (chimpanzees, gorillas, orangutans, gibbons) should receive 3 to 5 ml IG every 4 to 6 months.[8]

Post-Exposure Prophylaxis. Transmission of HAV is not common to casual contacts of a single case in schools, offices, factories, and hospitals. IG is not recommended in these settings unless an epidemic develops. It is not recommended that IG be administered routinely in common source outbreaks, especially after clinical hepatitis has appeared in the exposed individual, because the 2-week period during which IG is effective has usually elapsed (Table 17–1).

Postexposure prophylaxis of type A hepatitis after identification of an index case requires that IG be given intramuscularly in a dose of 0.02 ml/kg. Serologic testing for index cases suspected of having acute hepatitis A is recommended, because only 38% of cases of acute hepatitis in the United States are caused by HAV. Contacts of index cases need not await serologic testing, however, because it is not cost-effective and only delays prompt administration of IG.

Vaccines

Vaccines against HAV, including inactivated, whole virus vaccine, analogous to the Salk polio vaccine, and live, attenuated vaccine, analogous to the Sabin oral polio vaccine, although actively being developed,[9] are presently unavailable for clinical use. A safe and effective vaccine can be useful in preventing HAV infection in those in high-risk groups. These include children attending day care centers, overseas travelers, homosexual men, military population, and institutionalized individuals.[3]

HEPATITIS B

Worldwide, about 200 million people are carriers of hepatitis B virus (HBV).[10] The total number of those with HBV infection in the United States is estimated to be 300,000 annually, with approximately 75,000 (25%) of those infected actually developing acute hepatitis.[1]

Of these individuals, 6 to 10% become HBV carriers at risk for developing chronic liver disease, including cirrhosis and hepatocellular carcinoma.[1] A large reservoir of potentially infectious patients exists. Up to 1 million HBV carriers may be in the United States alone.[11] HBV is not directly cytopathic. Interactions between HBV and the host's immune system are important in determining the outcome in HBV infection.[12]

TABLE 17–1. POSTEXPOSURE PROPHYLAXIS OF TYPE A HEPATITIS: SPECIFIC

Nature of Exposure	Immune Globulin (0.02 mg/kg)
Close personal contacts, day care centers	All household and sexual contacts; all staff and attendees if one or more cases are recognized among children or employees, or cases are recognized in two or more households of center attendees
Schools	Routine use not indicated; only those who have close personal contact with patients in a school- or classroom-centered outbreak
Institutions for custodial care	Residents and staff with close contact with patients with hepatitis A
Hospitals	Routine use not indicated except in outbreaks, persons exposed to infective feces
Offices and factories	Routine use not indicated
Common source exposure	Patrons if infected person is directly involved in handling of foods that are not to be cooked before they are eaten, poor hygiene of food handlers, identified within 2 weeks of exposure

From the Centers for Disease Control: Recommendations for protection against viral hepatitis. MMWR, 34:313, 1985.

TRANSMISSION AND RISK FACTORS

Perinatal Transmission

Perinatal hepatitis B deserves important consideration in the context of hepatitis B immunoprophylaxis for several reasons. First, most infants exposed to HBsAg infection in the perinatal period become chronic carriers.[13] Second, hepatic malignancy can occur. The relative risk of developing hepatocellular carcinoma is 100 times greater in an HBV carrier.[14] Third, perinatal hepatitis B is preventable through the timely use of hepatitis B immune globulin (HBIG) and hepatitis B vaccine.[15]

Prophylaxis against HBV in the newborn is effective because infants acquire HBV infection at or near the time of delivery, and not in utero. Administration of HBIG and of hepatitis B vaccine within 12 hours of delivery reduces the carrier rate from an expected 70 to 90% to only 5 to 10%, for an efficacy rate of 85 to 95%.[15]

It is recommended that infants born to mothers who are HBsAg-positive be given HBIG within 12 hours of birth. The first dose of vaccine should also be given within that time, but at a different site.

Role of HBeAg

The degree of infectivity is modified by the presence of hepatitis B e antigen (HBeAg) or its antibody (anti-HBe). Approximately 95% of the offspring of an HBeAg-positive mother are infected during the perinatal period,[16] and 90% eventually progress to chronicity.[17] It is estimated that more than 25% of these carriers die from hepatocellular carcinoma or cirrhosis. The rate of perinatal transmission of HBV is between 0 and 12% if the mother is anti-HBe–positive.[11]

The importance of starting effective immunoprophylaxis underscores the need for proper identification of infants at risk of perinatal hepatitis B. Serologic screening for HBsAg can identify mothers who may transmit HBV to the infant.

Prenatal Screening

In the past, the Advisory Committee on Immunization Practices (ACIP) recommended that HBsAg screening be limited to women in specified high-risk categories (i.e., women of Asian, Pacific Island, or Alaskan Eskimo descent, whether immigrants or born in the United States). It was thought that 80 to 90% of infants at risk could be identified and effective prophylaxis instituted. Problems were encountered, however, in the implementation of limited prenatal screening of pregnant women for HBsAg. For example, following previous ACIP guidelines, it was found that only 35 to 65% of HBsAg-positive mothers would have been identified. In addition, persons providing health care to pregnant women were often not aware of the risks of perinatal transmission of HBV and of the recommended screening and treatment guidelines.[19]

HBsAg screening has been broadened to include all pregnant women. It is the only strategy that provides acceptable control of perinatal HBV transmission. In the United States, screening approximately 3.5 million pregnant women annually for HBsAg would identify 16,000 HBsAg-positive mothers and allow treatment to prevent HBV infection.[19]

It is recommended that HBsAg screening be routinely carried out during early prenatal visits.

Health Care Workers and HBV Infection

It has been established that health care personnel are at an increased risk of developing viral hepatitis, especially hepatitis B. Exposure to HBV is common for the hospital worker. About 1% of patients admitted to the hospital carry the virus.[20] In the health care setting, HBV may be transmitted by percutaneous inoculation or by contact of an open wound, nonintact skin, or mucous membranes to blood or blood contaminated body fluids.[21]

Blood is the most important source of HBV in this context. It has been established that blood contact, rather than patient contact, is associated with an increased prevalence of HBV markers.[22] Of those who receive a needle stick exposure from HBsAg-positive individuals, 6 to 30% become infected.[21] This is not surprising, because serum positive for HBsAg diluted to 10^8 is still infective.[23]

It is estimated that 12,000 health care workers become infected with HBV annually that 700 to 1,200 of those infected become HBV carriers, and that 10 to 30% of health care personnel show evidence of past or present HBV infection.[21] In a survey of 434 oral surgeons, 26% demonstrated serologic evidence of past or current infection with HBV.[24]

Although most health care workers tend to focus on the icteric patient, all patients should be assumed to be infective for HBV and other blood-borne contaminants. Universal blood and body fluid precautions should be observed.

Vaccines

Plasma-Derived Vaccine. Plasma-derived vaccine to prevent hepatitis B was introduced in 1982. It is safe, effective, and immunogenic.

The first-generation vaccine was derived from the plasma of persons with the same risk behaviors as those affected with AIDS. The plasma undergoes ultracentrifugation and is further processed through three inactivation steps using pepsin, urea, and formalin. This inactivation process renders the plasma free of viral contaminants, including HIV.

No serious, adverse side effects have been associated with the use of the plasma-derived hepatitis vaccine. Introduction of the vaccine coincided with growing awareness regarding AIDS, and acceptance of the vaccine may have been lukewarm because of this concern.

Recombinant Vaccine. The recombinant hepatitis B vaccine is the first recombinant-derived human vaccine ever made available for use. It is the first medical product derived from common bakers' yeast (Saccharomyces cerevisiae).[25] By recombinant DNA technology, HBsAg is expressed within yeast cells. The recombinant vaccine is highly immunogenic. It was licensed for use by the FDA in 1986.

No apparent difference has been seen in the immune response to plasma-derived and recombinant vaccine. The antibody response seems to be directed against a common determinant that is present in both vaccines. They can be used interchangeably during the course of vaccination, except for hemodialysis patients, in whom the present formulation of recombinant vaccine entails using a larger volume (4.0 ml) and more aluminum hydroxide (2.0 mg) than currently recommended as adjuvant in vaccines. Both plasma-derived and recombinant vaccines stimulate active antibody production against HBV infection, and provide protection against HBV for several years.

Intradermal Hepatitis B Vaccination. In the United States, a complete course of three intramuscular injections of hepatitis B vaccine for an adult costs about $100 to 130. The expense of plasma-derived and recombinant vaccine has prompted re-evaluation of the use of intradermal vaccination against HBV.

It is important that inoculation be intradermal and not subcutaneous because of inadequate antibody response in the latter. Seroconversion following inoculation is slower compared to intramuscular injection, and antibody titers are relatively lower. Despite these disadvantages, the intradermal approach remains a valid option in making extensive vaccination cost-effective. Intradermal inoculation allows dosage reduction to 10% of the intramuscular dose.[26]

Low Impact of Hepatitis B Vaccination on Incidence. In spite of the hepatitis B vaccine being available since 1982, it has had little or no impact on the incidence of HBV in the United States. Only 36% of the identified high-risk population have been vaccinated.[27] The reasons are varied. First, it is expensive. Second, it requires multiple injections several months apart. Third, the medical profession is not well informed about the indications for hepatitis B vaccine. Lastly, persistent although unfounded doubts exist among the poorly informed about the safety of the vaccine, especially in regard to HIV transmission.[28]

During the 5-year period following introduction of the plasma-derived vaccine, vaccine use centered primarily on the following: (1) persons who work in the health care professions; (2) staff and clients of institutions for the developmentally disabled; and (3) staff and patients of hemodialysis units. The vaccination programs have failed to reach those in other high-risk groups, however, including parenteral drug abusers, homosexual men, and homosexually active persons with multiple sexual partners.[27] Since 1985, though, a 52% decrease has been noted in the number of HBV cases in homosexual men, attributable to modifications of high-risk sexual behaviors that led to HIV infection.[29]

Low Responders and Nonresponders. An individual with a peak anti-HBs level less than or equal to 10 mIU/ml,* after a full course of hepatitis B vaccine, probably lacks protection against HBV. Low responders (anti-HBs, 10 to 100 mIU/ml) lose detectable anti-HBs within a few years. A good response is regarded as an anti-HBS level greater than or equal to 100 mIU/ml. This is followed by long-term immunity and protection against HBV infection.[30]

Low antibody levels are often seen in older and obese men. Age has a definite effect on the antibody response to vaccination, with older adults responding less vigorously than younger adults. Suboptimal response to HBV vaccine is also seen in homosexual men and hemodialysis patients. Although low antibody levels do not necessarily mean a complete lack of immunity, they are associated with a greater susceptibility to hepatitis B infection.

---

*10 milli-international units per milliliter (MIU/ml) of serum are equivalent to 10 sample ratio units (SRU).

The standard vaccine is a highly immunogenic preparation that induces a protective antibody response in 95% of healthy adults, 20 to 39 years of age, who complete the three-dose schedule.[27] In children, up to 99% are expected to be protected against HBV infection on completion of HBV vaccination program.

Anti-HBs and Level of Protection. Approximately 84% of adult vaccines still retain at least 10 mIU/ml anti-HBs for 2 years after vaccination. Continued protection may not depend on the persistence of antibody. Long-term follow-up studies of high-risk groups have suggested that, if the initial anti-HBs titer of 10 mIU/ml is achieved, those vaccinated are protected from clinical hepatitis, despite decreasing or absent titers. Among people who initially respond to vaccine, exposure may result in subclinical infection, but none develop chronic liver disease or carrier state. Revaccination of individuals when anti-HBs levels have fallen to less than 10 mIU/ml, or 5 years after the initial course of vaccination, has been recommended.[2,33] Of individuals who have less than or equal to 10 mIU/ml anti-HBs, 90% develop an anamnestic response to a booster dose.

Booster Dose and Revaccination. The proper timing of booster vaccination in persons who initially respond to vaccine but whose antibody levels subsequently decrease is unknown. Approximately 50% of persons who fail to respond initially acquire protective anti-HBs in response to revaccination. All low responders develop protective antibodies. Response, however, is usually transient, and anti-HBs peaks are generally moderate.

Measurement of anti-HBs 1 to 3 months after HBV vaccination is desirable to identify the subgroups of adequate responders, low responders, and nonresponders. Although it has been suggested that high-risk individuals (i.e., surgical residents) be tested yearly for anti-HBs, this may contribute significantly to the expense of a vaccination program.

Postexposure Prophylaxis. High-risk persons who should receive the vaccine are the following: (1) health care workers exposed to blood; (2) clients and staff of institutions for the developmentally disabled; (3) hemodialysis patients; (4) homosexually active men; (5) IV users of illegal drugs; (6) recipients of certain blood products; (7) household members and sexual contacts of HBV carriers; and (8) special high-risk populations (e.g., inmates of long-term correctional facilities, heterosexually active persons with multiple sexual partners, and international travelers to HBV epidemic areas). Approximately 30% deny belonging to these high-risk categories, and are therefore not considered for vaccination.[27]

For normal adults and children older than 10 years of age, 10 μg (1 ml) of the recombinant vaccine or 20 μg (1.0 ml) of the plasma-derived vaccine should be given in three intramuscular doses over 6 months. The second dose is administered 1 month after the first dose and the third dose is given 5 months after the second. The vaccine should be inoculated into the deltoid muscle. Pregnancy is not a contraindication in high-risk women.

Children younger than 11 years should receive 5 mcg (0.5 ml) by the same dosage schedule. Newborns of HBsAg carrier mothers should have a single dose of HBIG (0.5 ml) in addition to the standard HB vaccine schedule. Neonates and infants should receive the vaccine in the anterolateral thigh muscle.

For patients undergoing hemodialysis and other immunocompromised individuals, a 40-μg dose is recommended. As mentioned earlier, the present formulation of recombinant vaccine is not advisable in hemodialysis patients.[30]

For postexposure prophylaxis, passive immunization with HBIG is warranted. HBIG is prepared from plasma with high titers of anti-HBs (1:100,000).[8] It undergoes cold ethanol fractionation, which effectively inactivates blood-borne pathogens, including retrovirus (HIV). Although providing protection against HBV infection, its effect is temporary. Adverse reactions are uncommon when given intramuscularly. Because of the fear of inducing an immune complex disease, it should not be given to an HBV carrier.

Postexposure prophylaxis is indicated in major instances: (1) perinatal exposure of an infant born to an HBsAg-positive mother; (2) accidental percutaneous or permucosal exposure to HBsAg-positive blood; and (3) sexual exposure to an HBsAg-positive person.[27] In each situation, the exposed person should receive passive immunization with HBIG and active immunization with hepatitis B vaccine.

For perinatal exposure to an HBsAg-positive mother, a regimen combining 0.5 ml (10 μg) of HBIG and 0.5 ml (10 μg) of hepatitis B vaccine is recommended. They should be administered intramuscularly at different sites as soon as possible after birth, preferably within 12 hours of exposure.

Recommendations for hepatitis B prophylaxis following percutaneous exposure are listed in Table 17–2. Any person who sustains an accidental needle stick exposure is identified as at risk for acquiring hepatitis B, and should therefore be considered a candidate for hepatitis B vaccine.

Prophylaxis against hepatitis D (delta) virus (HDV) infection depends on adequate protection against hepatitis B, because HDV is an incomplete virus that requires HBsAg to replicate.

Hepatitis B is a disease of worldwide distribution. It is an established cause of chronic liver disease, including chronic active hepatitis and cirrhosis. It is second only to tobacco among known human carcinogens, accounting for 80% of cases of hepatocellular carcinoma.[31] The development and licensing of safe, effective, and immunogenic vaccines should make it possible to prevent hepatitis B and its chronic sequelae.

NON-A, NON-B HEPATITIS

Serologic testing for viral hepatitis has shown that at least two forms of hepatitis are distinct from viral A and B hepatitis. These were formerly called non-A, non-B (NANB) hepatitis.

NANB hepatitis occurs in two different epidemiologic settings, parenterally transmitted and enteric. Post-transfusion NANB hepatitis is the parenterally transmitted form of non-A, non-B hepatitis. It accounts for 25% of all recognized cases of viral hepatitis in the United States.

TABLE 17–2. RECOMMENDATIONS FOR HEPATITIS B-EXPOSED PERSONS: PROPHYLAXIS FOLLOWING PERCUTANEOUS EXPOSURE

Source	Exposed Person: Unvaccinated	Exposed Person: Vaccinated
HBsAg-positive	One dose HBIG, immediately; initiate HB vaccine series	Test for anti-HBs; if inadequate antibody, give HBIG immediately, plus HB vaccine booster dose
Known source	Initiate HB vaccine series	Test source for HBsAg only, if exposed is vaccine non-responder; if source is HBsAg-positive, give HBIg x1 immediately plus HB vaccine booster dose
High risk, HBsAg-positive	Test sources for HBsAg; if positive, one dose HBIG	
Low risk, HBsAg-positive	Initiate HB vaccine series	Nothing required (?); IG for NANB
Unknown source	Initiate HB vaccine series	Nothing required (?); IG for NANB

From the Centers for Disease Control: Recommendations for protection against viral hepatitis. MMWR, 34:313, 1985.

Of those infected, 5 to 10% have a history of blood transfusion, 40% admit to a history of parenteral drug abuse, and approximately 3% relate an occupational exposure to blood. In 10%, heterosexual activity with multiple sexual partners and sexual exposure to a household member with known NANB hepatitis have been identified as risk factors.[32]

Approximately 750,000 NANB infections occur annually. Of these, 75,000 (10%) demonstrate evidence of chronic liver damage, and 7,500 to 15,000 have associated blood transfusion. NANB hepatitis is still the most common serious consequence of blood transfusion.[32] The risks for acquiring NANB after transfusion approaches 7 to 12%. Of infected individuals, 40 to 70% demonstrate persistent liver function abnormalities, and 10 to 25% of these eventually develop cirrhosis. A carrier state exists.

Parenterally transmitted non-A, non-B hepatitis virus has been cloned from nucleic acid extracted from chimpanzee plasma, and has been provisionally named the hepatitis C virus. A serologic assay for detecting antibody to an epitope of the virus has been developed.[33]

Before this technologic advance, indirect screening using anti-HBc and elevated serum alanine aminotransferase levels (surrogate testing) was used to identify possible NANB carriers. Prevention of NANB hepatitis in the United States relies on judicious use of blood and its components, as well as on careful donor selection. In fact, the single most important intervention in the prevention of NANB hepatitis appears to be the replacement of paid, commercial blood donors by all-volunteer, repeat blood donors.

Specific prophylaxis for NANB hepatitis is not available. Attempts to prevent hepatitis C have mostly involved the use of IG, but solid data are lacking. IG is recommended at a dose of 0.06 ml/kg, however, for percutaneous exposure to persons with known NANB hepatitis.[1]

Enterically transmitted non-A, non-B hepatitis (ET-NANB) is epidemiologically similar to hepatitis A. It is transmitted by the fecal-oral route. It was first described in an epidemic in New Delhi, where 29,000 cases of icteric hepatitis occurred in 1955 to 1956.[2] Subsequently, large outbreaks have been reported, mainly in developing countries. A 20% case fatality rate has been found in pregnant women infected with ET-NANB.

As with hepatitis A, clinical illness is more common in adults than in children. The occurrence of epidemic hepatitis in a population suspected to be immune to hepatitis A should alert authorities to consider ET-NANB hepatitis.

The diagnosis of ET-NANB hepatitis is based on exclusion of hepatitis A and B virus, epidemiologic characteristics of the outbreak, and the identification of 20- to 34-nm virus-like particles in stools of acutely ill patients. Persons traveling to high-risk areas are advised to avoid possibly contaminated food or water.[34]

REFERENCES

1. Centers for Disease Control: Recommendations for protection against viral hepatitis. MMWR, 34:313, 1985.
2. ________: Progress in the control of viral hepatitis: Memorandum from a WHO meeting. Bull WHO, 66:443, 1988.
3. Lemon SM: Type A viral hepatitis: New developments in an old disease. N Engl J Med, 313:1059, 1985.
4. Balistreri WF: Viral hepatitis. Pediatr Clin North Am, 35:375, 1988.
5. Francis DP, Hadler SC, Pendergast TJ, et al: Occurrence of hepatitis A, B, and non-A/non-B in the United States: CDC Sentinel County Hepatitis Study, I. Am J Med, 76:69, 1984.
6. Stiehm ER (moderator): Intravenous immunoglobulin as therapeutic agents. Ann Intern Med, 107:367, 1987.
7. Mosley JW, Reister DM, Brachott D, et al: Comparison of two lots of immune serum globulin for prophylaxis of infectious hepatitis. Am J Epidemiol, 87:539, 1968.
8. Seeff LB, Hoofnagle JH: Immunoprophylaxis of viral hepatitis. Gastroenterology, 77:161, 1979.
9. Karron RA, Daemer R, Ticehurst J, et al: Studies of prototype live hepatitis A virus vaccines in primate models. J Infect Dis, 157:338, 1988.
10. Murray-Lyon IM: Strategies for preventing hepatitis B. Q J Med, 264:277, 1989.
11. Zimmerman FH, Wormser GP: Exposure to hepatitis B: Review of current concepts. Bull NY Acad Med, 65:741, 1989.
12. Villanueva SY, Danzi JT: The immunological aspects of acute and chronic liver disease. Guthrie J, 59:51, 1990.

13. Stevens CE, Beasley RP, Tsui J, Lee WC: Vertical transmission of hepatitis B antigen in Taiwan. N Engl J Med, 292:771, 1975.
14. Beasley RP, Hwang LY, Lin CC, Chien CS: Hepatocellular carcinoma and hepatitis B virus: A prospective study of 22,707 men in Taiwan. Lancet, 2:1129, 1981.
15. Stevens CE: Perinatal hepatitis B virus infection: Screening of pregnant women and protection of the infant. Ann Intern Med, 107:412, 1987.
16. Stevens CE, Neurath RE, Beasley RP, et al: HBeAg and anti-HBe detection by radioimmunoassay: Correlation with vertical transmission of hepatitis B virus in Taiwan. J Med Virol, 3:237, 1979.
17. Shikata T, Yano M, Shiraki K, Oda T: Efficacy trial of HBIG and hepatitis B vaccine for the prevention of perinatal HBV transmission. *In* Viral Hepatitis and Liver Disease. Edited by GN Vyas, JL Dienstag, and JH Hoofnagle. Orlando, Grune & Stratton, 1984, pp 593–606.
18. Beasley RP, Hwang LY: Epidemiology of hepatocellular carcinoma. *In* Viral Hepatitis and Liver Disease. Edited by GN Vyas, JL Dienstag, and JH Hoofnagle. Orlando, Grune & Stratton, 1984, pp 209–224.
19. Centers for Disease Control: Prevention of perinatal transmission of hepatitis B virus: Prenatal screening of all pregnant women for hepatitis B surface antigen. MMWR, 37:341, 1988.
20. Maynard JE: Nosocomial viral hepatitis. Am J Med, 70:439, 1981.
21. Centers for Disease Control: Guidelines for prevention of transmission of human immunodeficiency virus and hepatitis B virus to health care workers and public safety workers. MMWR, 38(Suppl 6):1, 1989.
22. Dienstag JL, Ryan DM: Occupational exposure to hepatitis B virus in hospital personnel: Infection or immunization. Am J Epidemiol, 115:26, 1982.
23. Shikata T, Karasawa T, Abe K, et al: Hepatitis HBe antigen and infectivity of hepatitis B virus. J Infect Dis, 136:571, 1977.
24. Reingold AL, Kane MA, Hightower AW: Failure of gloves and other protective devices to prevent transmission of hepatitis B virus to oral surgeons. JAMA, 259:2558, 1988.
25. Ellis RW, Gerety RJ: Plasma-derived and yeast-derived hepatitis B vaccines. Am J Infect Control, 17:181, 1989.
26. Wahl M, Hermodsson S: Intradermal subcutaneous or intramuscular administration of hepatitis B vaccine: Side effects and antibody response. Scand J Infect Dis, 19:617, 1987.
27. Immunization Practices Advisory Committee: Update on hepatitis B prevention. MMWR, 36:353, 1987.
28. Hoofnagle JH: Toward universal vaccination against hepatitis B virus. N Engl J Med, 321:1333, 1989.
29. Centers for Disease Control: Changing patterns of groups at high risk for hepatitis B in the United States. MMWR, 37:429, 1988.
30. Immunization against hepatitis B. Lancet, 1:875, 1988.
31. Maynard JE, Kane MA, Hadler SC: Global control of hepatitis B through vaccination: Role of hepatitis B vaccine in the expanded program of immunization. Rev Infect Dis, 2:S574, 1989.
32. Alter M, Sampliner RE: Hepatitis C: And miles to go before we sleep. N Engl J Med, 321:1538, 1989.
33. Kuo G, Choo QL, Alter HJ, et al: An assay for circulating antibodies to a major etiologic virus of human non-A, non-B hepatitis. Science, 244:362, 1989.
34. Centers for Disease Control: Enterically transmitted non-A, non-B hepatitis: Mexico. MMWR, 36:597, 1987.

chapter

18

THE OFFICE MANAGEMENT OF COMMON PERIANAL DISEASES

James Ferenzi
Joseph A. Scopelliti

Perianal disease, including hemorrhoids and fissures, is a common office complaint seen by family practitioners, internists, and gastroenterologists. Various perianal diseases are discussed in this chapter. Most of these can be evaluated thoroughly in the office setting, without a need for any other investigation and most, if not all, can also be treated in the office.

HEMORRHOIDS

Hemorrhoids consist of the submucosal tissue cushions that line the anal canal. They are composed primarily of veins, venules, arterioles, and smooth muscle fibers. Three main hemorrhoidal veins are located in the left lateral, right anterior, and right posterior positions when the patient is in the usual proctoscopic position. The major function of hemorrhoids seems to be in aiding anal continence and sphincter sealing, but they may also serve as a cushion during defecation. Hemorrhoids are generally divided into internal and external types, depending on the locale of enlargement.

EXTERNAL HEMORRHOIDS

External hemorrhoids are dilated veins of the inferior hemorrhoidal plexus, located distal to the dentate line. External hemorrhoids typically present with painful bleeding on bowel movement. They are prone to thrombosis, which results in an acute and significant discomfort. The patient often then notes a hard lump, which develops concomitant with the thrombosis.

On examination external hemorrhoids can be identified without the use of a proctoscope. The presence of a thrombosed hemorrhoid can easily be felt.

Treatment for a thrombosed external hemorrhoid involves incision and removal of the clot. This must be carried out within 48 hours of onset of symptoms. Patients seen after 48 hours should be treated conservatively, because excision and removal of the clot are not then generally successful. Removal of a thrombosed hemorrhoid can be carried out in the office setting using a local anesthetic. After excision, the patient should be instructed to maintain a soft bowel movement through the use of bulk-forming agents. In addition, sitz baths, three to four times daily for the week following excision, are recommended. Thus, if the patient is seen after 48 hours, conservative therapy should include the use of stool-softening agents, sitz baths, and cortisone-containing creams.

External hemorrhoids must be differentiated from external skin tags. These are composed of redundant and fibrotic skin that develops at the anal verge. They are the result of previously thrombosed external hemorrhoids, or might even represent chronic enlargement of the external hemorrhoidal veins. Often, these are noted by the patient as a soft nodularity protruding from the anal canal. The most common symptoms associated with external skin tags are pruritus and difficulty in cleansing the area.

On examination, external skin tags are characterized by typically redundant skin, with little submucosal tissue. Treatment of these is limited, because they rarely cause problems. Treatment for pruritus is discussed below (see Pruritus Ani). Excision of these is rarely needed, and should only be performed if the patient has significant irritation as the result of poor perianal hygiene.

INTERNAL HEMORRHOIDS

Internal hemorrhoids are the vascular plexus that is located above the dentate line. These present with painless, bright red rectal bleeding associated with bowel movements. Generally, this occurs in the patient who has a history of chronic constipation. Pain may also accompany the bowel movement, but this is more typical of an anal fissure. The patient describes the blood as bright red, and usually located externally on the stool surface. The finding of blood after completion of defecation on toilet tissue also indicates internal hemorrhoids. Patients may occasionally note spontaneous bleeding, which they become aware of while sitting, but this is not associated with any bowel movement or other activity. Finally, the bleeding may be substantial in appearance, and the patient notes that the blood "turned the toilet bowl red."

Digital anal examination can occasionally define the presence of hemorrhoids. They can usually be palpated when they are larger. Usually, an anoscopic or proctoscopic examination is incorporated into the evaluation to define the pathology completely. An anoscopic examination is particularly helpful, and attention must be paid to the degree of prolapse into the lumen by hemorrhoidal veins to determine their severity (see below). When flexible sigmoidoscopy is done, a retroflexed view in the rectum must be used to define the extent of hemorrhoids clearly.

Internal hemorrhoids are divided into four types. First-degree hemorrhoids are those that are identified as larger than normal on proctoscopic examination. They do not extend beyond the dentate line on straining, and may be associated with periodic bleeding. The treatment of these hemorrhoids usually involves the addition of bulk-forming agents to the diet to avoid constipation. The use of a hydrocortisone-containing suppository may also be beneficial. This probably serves as a lubricant to prevent a traumatic bowel movement. More aggressive therapy is not needed for this level of problem.

Second-degree hemorrhoids can be noted to prolapse with straining, but reduce spontaneously. They are most often seen on anoscopic examination as prolapsing into the lumen. Third-degree hemorrhoids prolapse on straining or walking and require manual replacement. They are seen prolapsed into the lumen on anoscopic examination without straining. Fourth-degree hemorrhoids are a large prolapsing plexus of internal hemorrhoids. They are generally always prolapsed, and are prone to strangulation.

Therapy for second-, third-, and fourth-degree hemorrhoids is variable, depending on the severity of the problem and the patient's desires. Conservative therapy includes maintaining a soft, bulky stool that requires no straining on bowel movements. Topical therapy should include a hydrocortisone-containing suppository used once daily for 2 to 4 weeks, preferably applied at night. Avoiding local irritation by maintaining clean, dry perianal skin is helpful. Talcum powder or a witch hazel preparation to cleanse the perianal skin after bowel movements and baths is helpful. Harsh soaps and vigorous scrubbing of the perianal skin should be avoided. Tight undergarments and clothing should be avoided; cotton undergarments are preferable. Dietary measures are usually helpful if the patient can clearly identify a bothersome food, but a strict diet is not indicated.

Other topical treatments or suppository medications are generally not helpful. Specifically, topical or suppository medications containing anesthetics of the "-caine" type should be avoided because of the potential for allergic reactions.

Specific therapies that can be carried out in the office include rubber band ligation, cryotherapy, infrared coagulation, and laser therapy. Rubber band ligation is the most widely used of these techniques. It can be used for second- and third-degree internal hemorrhoids that are symptomatic. It may be carried out during a routine sigmoidoscopy with a rigid sigmoidoscope. The rubber bands are applied around the hemorrhoid while it is grasped. It adheres to the hemorrhoid for about 48 hours, during which time the hemorrhoid strangulates and then sloughs off. Repeat treatments at 3- to 4-week intervals are required until all major hemorrhoids have been eradicated. Complications include prolonged pain and recurrent bleeding at the site of the hemorrhoidal slough.[1]

Cryotherapy is another technique that has been used for more than 15 years. It involves the use of liquid nitrogen, along with a probe, to achieve rapid freezing of the hemorrhoidal vein. Complications are essentially the same as those for rubber band ligation, but it has a lower success rate.[2]

Infrared coagulation has proven to be a rapid and useful technique for the obliteration of internal hemorrhoids. It can easily be used on first- and second-degree hemorrhoids. It has been used in third-degree hemorrhoids with lesser success, but is still an option before surgery. The infrared coagulator is a wand-shaped device that allows controlled heat to be applied to the base of the hemorrhoid. The hemorrhoidal veins are coagulated individually. The patient requires repeat treatments at 2- to 3-week intervals, usually require three or four treatment sessions in all. A success rate of 80 to 90% can be expected.[1,3]

The most expensive nonsurgical method for the treatment of hemorrhoids is laser therapy. Laser light produces an intense focus of heat, and it can be used to treat all four types of internal hemorrhoids. The major drawback is the expense of this technology. Complications include postoperative bleeding, stenosis, and a discharge from hemorrhoidal necrosis. Laser therapy has little advantage over infrared coagulation at this time.

Fourth-degree hemorrhoids almost always require surgical correction. Unless the patient is an extremely high-risk surgical candidate, this is the therapy of choice for all patients. The success rate of surgical hemorrhoidectomy is 85 to 90%, although it is possible that the hemorrhoids may recur. Patients should be strongly advised after all forms of therapy to maintain a high-fiber diet to avoid such recurrences.[4]

Finally, and most importantly, it cannot be stressed enough that hemorrhoidal bleeding is a diagnosis that necessitates the exclusion of other causes of bleeding. A complete evaluation of the colon is necessary in any patient in whom the source of bleeding is questionable to rule out neoplasms. Many patients complain that their "hemorrhoids are always bleeding," but this should not preclude a thorough investigation of the lower gastrointestinal tract.

ANAL FISSURE

An anal fissure is a longitudinal tear that traverses the anal canal. It may occur within the anal canal above the dentate line, in which case the tear only penetrates the mucosa of the rectum. The tear may also extend below the dentate line into the skin-lined part of the anal canal. The tear is usually a few millimeters wide, and may be as long as 1 cm.

Symptoms from an anal fissure are primarily pain on defecation and rectal bleeding. Depending on the locale of the tear, either or both of these symptoms can be present. When the tear extends into the squamous-lined portion of the anal canal, the patient has distinct pain with defecation that can be described as a sharp or burning sensation with bowel movements. When the tear extends primarily proximally into the rectal mucosa, bright red bleeding with bowel movements is noted. This is a result of tearing into the submucosal hemorrhoidal vein plexus.

Anal fissures are generally the result of a traumatic event, usually the passage of a large, hard stool. They may be the result of a fibrotic anal canal that is not distensible.

Most anal fissures occur in the posterior midline, but may also be found in the right or left side of the anal canal anteriorly.

It is occasionally possible to feel the anal fissure by digital examination. This reveals a linear area of induration and tenderness that might be rather narrow.

Proctoscopic examination is usually diagnostic. This should be carried out carefully, because anal fissures can sometimes be difficult to see in the creases of the anal canal. Special care should be taken at this time to examine the mucosa of the rectum to ensure that this does not represent inflammatory bowel disease.

Therapy of an anal fissure involves the addition of bulk-forming agents to the diet to maintain soft bowel movements. Warm sitz baths and good anal hygiene aid in symptomatic relief. Finally, the use of a hydrocortisone-containing suppository medication may speed healing, although this has not been proven definitively at present.

Because of the fibrosis that results from the anal fissure, a number of patients with this problem find it to be chronic in nature. The fibrosis caused by anal fissure results in loss of elasticity and recurrence of the fissure. If this becomes refractory to stool-softening agents and local measures, surgical intervention should be considered. Lateral internal sphincterotomy alone or in conjunction with excision of the anal fissure are the surgical choices.[4]

FISTULA IN ANO

Fistula in ano is an inflammatory tract with its secondary or external opening in the perianal skin and the primary or internal opening of the anal canal at the dentate line. It generally produces an abscess in the intersphincteric space of the anal canal.

These fistulas follow what is called Goodsall's rule:

1. The external opening is anterior to an imaginary line drawn across the midpoint of the anus; therefore, the fistula usually runs directly into the anal canal.
2. The external opening is posterior to that line, and the tract usually occurs at the posterior midline of the anal canal.
3. An exception is when the external opening is anterior and more than 3 cm from the anus; the tract may then occur posteriorly and end in the posterior midline.[4]

The patient's complaints generally pertain to the development of pain, particularly on defecation, which is often a constant throbbing discomfort. It is usually associated with a clear or serous drainage from the opening. Patients occasionally have drainage without pain. It is rare for the patient to have bloody drainage spontaneously, although this may be created when external pressure is applied. Patients often have a previous history of anorectal abscesses, with intermittent drainage of a fistula.

The major significance of fistulas is the possibility of inflammatory bowel disease, specifically Crohn's disease. Any patient who has a recurrent perianal fistula needs to have a thorough work-up to rule out the presence of inflammatory bowel disease. Ileocolonic Crohn's disease is the most frequent cause of perianal fistulas secondary to inflammatory bowel disease. Other disorders that may cause a perianal fistula include sigmoid diverticulitis, hidradenitis suppurativa, pilonidal cysts, and low rectal and anal carcinomas.

Therapy involves identifying the primary opening. This usually requires anesthesia, and is often done in an operating room. The fistula can be identified and unroofed with healing by secondary intention. Fistulectomy is rarely necessary. The placement of a seton through the fistula often aids in the maturation of the fistula so that it can be adequately controlled by surgery.

CONDYLOMATA ACUMINATA

Condylomata acuminata are sexually transmitted warts that are the result of infection with a papillomavirus. They produce a soft, villiform growth in the perianal skin or squamous epithelium of the anal canal. Occasionally, they can extend into the upper anal canal, or even the lower rectum. They usually present with bleeding and itching as a result of the irritation.

Their soft papillary appearance is almost always diagnostic. Biopsy confirms their exact nature. Occasionally, squamous cell carcinoma can be mistaken for this illness.

Diagnosis is usually made by visual inspection. Sigmoidoscopy should be performed in all cases to document the extent of the warts, because those in the anal canal that are not treated serve as a focus for recurrence.

Small warts can be treated with a topical solution of 25% podophyllin. More extensive warts require excision or fulguration under anesthesia. A more efficacious method of managing these warts is excision by carbon dioxide laser. Patients should be aware of the high recurrence rate with all forms of treatment. In women, a vaginal examination to determine extension of the warts into the vaginal vault is necessary.

PROCTALGIA FUGAX

Proctalgia fugax a severe, spasmodic rectal pain, lasting a few seconds to a few minutes. It is generally described by the patient as a sensation of sitting on a knife. The patient notes that the pain comes on for no apparent reason, and it can occasionally be provoked by prolonged periods of sitting. The pain often disappears spontaneously, without any residual symptoms.

The pain appears to be caused by spasms of the levator ani muscles. It is important to ensure that no perianal inflammatory process is present.

The examination should include a digital rectal examination to observe any perianal tenderness. A proctosigmoidoscopic examination should also be performed to rule out the presence of proctitis and any intra-anal pathology, such as an anal fissure, which may be causing the problem.

Acute attacks can be treated with sitz baths and stool softeners. Occasionally, patients with profound symptoms can be managed with belladonna and opium suppositories, but these should be reserved for the most severe cases. Any perianal or rectal pathology should be promptly treated to alleviate relapses.

PRURITUS ANI

Pruritus ani is a frequent complaint seen in the office setting. Patients are often somewhat reluctant to discuss it, however, and it is necessary to obtain a history. Patients are often shy about their personal hygiene habits so this may seem trivial, but it can be of considerable importance to the patient.

Patients note that their pruritus often improves immediately after bathing and is worse during the daytime. It is common to see it exacerbated by long periods of sitting. It is important to question the patient about other perianal diseases, particularly chronic hemorrhoidal disease.

The physical examination begins with close scrutiny of the perianal skin. Areas of excoriation and perianal dermatitis should be noted. The presence of excessive moisture in this area should also be sought. An anoscopic examination is also important to determine whether other perianal disease is present.

A wide variety of disorders can cause perianal dermatitis. These include anorectal disease, such as hemorrhoids and anal fistulas. Dermatologic disorders, such as psoriasis and contact allergies, are important, and other infectious agents, particularly worms, need to be considered.

The most important cause is probably the patient's hygiene pattern. Most patients with pruritus find this to be a intense symptom that they try to correct by vigorous cleansing, which results in a macerated and overly sensitive perianal skin. In addition, the presence of soap residue only exacerbates the itching. The first step in the treatment of this condition, therefore, is strict avoidance of vigorous scrubbing with soap. Patients should be instructed to cleanse the area gently with a cool, moist washcloth, and using a witch hazel solution this is often beneficial.

Specific treatment is based on the history and physical examination findings. Patients with primary anorectal diseases need to have those treated directly. Dermatologic diseases, such as psoriasis, have specific treatment plans, which should be followed. The patient should be inspected closely for the presence of any infections, and these should be treated appropriately. Finally, for the patient with no obvious source for the pruritus, who does not respond to these conservative measures, a short course of topical hydrocortisone cream can be helpful. This should not be used on a long-term basis, because anal dermal thinning can result. Finally, zinc oxide ointment over the long term can be used for those patients refractory to all other forms of treatment.

REFERENCES

1. Keighley RB: A randomized trial to compare photocoagulation with rubber band ligation for treatment of hemorrhoids. Colo-Proctol, 5:310, 1981.
2. Williams JA: The management of piles. Br Med J, 285:1137, 1982.
3. Frank WL: A comparison of methods of thermal treatment of hemorrhoids. Colo-Proctol, 5:311, 1981.
4. Goligher JC: Surgery of the Anus, Rectum and Colon. 5th Ed. Philadelphia, WB Saunders, 1984, pp 178–220.

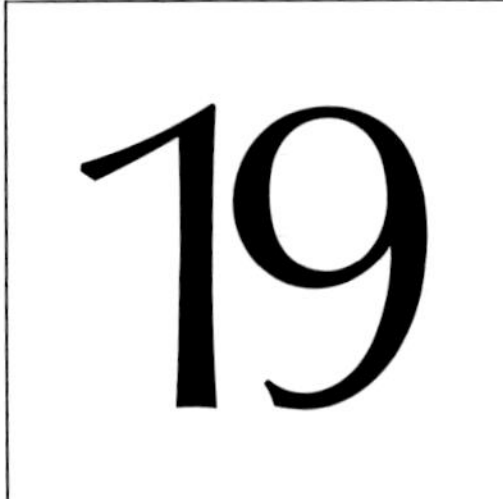

RECOGNITION AND MANAGEMENT OF PREMALIGNANT GASTROINTESTINAL LESIONS

Romulo Bunao

A precancerous lesion or disease is a condition that is more likely to be associated with the development of a particular cancer that would not be diagnosed in a matched population lacking that disorder.

SURVEILLANCE

Mass screening and the more specific at-risk patient surveillance require the clinician to assess cancer risks based on a personal and family history and physical signs, and to apply the most cost-effective, acceptable, and noninvasive diagnostic testing system. Although epidemiologic studies have established a close association between the occurrence of cancer and infection, many environmental carcinogens have been implicated in human gastrointestinal cancers. Heredity has been incriminated in the pathogenesis of the disease, and exciting discoveries have shown that important oncogenes may cause cancer and other genes may suppress it.

GASTROINTESTINAL ONCOLOGISTS AND PRIMARY PHYSICIANS

Because the primary physician bears most of the responsibility in cancer detection, gastrointestinal oncologists should be consulted for their expertise and advice. Regional cancer centers should offer training programs in gastrointestinal oncology to educate primary or referring physicians. Foremost is the role of endoscopy in the surveillance of premalignant conditions. This technology provides extraordinary insights in regard to cancer detection and prevention.

PREMALIGNANT GASTROINTESTINAL CONDITIONS

ESOPHAGEAL DISEASES

Achalasia. This is an esophageal motor dysfunction characterized manometrically by aperistalsis of the body, usually elevated lower esophageal sphincter (LES) pressure, and impaired LES relaxation. Clinically, more than 90% of patients have dysphagia, 70% have reflux or regurgitation, often on recumbency, and noncardiac chest pain is observed in less than 30% of patients. Odynophagia, pulmonary complications, weight loss, and malignancy are late symptoms. Radiographically, the esophagogram shows a dilated body of the esophagus, with a birdbeak tapering of the distal esophagus. Secondary achalasia caused by tumor of the esophagogastric junction can simulate these typical roentgenographic features. Treatment includes the use of calcium-blocking agents such as nifedipine and pneumatic dilation and esophagomyotomy in patients failing medical therapy.

The incidence of squamous cell carcinoma increases threefold to tenfold in chronic achalasia, usually occurring in the middle or lower third of the esophagus.[1] The mean interval from the diagnosis of achalasia to the diagnosis of the cancer is 15 years. An endoscopic surveillance program including both biopsy and cytology approaches 100% sensitivity in the diagnosis of this cancer. If early stage malignancy is to be detected for surgical cure, annual endoscopy is recommended.

Barrett's Esophagus and Chronic Gastroesophageal Reflux Disease. The metaplastic changes from squamous to columnar epithelium of the distal esophagus develop in about 10% of patients with chronic gastroesophageal reflux disease (GERD), with a white male predominance.[2] Clinically, 90% of patients with a Barrett's esophagus (BE) present with heartburn (pyrosis), but some patients are asymptomatic. Patients with a BE are at increased risk for developing an associated complication, such as peptic ulcer, perforation, stricture, bleeding, or malignancy. Radiographically, 72% of BE patients do not demonstrate the classic hiatal hernia with midesophageal ulcer.[3] Patients with a BE are at increased risk of developing an esophageal cancer, which occurs in 10 to 15% of patients.[4] Associated factors such as smoking and alcoholism raise the cancer risk by 30- to 40-fold.[4]

Therefore, a surveillance program is imperative. An endoscopic surveillance every 1 to 2 years is recommended. It is known that high-grade dysplasia is the precursor of an invasive esophageal malignancy. Flow cytometric DNA aneuploidy reportedly has a 60 to 80% sensitivity in the diagnosis of this cancer. High-grade dysplasia, if reconfirmed, warrants consideration of an esophagectomy in low-risk patients. The presence of low-grade dysplasia mandates vigorous medical therapy for 8 to 12 weeks, with repeat biopsies being done at 3-month intervals until two consecutive biopsy specimens have shown no dysplasia. Although antireflux surgery may rarely lead to regression of the columnar-lined lower esophagus, it does not decrease the cancer risk.

Lye Stricture. Squamous cell cancer that occurs in a lye-injured esophagus comprises 7.2% of all esophageal cancers.[4] The average interval between the acute caustic burn and the malignant transformation is about 20 to 46 years.[5] The incidence of squamous cell carcinoma in this type of patient is 0.8 to 4%.[4] A surveillance program with endoscopy should begin 10 years postinjury. A good prognosis is associated, because the carcinoma is surrounded by rigid scar that allows only intraluminal growth and prevents early, extraesophageal dissemination. An esophagectomy is the operation of choice, rather than bypass, because another malignancy could develop years after the first operation in the remaining esophagus.

Plummer-Vinson Syndrome. Also known as Paterson-Kelly-Brown syndrome, this cervical dysphagia is secondary to a cervical esophageal web associated with iron-deficiency anemia. It carries a 30% increased risk of squamous cancer of the hypopharynx and the upper third of the esophagus. A female preponderance occurs in this disease. A yearly endoscopic surveillance program is recommended.

Tylosis. This is inherited autosomal dominant focal palmoplantar-gingival hyperkeratosis syndrome. The chance of development of squamous cancer of the skin and esophagus increases to 95% after 60 years of age, with the cancer occurring in the distal esophagus in about 40% of cases.[6] A semiannual surveillance interval is recommended for life after establishment of the diagnosis.

DISEASES OF THE STOMACH

Pernicious Anemia and Atrophic Gastritis (Type A). These predispose to benign and malignant glandular tumors of the gastric fundus and antrum. In pernicious anemia a three-fold increase in the incidence of both cancer and carcinoid tumor is seen.[7,8] Hypergastrinemia results from the unopposed feedback mechanism, which involves hydrochloric acid and gastrin. This causes argyrophil cell hyperplasia in the chronic atrophic gastritis, and finally produces microcarcinoids and invasive carcinoid neoplasia.[9] The intestinal metaplasia that results as a consequence of the chronic atrophic gastritis is considered precancerous, but gastric dysplasia occupies a place intermediate between intestinal metaplasia and early malignancy. In the presence of dysplasia, an endoscopic surveillance should be carried out every 6 months for moderate dysplasia and every 3 months with associated severe dysplasia. The incidence of cancer associated with atrophic gastritis is 4.2%, whereas it increases to 5.2% in the presence of a gastric ulcer.[8] A periodic surveillance program is recommended for patients with either gastric condition, with an endoscopy being done at least every 2 years.[10]

Recently, patients with chronic gastritis infected with Helicobacter pylori and increased antibody levels are found at risk for gastric carcinogenesis. Retrospective studies show that H. pylori maybe a co-factor in the development of intestinal-type of gastric carcinoma.[11,12,13]

Menetrier's Disease. This is hypoproteinemic hypertrophic gastropathy that is usually diagnosed after the sixth decade of life. A diagnosis of gastric cancer can be established 10 years after this diagnosis, and can be associated with a hypercoagulable state and gastric hemorrhage.[14] A total gastrectomy is the treatment of choice for Menetrier's disease. The rationale is to stop the protein loss, prevent the development of malignancy, and permit anastomotic reconstruction between the normal esophagus and intestine.

Gastric Ulceration. It is estimated that about 25% of stomach ulcerations are diagnosed as being associated with an adenocarcinoma of the stomach. These ulcerations occur in a gastric cancer and do not occur de novo in benign gastric ulcerations. The symptoms of an early gastric carcinoma are vague but include dyspepsia, early satiety, and anorexia. Any patient with these symptoms above the age of 40 years should have an endoscopic evaluation to exclude a gastric cancer. All gastric ulcerations require endoscopic biopsy and cytologic evaluation to exclude malignancy. Once the diagnosis of a gastric ulceration has been established, even with negative histologic or cytologic review, it is imperative to prove total healing of the ulcer by endoscopic follow-up. The presence of dysplasia as determined histologically mandates confirmation by repeat biopsy because of the association of dysplasia with inflammation, rather than a malignant process.

An ulceration can occur in a gastric lymphoma, which is usually located in the fundus or cardia of the stomach. The endoscopic, histologic, and radiologic features usually distinguish a gastric lymphoma from an adenocarcinoma of the stomach. A confirmed histologic diagnosis of pseudolymphoma should be considered a precursor lesion of malignant potential.[15] Resective therapy is justified to establish a diagnosis and to render therapy.

Gastric Polyp. An adenoma of the stomach is the second most common type of gastric polyp, accounting for approximately 10 to 25% of all stomach polyps.[7,16] It is invariably associated with atrophic gastritis and intestinal metaplasia. As with its colonic counterpart, a gastric adenoma is associated with malignant transformation in 6 to 50% of cases, and 50% of gastric adenomas occur in association with cancer elsewhere in the stomach.[7] The recognition of a gastric adenoma requires histologic identification of the presence of dysplasia. Close clinical and endoscopic follow-up are required. A premalignant adenomatous polyp almost always occurs as a solitary lesion. Fundic gland polyposis is considered nonmalignant, but patients with familial colonic polyposis with gastroduodenal adenomatous polyps are at high risk for developing periampullary cancer in these adenomatous polyps.[13]

Gastric Remnant. Patients with a gastric remnant have a higher tendency for developing cancer (8.6%) than individuals with an intact stomach (3.9%).[17] The average "free interval" from surgical resection until a malignancy is diagnosed is more than twenty years postgastrectomy. Annual routine gastroscopic surveillance leads to an earlier detection rate and a higher rate of resectability if a gastric remnant cancer is found. Beginning 10 to 15 years postgastrectomy, a yearly surveillance program is highly recommended.[16]

SMALL BOWEL MALIGNANCIES

Primary Cancers. These are surprisingly rare—about 40 to 60 times less common than those of the colon. High-risk patients are found with these conditions, however, and they should be placed under surveillance.

Gluten-Sensitive Enteropathy or Celiac (Nontropical) Sprue. Small intestinal lymphoma and carcinoma can occur, as can carcinoma, in other sites, such as the pharynx, esophagus, rectum, skin, lungs, and ovaries. Clues suggestive of a small intestinal lymphoma usually include steatorrhea, a rising IgA titer, and failure to respond to a gluten-free diet.[19] A small intestinal lymphoma has been reported in patients with dermatitis herpetiformis associated with gluten-sensitive enteropathy (GSE).

Crohn's Disease. In long-standing disease of the small intestine, adenocarcinoma of the jejunum or ileum can develop. This is diagnosed more often in younger patients. This type of malignancy usually occurs in areas of stricture or in segments of the small intestine that have been surgically bypassed.[20] The cancers tend to be poorly differentiated, and have a poor prognosis. Surveillance is difficult and impractical, except in areas accessible to endoscopic examination or enteroscopy. Dysplasia develops in 23 to 58% of cases with a known malignancy, but it appears less useful as a surveillance marker.[21] Nonetheless, intestinal dysplasia should alert one to the possibility of a coexistent, invasive malignancy.

Immunodeficiency Syndromes. AIDS patients and transplant recipients are at high risk for developing neoplasias, such as Kaposi's sarcoma and non-Hodgkin's lymphoma. A high index of suspicion should always be a prime consideration.

COLON CONDITIONS

The colonic adenoma-cancer sequence, polyposis syndromes, family cancer syndrome, inflammatory bowel disease, and prior colon cancer have been discussed in Chapter 9, along with recommended surveillance measures for each disease group. Three conditions are discussed here because of their premalignancy potential for the development of colon cancer.

Postureterosigmoidostomy. Colonic adenoma and cancer can develop near the ureteral implantation site within the colon.[22] Annual fecal hemoccult testing is recommended along with flexible sigmoidoscopy every third year for surveillance of the site.

Chronic Radiation Enteritis-Colitis. With the aggressive use of radiotherapy cancer control, radiation-induced sequelae has become a common problem. Patients who survive abdominopelvic malignancies have a 2 to 3.6% risk of developing secondary cancer within 10 years after radiotherapy.[23] Reports of synchronous small and large bowel cancer developing after abdominopelvic irradiation supports the causal relationship between therapeutic irradiation and subsequent radiogenic cancer.[24] Therefore, secondary tumor screening should be integrated into primary tumor follow-up, as recommended.[25]

Bowen's Disease. This condition is characterized by severe dysplasia or carcinoma-in-situ within the rectal canal. It has a 70% conversion rate to squamous cell cancer of the anus.[26] This premalignant condition can be diagnosed in patients with venereal warts or herpes simplex type II infection, or in HIV-seropositive individuals.

Immunodeficiency Syndromes. Organ transplant recipients and other immunosuppressed patients have a dramatically increased incidence of vulvar and anal carcinoma, and should be enrolled in an anal cancer surveillance program.[27] In addition, AIDS patients can develop either a Kaposi's sarcoma or lymphoma of the anorectal area.[28,29]

LIVER AND PANCREAS DISORDERS

Liver Cancer. The risk of a cirrhotic patient developing a hepatocellular carcinoma (HCC) is about 40 times that of persons with a normal liver.[30] In idiopathic hemochromatosis (IHC), a hepatoma occurs in about one-third of patients with advanced cirrhosis, and the progression to cancer cannot be prevented by vigorous phlebotomy treatment.[30] Statistically, hepatoma is now the most common cause of death in patients with IHC. Early diagnosis of IHC is the most important consideration, so that phlebotomy therapy can prevent the progression to cirrhosis and cancer. Patients with known IHC and cirrhosis should be considered for liver transplantation to prevent the development of a hepatoma.[31]

Patients with chronic liver disease associated with the hepatitis B virus have a risk of developing HCC that is 200 times that of normal individuals.[32] Many epidemiologic studies have established a close association between HCC and chronic HBV infection, with 10% of patients with posthepatic or postnecrotic cirrhosis eventually being diagnosed with HCC.[33] The male prevalence of HCC is a result of the fact that a hepatoma is an androgen-dependent tumor.

Hepatocarcinogen Exposure. Certain chemicals are associated with an increased risk for the development of a hepatoma. Thoratrast, formerly used as an angiographic agent, has an increased risk for HCC development of 47 times that of people without an exposure.[30] In addition, the prolonged use of androgens and exposure to aflatoxin B-1 have been incriminated in the development of a hepatoma. People exposed regularly to vinyl chlorides or arsenicals have an increased risk of developing an angiosarcoma of the liver, more than 3000 times that of normal people, and an increased risk for being diagnosed with a HCC, which is 20 times that of individuals without any exposure to these agents.[30]

Patients with cirrhosis and a known premalignant condition require annual physical examinations, abdominal ultrasound evaluations, and α_1-fetoprotein serology in an attempt to diagnose a hepatoma in its earliest stages.[34] The use of selective angiography is helpful in the diagnosis of HCC and in determining the feasibility of resection.

Cholangiocarcinoma. An association has been noted with parasitic infections such as schistosomiasis and with infection by Clonorchis sinensis or other liver flukes. Patients with inflammatory bowel disease are rarely diagnosed with a cholangiocarcinoma.

Pancreatic Cancer. This is a disease of the elderly, with the average age being 68.5 years. It occurs predominantly in males and is more commonly diagnosed in those with chronic pancreatitis and diabetes.[35] The diagnosis of insulin-dependent diabetes in a middle-aged person with associated abdominal pain, however, should alert the clinician to the possibility of a cancer of the pancreas.

The incidence of pancreatic carcinoma varies from 0.8 to 25% in patients with chronic calcifying pancreatitis (CCP), and close surveillance is therefore needed for the detection of early malignant change. Clinically, none of the presently available endoscopic or radiologic diagnostic tests can make the diagnosis of pancreatic cancer in patients with CCP before it is unresectable. A strong index of suspicion is required to achieve an early diagnosis.

Many new diagnostic tests, including the serologic marker CA 19-9, endoscopic ultrasound, and percutaneous needle aspiration, have a high degree of sensitivity and specificity in the diagnosis of pancreatic cancer. None of these tests, however, have improved the clinical ability to diagnose resectable or curable pancreatic cancer.[36]

REFERENCES

1. Feldman M: Esophageal achalasia syndromes. Am J Med Sci, 295:60, 1988.
2. Reid BJ, Haggitt RC, Rubin CE, Rabinovitch PS: Barrett's esophagus: Correlation between flow cytometry and histology in detection of patients at risk for adenocarcinoma. Gastroenterology, 93:1, 1987.
3. Spechler SJ, Goyal RK: Barrett's esophagus. N Engl J Med, 315:362, 1986.
4. Lightdale C, Winawer S: Screening diagnosis and staging of esophageal cancer. Semin Oncol, 11:101, 1984.
5. Moore WR: Caustic ingestions: Pathophysiology, diagnosis, and treatment. Clin Pediatr, 25:192, 1986.
6. O'Mahony MY, Ellis JP, Hellier M, et al.: Familial tylosis and carcinoma of the esophagus. J R Soc Med 77:514, 1984.
7. Haentjens P, Willems G: Precancerous lesions in the stomach. Acta Chir Belg 84:277, 1984.
8. Tittobello A, Testoni PA, Masci E, et al.: Gastric cancer in chronic atrophic gastritis. Clin J Gastroenterol 9:298, 1987.
9. Moses RE, Frank BB, Leavitt M, Miller R: The syndrome of type A chronic atrophic gastritic, pernicious anemia, and multiple gastric carcinoids. J Clin Gastroenterol, 8:61, 1986.
10. Allum WH, Hallissey MT, Dorrell A, et al.: Programme for early detection of gastric cancer. Br Med J (Clin Res), 293:541, 1986.

11. Wyatt J: Gastritis and its relation to gastric carcinogenesis. Semin Diagn Pathol, 8:137, 1991.
12. Namura A, Stemmermann G, et al.: Helicobacter Pylori infection and gastric carcinoma among Japanese Americans in Hawaii. N Engl J Med, 325:1132, 1991.
13. Parsonnet J, Vandersteen D, Goates J, et al.: Helicobacter Pylori infection in intestinal- and diffuse-type gastric adenocarcinomas. J Natl Cancer Inst, 83:640, 1991.
14. Cooper BT, Menetrier's disease. Dig Dis Sci, 5:33, 1987.
15. Scoazec JY, Brousse N, Potet F, Jeulain JF: Focal malignant lymphoma in gastric pseudolymphoma: Histologic and immunohistochemical study of a case. Cancer, 57:1330, 1986.
16. Harju E: Gastric polyposes and malignancy. Br J Surg, 73:532, 1986.
17. Loscos JM, Gutierrez del Olma A, Nisa E, et al.: Cancer of the gastric stump. Gastrointest Endosc, 32:75, 1986.
18. Pointer R, Schwab G, K'Onigsrainer A, et al.: Early cancer of the gastric remnant. Gut, 29:298, 1988.
19. Selby WS, Gallagher ND: Malignancy in a 19-year experience with celiac disease. Dig Dis Sci, 24:684, 1979.
20. Neoplasia and gastrointestinal malignancy in IBD. *In* Inflammatory Bowel Disease, 3rd Ed. Edited by JB Kirsner and RG Shorter. Philadelphia, Lea & Febiger, 1988, pp 281–298.
21. Stein JH: Internal Medicine, 2nd Ed. Boston, Little Brown & Co., 1986, pp. 156-164.
22. Berg NO, Fredlund P, M'ansson W, Olsson SA: Surveillance colonoscopy and biopsy in patients with ureterosigmoidoscopy. Endoscopy, 19:60, 1987.
23. Sandler RS, Sandler DP: Radiation induced cancer of the colon and rectum: assessing the risk. Gastroenterology, 84:51, 1983.
24. Gajroj H, Davies DR, Jackson BT: Synchronous small and large bowel cancer developing after pelvic irradiation. Gut 28:126, 1988.
25. DeCarli A, Heer M, Espinosa N, et al.: Colorectal carcinoma following radiotherapy of gynecological carcinoma. Schweiz Med Wochenscher, 118:716, 1988.
26. Scoma JA, Levy EI: Bowen's disease of the anus. Dis Colon Rectum, 18:137, 1975.
27. Sheil AG: Cancer in organ transplant recipients: Part of an induced immune deficiency syndrome. Lancet, 1:559, 1984.
28. Friedman SL, Wright TL, Altman DF: Gastrointestinal Kaposi's sarcoma in patients with AIDS: Endoscopic and autopsy findings. Gastroenterology 89:102, 1985.
29. Zeigler JL, Beckstead JA, Volberding PA, et al.: Non-Hodgkin's lymphoma in 90 homosexual men. N Engl J Med 311:565, 1984.
30. Rustgi VR, Hoffnagle JH, Lotze MT, et al.: Epidemiology of hepatocellular carcinoma. Ann Intern Med 108:390, 1988.
31. Iwatsuki S, Gordon RD, Starzl TE, et al.: Role of liver transplantation in cancer therapy. Ann Surg, 202:401, 1985.
32. Johnson PJ, Williams R: Cirrhosis and the etiology of hepatocellular carcinoma. J Hepatol 4:140, 1987.
33. Beasley RP, Hwang Lu-Yu: HCC and HBV. Semin Liver Dis, 4:113, 1984.
34. Arrigori A, Andriulli A, Gindro T, et al.: Pattern analysis of AFP in early diagnosis of HCC in cirrhosis. Int J Biol Markers, 3:172, 1988.
35. Wynder EL, Maruchi K, Maruchi SN, et al.: Epidemiology of cancer of the pancreas. J Natl Cancer Inst 50:645, 1973.
36. Haglund C: Tumor marker antigen CA 125 in pancreatic cancer: A comparison with CA 19-9 and CEA. Br J Cancer 54:897, 1986.

chapter

20

EVALUATION OF THE PATIENT WITH ABNORMAL LIVER CHEMISTRIES

Talley Parker, M.D.
Eugene R. Schiff, M.D.

The patient who presents with "abnormal liver function tests" confronts us with a vast array of diagnostic possibilities and a potentially broad range of liver dysfunction. For example, a patient with acute hepatitis A may be severely symptomatic with abnormal chemistries, yet have a good prognosis and good residual liver function, whereas one with advanced cirrhosis may complain of few symptoms and have essentially normal chemistries, but have minimal residual hepatocyte function and a rather dismal prognosis. Among patients with abnormal liver chemistries are those with medically treatable but potentially fatal liver disease (Wilson's disease, autoimmune hepatitis, hemochromatosis), with surgical disease (cholelithiasis), with oncologic disease (hepatoma, metastases) and without disease (Gilbert's syndrome). Some present in the emergency room nauseated, vomiting, icteric, and acutely ill, whereas others are detected during routine medical check-ups or when they donate blood. Although the acutely ill patient usually undergoes appropriate diagnostic work-up and treatment, the patient who is asymptomatic, with minimal abnormalities, is often investigated inadequately because it is assumed that his disease is not significant. It is our hope to present an efficient plan for sorting out the various possibilities, with special emphasis on outpatient management and detection of treatable disease.

One of the first considerations is determination of the urgency of the evaluation. In general, if the transaminase levels are greater than 2.5 times the upper limit of normal, evaluation should be rapid. A patient who has physical or chemical evidence of chronic liver disease should be evaluated without delay. It is not necessary to follow the chemistries for 6 months, awaiting a return to normal, before performing a diagnostic biopsy. Severely ill patients should have a battery of diagnostic tests performed concurrently, sacrificing elegance for expedience in the hope of diagnosing treatable liver disease. It is not our purpose here to discuss the management of patients with acute hepatic decompensation once a diagnosis has been made, but some brief guidelines are mentioned. Markedly elevated transaminase levels should suggest viral hepatitis or toxic hepatitis, such as acetaminophen overdose. Altered mental status, prothrombin time greater than 3 seconds prolonged, or intractable nausea and vomiting indicate the need for hospitalization and expeditious diagnostic work-up. Other patients can be assessed as outpatients, with the urgency dictated by the degree of hepatic decompensation and the suspected diagnosis.

HISTORY

The most important aspect of the evaluation of the patient with liver disease is a thorough history and physical examination. Usually, the differential diagnosis is greatly limited by this exercise. Many of the questions that one must ask are personal and often embarrassing for the patient and uncomfortable for the physician but, because of liver disease are frequently infectious and are related to lifestyle, neither diagnosis nor appropriate counseling can be accomplished without openness and honesty on the part of the physician and patient.

A mental checklist is helpful in eliciting the history. Certain elements are fundamental. One must seek a history of surgery and possible transfusions. Many patients present years after hysterectomy or coronary artery bypass with chronic post-transfusion hepatitis and cirrhosis. A history of diabetes mellitus, obesity, or hyperlipidemia may explain fatty liver infiltration, probably the most common cause of mild liver chemistry abnormalities. Less well recognized is the glycogen-laden liver of a diabetic with recent tight control because of the use of an insulin pump.

Another common cause of abnormal liver function tests (LFTs) is medications. One should obtain a complete list of all prescription and over-the-counter medicines and vitamins including any recently discontinued. We have found it helpful to ask the patient or a family member to empty the medicine cabinet and bring all the medicine vials to the clinic. Literally hundreds of drugs cause hepatotoxicity, either producing a cholestatic or hepatocellular pattern of injury. Many types of drugs have been implicated (Table 20–1). The importance of nonprescription drugs should be emphasized, because they are frequently not mentioned by patients without direct inquiry. A well-advertised cold remedy containing the hepatotoxin acetaminophen and alcohol, which potentiates acetaminophen's conversion to a toxic metabolite, has been implicated in acetaminophen hepatotoxicity when taken in excessive amounts. Many nonsteroidal anti-inflammatory drugs (NSAIDs) have been implicated as causes of hepatitis. Niacin, a vitamin in vogue for the control of serum lipid levels, has been implicated in acute toxic hepatitis. Vitamin A, when taken in large

TABLE 20–1. CLASSES OF DRUGS IMPLICATED IN HEPATOTOXICITY
Analgesics and anesthetics
Anti-anginals
Anti-arrhythmics
Anticonvulsants
Antidepressants
Antihypertensives
Anti-inflammatories
Antimicrobials
Antineoplastics
Diuretics
H_2 blockers
Laxatives
Oral hypoglycemics
Psychotropics
Salicylates
Steroids, anabolic and contraceptive
Sulfa-containing drugs

doses (40,000 units/day) may lead to cirrhosis. Another hepatotoxin widely ingested and less frequently acknowledged is alcohol. According to Sherlock, the "danger" dose of alcohol is 80 g/day.[1]

Any previous history of cancer is pertinent, and metastatic lesions to the liver must be ruled out. Epidemiologic data are sought. One must rule out intravenous drug use, male homosexual encounters, and sexual contact with partners at risk for viral hepatitis and promiscuous behavior. If one suspects viral hepatitis and none of these factors is present, consider any activity involving parenteral exposure, such as dental care, ear piercing, employment in health care professions, or in the care of the institutionalized mentally impaired. Evidence of any previous liver abnormalities, such as previous abnormal liver screens or any diagnostic tests, such as abdominal ultrasound, CT scans, or liver-spleen scans, which might be compared to current studies, should be sought.

The patient should then be questioned about symptoms. Various constellations of symptoms indicate different categories of hepatobiliary disease. Pain, with careful characterization, is a useful symptom. An exquisitely tender liver suggests congestion, either secondary to right-sided heart failure and increased right atrial pressure, or Budd-Chiari syndrome (hepatic vein thrombosis). In contrast, hepatitis is associated with a dull, constant ache of a stretched Glisson's capsule. Biliary colic is frequently severe but episodic, postprandial, or nocturnal, and causes extreme restlessness. Absence of pain with jaundice, but without signs of chronic liver disease, suggests the need to rule out pancreatic or biliary cancer. Biliary colic with melena suggests hematobilia and a history of trauma, surgery, or liver biopsy should be sought. Nausea and vomiting accompany acute hepatitis or biliary tract disease, such as choledocholithiasis. Fatigue is a nonspecific complaint that accompanies acute and chronic liver disease and many other illnesses. Fatigue and arthralgias, however, are frequently the only complaints in autoimmune hepatitis or chronic anicteric viral hepatitis. One should question the patient about fevers and sweats in consideration of entities such as disseminated tuberculosis or lymphoma. Weight loss and abnormal liver chemistries suggest a work-up for malignancy.

One should always question family members or close friends about symptoms such as changes in mental status. Irritability and personality changes may indicate stage I hepatic encephalopathy. Frequently, the patient is unaware of this symptom. (Consider the corporate executive who has begun to doze during board meetings, is irascible with employees, or has been making questionable decisions.)

If Wilson's disease is a consideration, as it should be in any patient younger than 35 to 40 years old, family and associates should be asked about choreoathetoid movements and dysarthria. Skin color changes may be the initial clue to hemochromatosis. Photosensitivity may accompany porphyria. Pruritus often accompanies cholestasis, but often is also the first symptom of primary biliary cirrhosis (PBC). Loss of libido, impotence, or abnormal menses often accompany chronic liver disease, especially Laennec's cirrhosis.

Physicians in more rural locations need to be aware of a fact that is familiar to physicians in large cities and county hospitals: that infection with the HIV virus and attendant opportunistic infections are frequently associated with abnormal liver chemistries. Abnormalities range from a picture almost indistinguishable from sclerosing cholangitis related to infection of the biliary tree with cytomegalovirus or cryptosporidium to the more common fatty infiltration. Although occult HIV infection is a rare cause for liver chemistry abnormalities in an asymptomatic patient, it should certainly be considered in the differential diagnosis.

PHYSICAL EXAMINATION

The physical examination can provide evidence of chronic liver disease, cholestasis, biliary tract disease, or primary disease in other organ systems that result in hepatic abnormalities—for example, right-sided cardiac disease leading to hepatic congestion or pulmonary hypertension with "right-sided" congestion. A thorough physical examination should be done, including all organ systems.

Often, the first impression yields a large amount of information to the careful observer. The importance of assessing mental status cannot be overemphasized in the evaluation of the patient with liver disease. Are there subtle signs of encephalopathy, such as irritability, rambling thought processes, silly affect, or even frank disorientation, asterixis, or somnolence? Can one detect "fetor hepaticus," the odor of mercaptans frequently detectable on the breath of a patient with severely decompensated liver disease (or perhaps the patient's last drink)? Does the patient's nutritional status appear adequate, or is evidence of muscle wasting present? Is the patient's weight carried as ascites rather than as muscle mass? Does the skin show excoriations from pruritus, jaundice, ecchymoses, or spider angiomata? Does the patient appear ill?

Specifically, one should look for the signs of chronic liver disease: vascular spider angiomata, palmar erythema, splenomegaly, small, soft testes, decreased male body hair, and ascites or peripheral edema. Signs of cholestatic liver disease, such as jaundice, excoriations, and xanthelasma, are sought.

Liver size and texture are assessed. Tenderness over the liver is usually a sign of acute liver disease. Exquisite tenderness should suggest passive congestion or Budd-Chiari syndrome. The hepatojugular reflex should be elicited by steady pressure with the examiner's open hand over the liver, watching for any increased distention of the neck veins. Acute hepatitis with hepatomegaly may lead to moderate tenderness. Carcinoma, either primary hepatic or metastatic, may be painful or painless. One should attempt to elicit Murphy's sign, always remembering that abnormal liver chemistries may result from cholelithiasis, especially with choledocholithiasis and/or subsequent cholecystitis.

Several physical signs are specific to certain liver disease entities. A patient with Wilson's disease in the neurologic phase almost invariably has Kayser-Fleischer (KF) rings—brown, green, or gray rings visible in the cornea over the periphery of the iris. These are caused by copper deposition in Descemet's membrane of the cornea. Any young patient (less than 40 years old) with chronic liver disease or acute liver disease of uncertain cause should have a slit lamp examination done by an experienced ophthalmologist to rule out KF rings, because these are frequently present during pre-symptomatic stages of the disease. KF rings are sometimes seen in advanced stages of cholestatic liver disease, so they cannot be considered diagnostic of Wilson's disease. Xanthelasmas are frequently seen in PBC because of disordered lipid metabolism and hyperlipidemia. Brown skin pigmentation should suggest hemochromatosis.

THE CHEMISTRIES

At this point, the list of probable causes of the patient's liver dysfunction usually has been significantly reduced. The information gained from the history and physical examination is refined further by examination of the pattern of liver chemistries and by the addition of more specific biochemical and serologic tests and diagnostic procedures.

Further work-up should be tailored depending on whether the initial chemistries indicate cholestatic or parenchymal liver disease. Generally, aminotransferase, alkaline phosphatase, and bilirubin levels are determined initially, because these are contained in commonly available chemistry panels.

The aminotransferases, ALT (SGPT) and AST (SGOT), transfer α-amino groups of alanine and aspartic acid to α-ketoglutaric acid in amino acid metabolism. Both enzymes are found in many different tissues, including liver, cardiac muscle, skeletal muscle, kidney, brain, pancreas, lung, leukocytes, and erythrocytes, although ALT is considered more liver-specific. Their presence in serum usually indicates leakage through damaged cell membranes or cell necrosis of parenchymal cells. Selective elevation indicates parenchymal rather than cholestatic disease.

Alkaline phosphatase (AP) catalyzes the hydrolysis of organic phosphate esters at an alkaline pH. Its precise function is unknown. In addition to liver, APs are found in bone osteoblasts, small intestine brush border cells, proximal convoluted tubules, the placenta, and white blood cells. In the liver, they are produced in hepatocytes, canalicular membranes, and bile duct epithelium. Evidence has suggested that increased synthesis of AP, mediated by the action of bile acids on biliary epithelium, occurs in hepatobiliary disease. Normal values of AP vary, depending on age and gender. In adults (15 to 50 years old), AP is somewhat higher in men than in women. Over the age of 60, enzyme activity in women equals or exceeds that in men. Normal AP in adolescent males may triple that measured in adults. In late pregnancy, levels may double with the placental contribution. Evaluation of the source of an isolated, elevated AP level can be approached in several ways. Electrophoretic separation of isoenzymes has not been routinely available. Assays based on the heat sensitivity of AP from bone versus liver origin have been poorly reproducible. The best approach has been to assay 5′-nucleotidase, γ-glutamyl transpeptidase (GGTP), or leucine aminopeptidase (LAP), which are not elevated in bone disease. An increase in these enzyme levels in men and in nonpregnant women with an elevated AP level indicates the presence of hepatobiliary disease. 5′-Nucleotidase is primarily associated with canalicular and sinusoidal plasma membranes and parallels the activity of AP, so it can help clarify the significance of an elevated AP level in the presence of these other conditions. LAP is produced in large amounts by biliary epithelial cells. Therefore, values are highest in biliary obstruction, paralleling elevations in AP and 5′-nucleotidase levels. Unlike GGTP, LAP values are elevated by pregnancy.

Perhaps the only real "liver function tests" are those that measure the liver's synthetic function. These include determinations of serum protein levels, most importantly albumin and clotting factors.

Albumin is synthesized exclusively by the liver and tends to be normal in acute liver disease, such as viral hepatitis, toxic hepatitis, and obstructive jaundice. Heavy alcohol ingestion, chronic inflammation, and protein malnutrition all inhibit its synthesis. Causes of hypoalbuminemia unrelated to liver disease include protein malnutrition, protein-losing enteropathies, chronic infection, and nephrotic syndrome.

The prothrombin time (PT) indicates how fast prothrombin is converted to thrombin, as well as polymerization of fibrinogen by thrombin to fibrin. Factors I, II, V, VII, and X, all synthesized by the liver, are involved. Vitamin K, however, is required for γ-carboxylation of factors II, VII, IX, and X for calcium binding and activation. Vitamin K deficiency can be distinguished from hepatic insufficiency if the parenteral administration of vitamin K corrects the prothrombin time. PT is not a sensitive indicator of liver disease because coagulopathy indicates extensive liver damage, and a PT greater than 3 to 4 seconds prolonged, in the setting of chronic liver disease, is a poor prognostic sign.

Serum immunoglobulin levels are abnormal in many patients with chronic liver disease. This is thought to be secondary to decreased clearance by impaired reticuloendothelial cells. Certain patterns suggest particular disease entities. Striking increases in serum globulin levels, particularly IgG, suggest autoimmune hepatitis. Specific IgM increases suggest primary biliary cirrhosis, whereas increases in IgA suggest alcoholic liver disease. Chronic liver disease is associated with polyclonal increases in immunoglobulin levels.

Bilirubin is produced by the breakdown of hemoglobin, myoglobin, cytochromes, and other heme-containing proteins. Heme is initially oxidized in the reticuloendothelial cells of the liver and spleen. The heme ring is opened by the action of heme oxygenase, producing biliverdin and carbon monoxide. Biliverdin is then reduced to bilirubin, which is lipid-soluble. In this form, it is bound to albumin for carrier-mediated transport into hepatocytes, where it is solubilized by conjugation to glucuronic acid, a reaction that occurs in the endoplasmic reticulum of the hepatocyte. Another carrier-mediated membrane transport system moves conjugated or "direct" bilirubin into canalicular bile; this is considered the rate-limiting step in bilirubin excretion.

It is helpful to carry out fractionation into direct and indirect bilirubin, especially in isolated hyperbilirubinemia, because this limits the diagnostic possibilities. An increased unconjugated bilirubin level is usually caused by intravascular hemolysis or ineffective erythropoiesis, in which bilirubin turnover is increased, such as pernicious anemia, thalassemia, sideroblastic anemia, lead poisoning, or erythropoietic porphyrias. Deficiency of uridine diphosphate-glucuronyl transferase leads to unconjugated hyperbilirubinemia. The most common type is a benign condition called Gilbert's syndrome. The bilirubin concentration rarely exceeds 5 mg/dl and increases with fasting, fever, surgery, infections, excessive alcohol ingestion, and intravenous glucose. Diagnosis is made by checking a GGTP or serum bile salt level. If these are normal, the diagnosis is verified by placing the patient on a 300-kcal diet without lipids for 24 to 48 hours, at which time the bilirubin is increased by approximately 1.5 mg/dl.

Conjugated hyperbilirubinemia invariably means hepatic dysfunction or biliary obstruction. Causes of isolated increases in the conjugated bilirubin level, which are often forgotten, are sepsis leading to cholestasis, renal impairment, and hypotension or hypoxemia affecting oxygen sensitive central zones of the liver. In general, a bilirubin level greater than 30 mg/dl means hepatocellular dysfunction rather than extrahepatic obstruction, except in the setting of renal impairment. Because bilirubin must be in the conjugated form to be excreted renally, the presence of bilirubin in urine indicates hepatic dysfunction or obstruction.

Assays for serum bile acid levels, particularly cholylglycine (CG), are now available through reference laboratories. They have been disappointing in helping to narrow the differential diagnosis of liver disease. Their main usefulness lies in demonstrating the presence or absence of liver disease, if this is a consideration, such as in Gilbert's syndrome (CG level normal), or well-compensated cirrhosis (CG level elevated).

When initially confronted with a patient who has suspected liver disease, one should start with a standard battery of tests, including direct and total bilirubin, urinalysis for bilirubin, alkaline phosphatase, aminotransferases, prothrombin time, total protein and albumin, and possibly serum bile acids. On the other hand, if the patient is referred for abnormal chemistries, the initial step is to repeat the abnormal laboratory tests to rule out transient changes and to screen for hepatitis A, B and C (anti-HAV, IgM fraction, HBsAg, anti-HBC and antibody to hepatitis C). This is relatively cost-efficient and allows characterization of the dysfunction and direction of further evaluation. The chemistry profiles fit into one of several classifications: hyperbilirubinemia, cholestatic disease, and hepatocellular disease.

UNCONJUGATED HYPERBILIRUBINEMIA

The first and simplest category is isolated unconjugated hyperbilirubinemia. All other liver chemistries, including serum bile acids and GGTP, are normal. The diagnosis is usually Gilbert's syndrome. But before this syndrome is diagnosed, hemolysis should be ruled out with a hemoglobin, reticulocyte count, and serum LDH determination. A rare cause is Crigler-Najjar syndrome, type II, an autosomal dominant disorder characterized by a deficiency of glucuronyl transferase and producing an unconjugated bilirubin level in the range of 6 to 25 mg/dl.

Isolated bilirubin elevation of both the conjugated and unconjugated fractions, once other causes are ruled out and all other liver tests are normal, may be a result of Dubin-Johnson syndrome (a defect in transport of organic anions out of the liver into the bile) or Rotor's syndrome (a defect in the uptake and storage of conjugated bilirubin). The remainder of liver chemistry abnormalities can be divided into cholestatic disease and hepatocellular disease.

CHOLESTATIC DISEASE

Cholestatic disease is characterized by an elevation in the AP and GGTP levels out of proportion to the aminotransferase levels. Both bilirubin fractions are usually elevated. The aminotransferase levels are usually lower than 500 units. The albumin and globulin levels are usually normal, and the PT is normal or easily corrected with parenteral vitamin K. This group includes intrahepatic and extrahepatic cholestasis, and differentiation between the two cannot be made using standard laboratory tests. Patients with this profile should undergo ultrasound of the liver, gallbladder, and pancreas to rule out cholelithiasis, choledocholithiasis, dilated biliary tree, or a mass in the pancreas or liver. Those with biliary dilation but no obvious gallstones or pancreatic or hepatic mass need CT scan and endoscopic retrograde cholangiopancreatography (ERCP) or transhepatic

TABLE 20–2. CONDITIONS PRODUCING INTRAHEPATIC CHOLESTASIS
Viral hepatitis (cholestatic)
Alcoholic hepatitis
Pregnancy, including benign cholestasis of pregnancy and acute fatty liver pregnancy
Drugs
Cryptogenic cirrhosis
Sepsis
Hodgkin's disease
Benign recurrent cholestasis
Primary biliary cirrhosis
Sarcoidosis
Granulomatous infiltration
Amyloidosis
Neonatal problems: biliary artresia, bile plug syndrome, Byler's syndrome
Fatty infiltration of the liver

cholangiography (THC) to define the cause of the obstruction. Occult malignancy, sclerosing cholangitis, and choledochal cyst are considerations.

Those with a nondilated biliary tree most likely represent intrahepatic cholestasis (Table 20–2).

Further laboratory tests at this point include antimitochondrial antibody (AMA) and quantitative serum immunoglobulins, looking for an increased IgM titer and serologic evidence of primary biliary cirrhosis (PBC). It is assumed that possible toxic hepatitis, caused by drugs, has been ruled out by the history. All nonessential medicines should be discontinued. Serologic tests for hepatitis A and B should be done, if not done previously, because cholestatic forms of both of these have been documented. Liver biopsy should be considered, especially if the patient's condition is not improving and the diagnosis is still in question. If the diagnosis is not reached, the biliary tree must be visualized directly by ERCP or THC. THC should be used only if ERCP is not available for patients in whom the biliary tree is not dilated, because of the high rate of failure of THC in this setting.

Patients with an isolated elevated alkaline phosphatase level are sometimes difficult to separate from those with cholestasis. Initially, a GGTP, 5′-nucleotidase, or LAP test should be done to confirm the hepatic origin of AP. Again, AMA and IgM levels are checked to rule out early PBC. Ultrasound and CT scan may both be necessary if the ultrasound is negative. This category encompasses infiltrative diseases such as granulomatous, amyloidosis, and neoplasms, both primary and metastatic. The patient's medication history should again be reviewed, because many drugs cause granulomatous disease. Even minimal elevations in the alkaline phosphatase level should be investigated if present consistently because of the possibility of neoplasm with even subtle abnormalities in the AP level.

HEPATOCELLULAR DISEASE

Transaminase levels are elevated out of proportion to AP in hepatocellular disease. Both chronic and acute disease states are seen, and are sometimes difficult to distinguish at initial presentation. In general, markedly elevated transaminase and normal protein levels, without evidence on history or physical examination of chronic disease, suggest acute hepatocellular disease, particularly viral or toxic. Serologic tests for viral hepatitis, ANA, antismooth muscle antibodies, and quantitative serum immunoglobulins should be done to rule out viral hepatitis and autoimmune hepatitis. Toxic hepatitis must be reconsidered. A low ceruloplasmin or elevated 24-hour urine copper level suggests the diagnosis of Wilson's disease, an inherited disease of copper metabolism that is fatal if untreated. Wilson's disease should be ruled out in any patient younger than 40 years old with acute hepatitis of unknown cause, or with chronic hepatitis. Most patients with acute or chronic hepatocellular disease should have an ultrasound or CT scan visualization of the liver, biliary tree, and pancreas. Patients with severe hepatitis of unknown cause or chronic hepatitis should have a liver biopsy, either percutaneously or by laparoscopy, to determine the cause, stage of the disease, and prognosis. Laparoscopy is preferred if a mild coagulopathy is present or if sampling error is a consideration. Hepatitis is considered chronic after 6 months of elevated liver chemistries.

An AST:ALT ratio greater than 2 or 3, with an ALT less than 300, strongly suggests alcoholic liver disease or steatonecrosis. This ratio represents decreased activity of ALT caused by a deficiency of pyridoxal 5′-phosphate in patients who abuse alcohol. The synthesis of ALT requires greater amounts of pyridoxal 5′-phosphate than does that of AST. In future liver injury the abnormal ratio is preserved, even after cessation of drinking. Falsely depressed values of AST are seen in uremia, caused by a dialyzable inhibitor.

SUMMARY

One can direct the evaluation depending on whether the pattern of liver chemistry abnormalities suggests simple, unconjugated hyperbilirubinemia, cholestasis, or hepatocellular injury. In the first case, if the GGTP and cholylglycine levels are normal, one should rule out hemolysis and in most cases the work-up need go no further if the patient is asymptomatic. If the pattern is cholestatic or hepatocellular, further testing is necessary.

In a patient with a cholestatic pattern, the work-up should start with a right upper quadrant ultrasound to rule out biliary tree dilation. A dilated biliary tree suggests extrahepatic obstruction, and a CT scan and ERCP or THC should be done. Malignancy, sclerosing cholangitis, choledocholithiasis, and choledochal cyst should be considered. If the biliary tree is not dilated, toxic hepatitis should be reconsidered, all nonessential medicines stopped, viral hepatitis ruled out, AMA determined to rule out primary biliary cirrhosis, and liver biopsy and ERCP considered.

If the pattern shows a predominance of transaminase levels indicating hepatocellular damage, one should recheck the drug and alcohol history. Usually, repeat testing after complete abstention from alcohol or possible hepatotoxic drugs should reveal marked improvement in 1 month. If the alcohol and drug history is negative, if the hepatitis is acute or if abnormalities persist despite abstention, one should check viral serologies. If these are negative and the patient is asymptomatic, the patient can be observed. If abnormalities persist for 6 months, a chronic liver disease work-up is indicated, including the determination of AMA and quantitative immunoglobulins to rule out autoimmune hepatitis, iron and total iron-binding capacity and ferritin to rule out hemochromatosis, and ceruloplasmin and 24-hour urine for copper, if appropriate, to rule out Wilson's disease. An α-antitrypsin level should also be determined. A liver biopsy should be done, in most cases, after imaging by ultrasound or CT scan. One should remember that the presence of abdominal pain suggests the need for an imaging study as part of the initial evaluation.

If this approach is followed, a diagnosis can usually be obtained. In many cases, abnormalities are transient; in others, mild abnormalities are secondary to fatty infiltration or alcohol use. Liver chemistry abnormalities should not be ignored, because liver damage can progress without symptoms until impairment is significant. One should always remember to consider treatable causes of liver disease.

REFERENCES

1. Sherlock S: Diseases of the Liver and Biliary System. 7th Ed. London, Blackwell Scientific Publications, 1985.
2. Kaplan, Marshall M: Laboratory tests. *In* Diseases of the Liver. Edited by L Schiff and R Schiff. Philadelphia, JB Lippincott, 1987, pp 219–260.
3. Scharschmidt BF, Goldberg HI, Schmid R: Approach to the patient with cholestatic jaundice. N Engl J Med, 308:1515, 1983.
4. VanNiss MM, Diehl AM: Is liver biopsy useful in the evaluation of patients with chronically elevated liver enzymes? Ann Intern Med, 111:473, 1989.
5. Chapra S, Griffin PH: Laboratory tests and diagnostic procedures in evaluation of liver disease. Am J Med, 79:221, 1985.
6. McIntyre N: The limitations of conventional liver function tests. Semin Liver Dis, 3:265, 1983.
7. Bircher J: Quantitative assessment of deranged hepatic function: A missed opportunity? Semin Liver Dis, 3:275, 1983.

c h a p t e r

21

THE CARE AND DISINFECTION OF FLEXIBLE ENDOSCOPES AND ACCESSORIES

Melanie L. Swartz

The use of fiberoptic flexible endoscopic equipment and their accessories has advanced the field of gastroenterology by assisting in the diagnosis and treatment of gastrointestinal disorders. The use of this equipment, however, is not without associated risk, and demands special care and handling. Infection is one such risk. The thermolabile materials used in the construction of fiberoptic equipment creates problems when the issue of decontamination is addressed.[1]

Endoscopic-related infection may be transmitted in several ways. Bacterial infections may be associated with the use of contaminated endoscopic equipment. Bacterial infections from various organisms, including Pseudomonas aeruginosa, Serratia marcescens, Mycobacterium tuberculosis, and Salmonella spp. can be acquired in this manner by patients undergoing endoscopy.[1,2] Endoscopic cross infection has been demonstrated in two ways: (1) direct patient-to-patient transmission; and (2) indirect transmission through inoculation of opportunistic organisms into patients following colonization in endoscopic equipment.[1] A warm, moist environment provides the proper conditions for opportunistic bacteria to multiply quickly. These conditions make endoscopic equipment such as the endoscopic water bottle and other accessories susceptible to colonization of bacteria.

Bacteria may also be spread, and possibly result in infection, from the gastrointestinal tract through the bloodstream to potentially susceptible tissues (e.g., heart valves) or prostheses (e.g., total hip replacements) during endoscopy.[2] Special consideration must be given to the increased risk of infectious organisms being transmitted during endoscopy to patients with severe neutropenia or immunodeficiency syndromes, or to those receiving immunosuppressive chemotherapy. Additional intervention in regard to the decontamination of endoscopic equipment is required prior to its use on these patients.

Finally, the transmission of infection must also be considered a risk for endoscopy personnel. Infected patients may transmit disease to those involved with the procedure as well as to those involved with the care and handling of the equipment following the procedure. Personnel can be exposed to infectious materials directly or indirectly through the contamination of the endoscope with blood, body fluids, and stool.

The category I recommendation from the Centers for Disease Control regarding the cleaning, disinfection, and sterilization of patient care equipment has stated that "Equipment that touches mucous membranes, e.g., endoscopes, endotracheal tubes, anesthesia breathing circuits, and respiratory therapy equipment, should receive high-level disinfection."[3] To achieve high-level disinfection, the endoscope must first be cleaned meticulously to remove adherent patient material from the external surfaces and from the internal surfaces and channels. This is done through the use of soap, water, and brushes. Following this, these surfaces must be exposed to a germicidal chemical registered with the Environmental Protection Agency as a "disinfectant/sterilant."[3]

With regard to infection, identification of all at-risk individuals is not possible. Endoscopic equipment is used on patients with both recognized and unrecognized infections, so routine procedures should include cleaning and disinfecting the equipment in the same manner after being used on each patient.[3,4]

ENDOSCOPIC EQUIPMENT

CLEANING AND DISINFECTION

A major error in the cleaning, disinfecting, or sterilizing of the endoscopic equipment has been cited in almost every reported case of disease transmission associated with endoscopes.[3] Interpretive statements and rationale have been provided by the Association of Operating Room Nurses (AORN) in their Recommended Practice Statement VII, which states that "flexible and rigid endoscopes should be inspected, tested, and processed according to the design/type and manufacturer's instructions."[5] The AORN interpretive statements to the above include the following: "one, endoscopic equipment should be handled with care to prevent damage to lens, fiberoptic components, and delicate instruments and should be closely inspected at frequent intervals; and two, endoscopes should be disassembled, thoroughly cleaned and dried prior to decontamination by sterilization or disinfection." The rationale given for these statements are listed as the following: "one, the use of damaged instruments could possibly increase the risk of tissue trauma, infection, and the length of the operative procedure; and two, the prevention of dried secretions and organic material is imperative for proper cleaning, disinfection or sterilization; cleaning and drying of the endoscopes and accessories is essential to reduce the bioburden and minimize dilution of the disinfectant solution."[5]

Elimination of the risk of infection is the main objective of the cleaning and disinfection procedure. The contributing factors necessary to coexist for an endoscopic cross infection to occur are an index patient, a pathogenic organism, a susceptible host, and a contaminated endoscope or accessory.[1] In regard to these factors, the virulence of the organism and possibly the incubation time between procedures must also be considered.[1] Therefore, only thorough, aggressive cleaning and decontamination of the endoscopic equipment after each use can reduce the risk of endoscopic cross infection.

The care and handling of endoscopic equipment, including specialized cleaning and disinfection procedures, require personnel who are knowledgeable about the equipment and are properly trained in the cleaning and disinfecting procedures.

Before beginning any cleaning or disinfecting procedure, preparation of the cleaning area and of the personnel involved are important. Exposure of personnel to blood and body fluids can occur during the cleaning process. Gowns, gloves, masks, and protective eyewear should be available to be worn by individuals while performing the task of reprocessing the equipment.

Optimally, the cleaning and disinfecting procedure should be carried out in an area dedicated for equipment reprocessing, and this area should be separate from the patient procedure rooms. Separate clean and dirty utility rooms are recommended but, if this is not feasible, a minimum of separate clean and dirty areas must be maintained. These areas should also contain structural features such as special plumbing, drains, and pressurized air.

The immersibility of the endoscope must also be considered. At present, almost all endoscopes marketed are fully immersible, and their design allows for easier cleaning and disinfection. In addition to being totally immersible, another advantage of current endoscopes over earlier equipment is the ability to irrigate all channels with positive pressure.[4] Some units may still have some nonimmersible endoscopes in use. Differences in the construction of these endoscopes might include a "dead space" in the region of the valves, which may be difficult to irrigate, and a suction channel that extends from the handle of the instrument to the light source, which is less accessible.[4] With this type of instrument, the cleaning and disinfection procedures must be modified according to the manufacturers' instructions.

Manual Cleaning

Cleaning is defined as "the physical removal of organic material and/or soil from objects, usually using water with detergents to remove rather than to kill organisms."[2] The main objective of manual cleaning is to remove any gross organic contaminates and microorganisms from the endoscope.

Prior to the beginning of the manual cleaning procedure, and immediately following each endoscopic procedure, it is important to ensure the proper functioning of the air and water channels of the endoscope. This may be done in one of two ways. In the first method, while the light source is still on and the endoscope is plugged into it, the distal tip of the insertion tube is immersed in water and the air-water valve is lightly occluded with a finger. This allows air to flow from the distal tip if the air channel is not plugged, and bubbles can be seen in the water. Next, the distal tip is removed from the water and the air-water valve is depressed and held down. If the water channel is not plugged, a water spray or stream, depending on the scope, can be seen coming from the distal end of the insertion tube. Partial blockage of the channel is indicated by a slow drip of water rather than the full spray or stream, and consultation with the manufacturer may be necessary.

Another way of performing this same procedure involves disconnecting the water bottle from the endoscope while the endoscope is still connected to the light source and the power is turned on. Once the water bottle has been disconnected, the air-water inlet on the universal cord of the endoscope is blocked with a finger while the air-water valve is depressed. This allows all the water remaining in the channel to be pumped out; air can be pumped through the channel once it has been emptied of water.

Once the air-water channels are found to be free of debris, 150 to 200 ml of clean water should be immediately suctioned through the suction channel to flush through any remaining body fluids, and to remove any loose protein materials.

A leak test may now be performed if a leakage tester is available for use with the particular endoscope. This is helpful in detecting small leaks before major endoscope damage has occurred. The leakage tester provides a means of injecting air into the interstitial space of the light carrier and the insertion tube of the endoscope. Once the leakage tester is attached to the immersible endoscope, it is totally submerged in water and observed for any air bubbles. If air bubbles are detected, the integrity of the endoscope has been disrupted. The endoscope must then be sent out for repair. Immersing the endoscope once the integrity has been disrupted causes fogging or flooding of the lens system and/or damage to the fiberoptics. A potential for cross infection may also exist from pinholes by providing a path for microbial contamination of the interstitial space.[6]

Another piece of equipment is the maintenance unit. This may be obtained from some endoscope manufacturers and supplies the air and water functions of the light source necessary for the cleaning procedure. This allows the actual light source to be available to perform another procedure and provides convenience when establishing a separate, central cleaning area. The maintenance unit is relatively inexpensive.

The use of a nonabrasive detergent or cleaning solution or an enzymatic detergent to break down proteinaceous material is best for mechanical cleaning. Some endoscope manufacturers provide an air-water channel cleaning valve with the endoscope. Before cleaning begins, if this valve is

TABLE 21–1. SUPPLIES FOR MANUAL ENDOSCOPE CLEANING
Double sink or large basins (two)
Light source or maintenance unit
Suction pump
Syringe (30 to 50 ml)
Cleaning detergent and water
Manufacturer-supplied cleaning apparatus: channel cleaning adaptor; leak tester, if available
Gauze pads, 4″ × 4″
Channel cleaning brush
Soft-bristled toothbrush
Cotton-tipped applicators
70% ethyl alcohol
Protective attire: aprons or gowns, gloves, goggles, masks

available, the air-water valve from the endoscope should be removed and placed in the detergent solution, and the air-water channel cleaning valve should be inserted into the open port. This valve allows for a constant flow of air through the channel, without having to cover the valve opening with a finger. A full depression of the valve intermittently allows the water spray or stream to flow from the distal tip.

For the cleaning procedure, a double sink can be used in which one side is filled with the detergent solution and the other side is filled with clean water. This or a combination of sink and basin(s) may be used. The necessary equipment listed in Table 21–1 should be assembled in the cleaning area.

The manual cleaning procedure is as follows:

1. Connect the endoscope to the water bottle, light source, or maintenance unit, and suction pump and turn all power on.
2. If the full cleaning procedure has been delayed, the initial check for functioning and clearing of the air-water channel and suctioning of clean water, as described earlier, should have been performed directly after the procedure; otherwise, this becomes the first step in the cleaning process and should be performed now.
3. If available, the leak test should be carried out using a leak tester and following the manufacturers' instructions.
4. Following the leak test, connect any special cleaning adaptors supplied by the manufacturer to the endoscope, remove any hoods present on the distal end, and place in the detergent solution.
5. Reconnect the endoscope to the light source or maintenance unit, water bottle, and suction pump and turn all power on.
6. Suction approximately 150 to 200 ml of detergent solution through the endoscope suction channel by depressing the suction valve.
7. Flush any special channels (e.g., elevator, jet) through with detergent solution.

8. Remove the suction valve and place in the detergent solution to soak while angling the cleaning brush into the port, first through the universal cord and then through the insertion tube, so that the brush exits the endoscope at the distal tip.
9. Remove the biopsy valve and brush the small section of the biopsy channel at the forceps opening leading to the insertion tube.
10. Replace the biopsy valve and suction an additional amount of detergent solution through the endoscope.
11. Wipe the external surfaces of the control head, insertion tube, and universal cord with a soft cloth, sponge, or gauze dampened in the detergent solution.

    Note: For a nonimmersible endoscope, care must be used when brushing internal channels and wiping external surfaces, adapting the procedure appropriately.
12. Scrub the distal end of the insertion tube gently with a soft toothbrush.
13. Place the insertion tube of the endoscope in the clean water and suction copious amounts of clean water through all channels to rinse thoroughly.
14. Wipe the control head, insertion tube, and universal cord with a soft cloth, sponge, or gauze dampened in clean water, again using care if the endoscope is nonimmersible.
15. Turn the power off on the light source or maintenance unit and suction pump.
16. Remove all remaining valves and place in the detergent solution.
17. Clean the openings to the ports using a cotton-tipped applicator dipped in 70% alcohol. Repeat until the applicator remains clean.
18. Disconnect the endoscope from the light source or maintenance unit, water bottle, and suction pump.
19. Drain all channels of remaining water and dry the external surfaces in preparation for disinfection. Nonimmersible handles should be wiped with a cloth or gauze soaked in 70% alcohol, and dried.
20. Clean all valves, hoods, and port covers that have been soaking in the detergent solution with a soft toothbrush, rinse in clean water, and dry.
21. The endoscope is now prepared for disinfection or sterilization.

Disinfection

High-level disinfection is commonly achieved through the use of liquid germicides and involves killing all microorganisms, including pathogens (e.g., gram-negative and gram-positive bacteria, fungi, mycobacteria, and lipophilic and hydrophilic viruses), with the exception of high numbers of bacterial spores, when used according to manufacturers' instructions.[2,7] The Environmental Protection Agency (EPA) and the Public Health Service, Centers for Disease Control (CDC), use different definitions and classification schemes for chemical germicides.

The CDC investigates specific disease outbreaks and formulates recommendations for the use of chemical germicides in various patient care situations. The CDC uses a classification system that defines three levels of disinfection: high-level, intermediate, and low-level disinfection, depending on the amount and kind of microbial killing involved.[2]

The EPA approves products for disinfectant registration through the review of labeling and supporting data submitted by the registrants, but the EPA does not use the CDC classification of disinfection levels. The EPA-registered chemical germicide "sterilant" may be used for sterilization or high-level disinfection, depending on factors such as contact time and frequency of reuse.[2] The label of the individual product contains information on specific recommendations for disinfection.

Care must be used in the selection of a disinfectant. Glutaraldehyde-based products seem to be the most widely used germicides in the field of endoscopy today. The glutaraldehyde-based disinfectant should be EPA-registered for use and for reuse, if it is to be reused. The appropriate disinfectant must also be chosen after consideration is given to the type of instrument or surface on which it is to be used, and to the level of disinfection required. The disinfectant chosen should be effective against the worst expected microbial contamination, and the instrument manufacturers' specifications in regard to whether a particular disinfectant is safe to apply to the endoscope must be considered. Also, it is in violation of the law to use a disinfectant other than in accordance with the manufacturers' directions, as printed on the label. Effectiveness of the disinfectant varies with chemical composition, concentration, exposure time, temperature, and number of times used.[2]

The most practical and efficient means of minimizing the risk of infection through endoscopy seems to be high-level chemical disinfection, when properly performed.[1] Methods of cleaning and disinfecting endoscopes have been evaluated by Gerding and associates, and the results clearly indicated that mechanical cleaning alone is insufficient, because it does not adequately preclude the risk of transmitting infection.[1]

Certain environmental factors need to be considered when using chemical disinfectants. Suitable exhaust extraction facilities and adequate ventilation need to be provided in work areas in which these chemicals are used. Suitable eye protection must also be provided if splashing is a consideration.

The manual disinfecting procedure is as follows:

1. Disinfection may be accomplished through the use of manufacturer-supplied cleaning-disinfecting apparatus and disinfectant "boats."
2. Prepare the disinfectant for use as directed by the manufacturer.
3. Disconnect all valves, port covers, and hoods from the endoscope, and connect the manufacturer-supplied disinfecting apparatus according to instructions while the insertion tube of the endoscope is submersed in the disinfectant.
4. Using the attached disinfecting apparatus, fill all standard channels with disinfectant.

   Note: If the endoscope is the immersible type, the channels should be filled prior to immersion of the control head to avoid air locks from blocking flow (and filling) into the small air and water channels.[8]

5. If the endoscope is immersible, totally immerse the control head, insertion tube, and universal cord in the disinfectant, and continue filling the channels with several syringes of disinfectant until the disinfectant is observed exiting the channel openings at the end of the insertion tube and the universal cord.
   a. Any special channels should be filled with disinfectant.
   b. Submerse all valves, port covers, and hoods in the disinfectant.
6. If the endoscope is nonimmersible, introduce the disinfectant into the channels through the appropriate disinfecting apparatus supplied. The control head and universal cord are left outside the "boat" or container holding the disinfectant, and may be carefully wiped with gauze or a cloth dampened in the disinfectant.
7. As an alternative to filling the disinfectant manually, the endoscope, valves, hoods, and port covers may be inserted into a disinfector and the endoscope connected to the tubing for the air, water, and suction ports of the universal or umbilical cord. Once the disinfector is started, the disinfecting and rinsing of the endoscope and components are completed within the machine.
8. Soak the entire instrument in the disinfectant solution for the recommended length of time, as directed by the manufacturer's label. A bell or timer is useful in ensuring that the proper soak time has been observed.

   Note: The shortening of the soak time compromises the reliability of the disinfection process. Consistent lengthening of soak times, however, can lead to endoscope damage caused by prolonged exposure of the instrument seals to moisture.[8]
9. Rinse the instrument following disinfection with copious amounts (1500 to 2000 ml) of clean water using the manufacturer-supplied disinfecting apparatus to minimize the risk of introducing potentially irritating toxic residues into the patient.
   a. A second "boat" or container filled with sterile water is ideal for this purpose. If tap water is used, it should be followed with a 70% alcohol rinse and dried with compressed air.[7]
   b. On immersible endoscopes, the external portions of the endoscope and the valves, port covers, and hoods are also rinsed with copious amounts of water.
   c. On nonimmersible endoscopes, the insertion tube, channels, and valves are rinsed with copious amounts of water and the umbilical cord and control head are wiped with gauze or a cloth dampened with clean water, and then wiped with a fresh cloth dampened with 70% alcohol.
10. Blow air through or suction the channels and valves to remove water droplets and facilitate drying. Dry the external surfaces of the instrument.
11. Before storage, the channels should be flushed with 70 to 90% ethyl or isopropyl alcohol to facilitate drying and discourage growth of residual bacteria and fungi.[7]

Automatic Washer And Disinfectors

Several automatic washer-disinfectors are available commercially. Although they carry out the disinfecting process automatically, it is still necessary to clean the endoscope manually, prior to loading it into the machine to remove the gross solid, proteinaceous material.

These machines offer several advantages: (1) they ensure perfusion of the air channel as well as the water-suction channels of the instrument; (2) optimal time cycles are automatically followed for washing, disinfecting, and rinsing; (3) they free personnel from an important but tedious and repetive chore; (4) they offer the security of a consistent cleaning regimen, which is difficult to duplicate manually; and (5) if the plumbing for the machine is designed to be closed and contained, it minimizes staff exposure to the disinfectant, which may induce sensitivity reactions in some individuals.[1,4]

Some disadvantages to the washer-disinfector are the following: (1) they are relatively expensive; (2) they are complex and need care in use to avoid the possibility of the machine itself becoming a reservoir of bacterial infection; (3) the cycle length necessitates that at least two endoscopes be available for a busy endoscopy schedule; and (4) these machines are generally not mobile, and require adequate space for installation and use.[4]

STERILIZATION

The AORN Recommended Practice Statement VII states that sterilization, rather than disinfection, of endoscopes and accessories is a consideration for ensuring patient safety.[5] Cold gas (ethylene oxide) is effective for sterilizing flexible endoscopes. Gas sterilization has several disadvantages: (1) it may be impractical for routine use because it usually requires scheduling; (2) it is expensive; and (3) it is potentially damaging to the endoscope.[2,9]

Prior to sterilization with ethylene oxide, a fiberscope must be completely dry and the venting cap on fluid, air-tight instruments must be opened to avoid damage to the instrument.[10] Following gas sterilization, the instrument must be thoroughly aerated to remove all residual gas before it can be used again because of potential contact, inhalational toxicity, and mutagenic potential.[9] Aeration requires up to 7 days at room temperature, but the use of an aeration chamber can shorten this to 24 hours or less.[10] The manufacturer of the instrument should be consulted before sterilization with ethylene oxide.

Flexible fiberscopes are not heat-stable and autoclaving damages the equipment. Sterilization can be achieved by some liquid sterilants if the instrument is immersed completely for specified, prolonged exposure times, but endoscopes generally do not withstand prolonged immersion in liquid chemical germicides well, and this procedure could severely damage the instrument.[2,3] If using this procedure, the endoscope manufacturer should be consulted.

Flexible endoscopes that do not normally come into contact with sterile tissue do not require sterilization for safe endoscopy, although it may be a prudent measure.[2] Certain clinical situations are cause for concern, despite the acceptability of mechanical cleaning and disinfection. Ethylene oxide sterilization of endoscopes prior to examination of immunocompromised or chemotherapy patients is a sensible and cautious measure to ensure the highest level of safety for these patients.[3,4,7,9]

ACCESSORIES

Many different types of endoscopic accessories are available. These include such items as bite guards, endoscope valves, port covers, topical spray nozzles, cannulas, forceps, snares, injection needles, and brushes.

It has been noted that certain flexible accessories, such as reusable biopsy forceps and cytology brushes, may be more hazardous with respect to disease transmission than the actual endoscope.[3] Any accessories that break the mucosal barrier, such as biopsy forceps, are classified as critical instruments and require sterilization.[5,7,11]

Accessories that are nondisposable require meticulous cleaning prior to disinfection or sterilization. Adequate cleaning of a biopsy forcep is difficult because of its spring-like structural configuration and numerous crevices. The internal lumens of these spring-like devices become contaminated with patient material during use, and it has been shown to be extremely difficult, if not impossible, to remove this material during cleaning.[3] Salmonella newport transmission from an index patient to eight subsequent patients during colonoscopy has been linked to an inadequately disinfected biopsy forcep.[3] It is necessary to clean, and disinfect, and sterilize accessories between patients, unless a disposable item is used and discarded. With the exception of water bottles, all nondisposable accessories should be used only once in 24 hours.[8,12]

The cleaning and disinfecting procedure for accessories is as follows:

1. Place endoscopic accessories in a solution of a low-sudsing enzymatic detergent and water or hydrogen peroxide to soak immediately after use following a procedure.[8,10]
2. Hand clean any used accessories with a brush in fresh detergent solution at the end of the endoscopic procedure or schedule.
   a. All accessories should be dismantled as much as possible, removing all handles and withdrawing any inner parts from lumens.
   b. Any lumens must be flushed with detergent solution.
3. Place difficult to clean accessories, such as biopsy forceps and items with a spiral metal structure, in an ultrasonic cleaner for 15 minutes, if an ultrasonic cleaner is available.
4. Thoroughly rinse all accessories with clean water, flushing all lumens well.
5. Dry all accessories thoroughly. Compressed air must be used to dry any lumen, such as that of snares.

6. Perform sterilization and disinfection procedures according to the manufacturer's guidelines.
   a. Endoscopic accessories that are heat-stable, such as biopsy forceps, should be sterilized by autoclaving. Portable electric autoclaves are relatively inexpensive and practical.
   b. Endoscopic accessories that are not disposable or heat-stable may require ethylene gas sterilization. These accessories include sphincterotomes, snares, and cannulas, such as bipolar irrigating probes.
   c. Prolonged immersion of endoscopic accessories in an EPA-approved sterilant-disinfectant is an alternative. If this method is used, care must be taken to rinse the accessory well and to dry thoroughly.
7. Sterilize the water bottle and its connecting tubing at least daily, and use only sterile water to fill the bottle.[7]
   Note: Compressed air should be used to dry the two lumina of the water bottle cap and tubing.[8]
8. The use of disposable accessories may be safer, more efficient, and more economical over the long term.[5] Disposable items currently available include bite guards, cleaning brushes, cytology brushes, snares, sclerotherapy needles, and forceps.

FURTHER CONSIDERATIONS

STORAGE

Forced-air drying of the endoscope channels prior to storage is a critical part of the cleaning and disinfection procedure.[2] Thorough drying of the inner channels and the external surfaces of the endoscope minimizes the risk of opportunistic infection. Bacteria multiply in a moist environment. The drying process prevents proliferation of residual bacteria and fungi during storage, and is necessary following washing and disinfection in automatic machines.[2,7] Inner channel drying may be done using commercially available compressed air following manufacturer's recommendations, or by attaching suction to the distal tip of the endoscope.[1,7] To facilitate drying, 70–90% alcohol may be flushed through the channels prior to forced-air drying and storage.[2,7]

Following drying, endoscopes should be stored hanging and not coiled in the instrument case. Endoscopes should be hung in a storage closet that is clean, dry, and well ventilated.

QUALITY ASSURANCE

Certain factors concerning the care and handling of flexible endoscopes and accessories are worth noting in regard to quality assurance. The following steps allow early identification of a problem, the source of a problem to be traced when identified, and the appropriate changes in technique to be made, if necessary.[12]

1. Daily log books should be kept that include the identity of the endoscope used on a particular patient. This allows a problem to be identified if it is associated with a particular instrument.
2. Use of the disinfectant should be quality controlled.
   a. The date of activation and expiration should be recorded.
   b. The gluteraldehyde concentration should be tested for dilution regularly and recorded. Kits are commercially available for this purpose.

It is critical that the care and handling of the flexible endoscopic equipment be considered as an important feature of the procedure when performing endoscopy. Adequate cleaning, disinfecting, and sterilizing procedures require evaluation of factors such as space, personnel, finances, and quality assurance measures. Compromise in technique concerning the care and handling of flexible endoscopes and accessories may be equated with a compromise in patient care.

REFERENCES

1. Aliberti LC: The flexible sigmoidoscope as a potential vector of infectious disease, including suggestions for decontamination of the flexible sigmoidoscope. Yale J Biol Med, 60:19, 1987.
2. Infection control during gastrointestinal endoscopy: Guidelines for clinical application (ASGE Publ. No. 1018). Gastrointest Endosc, (Suppl), 34:37S, 1988.
3. Bond WW: Virus transmission via fiberoptic endoscope: Recommended disinfection. Epidemiology and disease control newsletter. Md State Med J, 37:497, 1988.
4. Cleaning and disinfection of equipment for gastrointestinal flexible endoscopy: Interim recommendations of a Working Party of the British Society of Gastroenterology. Gut, 29:1134, 1988.
5. Recommended practices: Care of instruments, scopes and powered surgical instruments. AORN J, 47:556, 1988.
6. Leak Testing Olympus Flexible Endoscopes. Steris Corp., 1989.
7. Recommended Guidelines for Infection Control in Gastrointestinal Endoscopy Settings. SGNA Infection Control Monograph, Rochester, NY, Society of Gastroenterology Nurses and Associates, Inc. 1990.
8. Protocol for Cleaning and Disinfecting Flexible Fiberoptic Endoscopes. Technical Bulletin 37H. St. Louis, Calgon-Vestal Laboratories.
9. Hughes CE, Gebhard RL: Forum: Gastrointestinal endoscopy—infection transmission and prevention. Asepsis 9:8, 1987.
10. Sivak MV, Spada IM: Gastroenterologic Endoscopy. Philadelphia, WB Saunders, 1987, pp 96–98.
11. Rutala WA: Draft guideline for selection and use of disinfectants. Am J Infect Control 17:24A, 1989.
12. Ott BJ: Infection Control Practices—GI Procedures. Mayo Medical Center Protocol-III. Rochester, MN, Mayo Clinic, 1988.

index

Page numbers in **boldface** indicate illustrations; numbers followed by "t" indicate tables.

F

M

R